T0226414

Consultations in Liver Disease

Editor

STEVEN L. FLAMM

CLINICS IN LIVER DISEASE

www.liver.theclinics.com

Consulting Editor
NORMAN GITLIN

February 2015 • Volume 19 • Number 1

ELSEVIER

1600 John F. Kennedy Boulevard • Suite 1800 • Philadelphia, Pennsylvania, 19103-2899

http://www.theclinics.com

CLINICS IN LIVER DISEASE Volume 19, Number 1
February 2015 ISSN 1089-3261, ISBN-13: 978-0-323-35443-1

Editor: Kerry Holland
Developmental Editor: Casey Jackson

Clinics in Liver Disease (ISSN 1089-3261) is published quarterly by Elsevier Inc., 360 Park Avenue South, New York, NY 10010-1710. Months of issue are February, May, August, and November. Business and Editorial Offices: 1600 John F. Kennedy Blvd., Ste. 1800, Philadelphia, PA 19103-2899. Customer Service Office: 3251 Riverport Lane, Maryland Heights, MO 63043. Periodicals postage paid at New York, NY and additional mailing offices. Subscription prices are $295.00 per year (U.S. individuals), $145.00 per year (U.S. student/resident), $401.00 per year (U.S. institutions), $395.00 per year (international individuals), $200.00 per year (international student/resident), $498.00 per year (international instituitions), $340.00 per year (Canadian individuals), $200.00 per year (Canadian student/resident), and $498.00 per year (Canadian institutions). Foreign air speed delivery is included in all *Clinics* subscription prices. All prices are subject to change without notice. **POSTMASTER:** Send address changes to *Clinics in Liver Disease*, Elsevier Health Sciences Division, Subscription Customer Service, 3251 Riverport Lane, Maryland Heights, MO 63043. **Customer Service: Telephone: 1-800-654-2452 (U.S. and Canada); 314-447-8871 (outside U.S. and Canada). Fax: 314-447-8029. E-mail: journalscustomer service-usa@elsevier.com (for print support); journalsonlinesupport-usa@elsevier.com (for online support).**

Reprints. For copies of 100 or more of articles in this publication, please contact the Commercial Reprints Department, Elsevier Inc., 360 Park Avenue South, New York, NY 10010-1710. Tel.: 212-633-3874; Fax: 212-633-3820; E-mail: reprints@elsevier.com.

Clinics in Liver Disease is covered in *MEDLINE/PubMed (Index Medicus)*, Science Citation Index Expanded, Journal Citation Reports/Science Edition, and Current Contents/Clinical Medicine.

Contributors

CONSULTING EDITOR

NORMAN GITLIN, MD, FRCP (LONDON), FRCPE (EDINBURGH), FACG, FACP
Formerly, Professor of Medicine, Chief of Hepatology, Emory University; Currently, Consultant, Atlanta Gastroenterology Associates, Atlanta, Georgia

EDITOR

STEVEN L. FLAMM, MD
Chief, Liver Transplantation Program; Professor of Medicine and Surgery, Northwestern Feinberg School of Medicine, Chicago, Illinois

AUTHORS

CHATHUR ACHARYA, MD
Department of General Medicine, Virginia Commonwealth University, Richmond, Virginia

NEZAM H. AFDHAL, MD
Professor of Medicine, Liver Center, Beth Israel Deaconess Medical Center, Harvard Medical School, Boston, Massachusetts

JOSEPH AHN, MD, MS, FACG, AGAF
Associate Professor of Medicine; Director of Clincal Hepatology, Division of Gastroenterology and Hepatology, Oregon Health & Science University, Portland, Oregon

ESTELLA M. ALONSO, MD
Professor, Department of Pediatrics, Northwestern University, Feinberg School of Medicine, Siragusa Transplantation Center, Ann & Robert H. Lurie Children's Hospital, Chicago, Illinois

SYED ABDUL BASIT, MD
Fellow, Section of Gastroenterology and Hepatology, University of Nevada School of Medicine, Las Vegas, Nevada

ALAN BONDER, MD
Instructor in Medicine, Liver Center, Beth Israel Deaconess Medical Center, Harvard Medical School, Boston, Massachusetts

NADIA K. BOZANICH, MD
Medicine, Indiana University School of Medicine, Indianapolis, Indiana

KIMBERLY BROWN, MD
Chief, Division of Gastroenterology and Hepatology, Henry Ford Hospital, Detroit, Michigan

ROBERT S. BROWN Jr, MD, MPH
Frank Cardile Professor of Medicine, Department of Medicine, Columbia University College of Physicians & Surgeons, New York, New York

CHALERMRAT BUNCHORNTAVAKUL, MD
Division of Gastroenterology and Hepatology, Department of Medicine, University of Pennsylvania, Philadelphia, Pennsylvania; Assistant Professor, Department of Medicine, Division of Gastroenterology and Hepatology, Rajavithi Hospital, College of Medicine, Rangsit University, Bangkok, Thailand

ATTASIT CHOKECHANACHAISAKUL, MD
Transplant Fellow Department of Surgery, Northwestern University, Chicago, Illinois

JONATHAN R. COGLEY, MD
Department of Radiology, VA Western New York Healthcare System, Buffalo, New York

ALBERT J. CZAJA, MD
Professor Emeritus of Medicine, Division of Gastroenterology and Hepatology, Mayo Clinic College of Medicine, Rochester, Minnesota

NARAYAN DHAREL, MD, PhD
Division of Gastroenterology, Hepatology and Nutrition, Virginia Commonwealth University, Richmond, Virginia

ROBERT GISH, MD
Division of Gastroenterology and Hepatology, Department of Medicine, Stanford University, Stanford, California

PRIYA KATHPALIA, MD
Division of Gastroenterology and Hepatology, University of California, San Francisco, San Francisco, California

LAURA M. KULIK, MD
Associate Professor in Medicine, Gastroenterology and Hepatology, Radiology and Surgery-Organ Transplantation, Northwestern University, Chicago, Illinois

PAUL Y. KWO, MD
Professor of Medicine; Medical Director, Liver Transplantation, Indiana University School of Medicine, Indianapolis, Indiana

ALISHA M. MAVIS, MD
Fellow in Transplant Hepatology, Department of Pediatrics, Northwestern University, Feinberg School of Medicine, Siragusa Transplantation Center, Ann & Robert H. Lurie Children's Hospital, Chicago, Illinois

FRANK H. MILLER, MD
Chief, Body Imaging Section and Fellowship Program and GI Radiology, Medical Director MRI, Professor, Department of Radiology, Northwestern Memorial Hospital, Northwestern University, Feinberg School of Medicine, Chicago, Illinois

ERIN K. O'NEILL, MD
Department of Radiology, Northwestern Memorial Hospital, Northwestern University, Feinberg School of Medicine, Chicago, Illinois

K. RAJENDER REDDY, MD
Division of Gastroenterology and Hepatology, Department of Medicine, University of Pennsylvania, Philadelphia, Pennsylvania

REENA J. SALGIA, MD
Senior Staff Physician, Division of Gastroenterology and Hepatology, Henry Ford Hospital, Detroit, Michigan

RICHARD K. STERLING, MD, MSc
VCU Hepatology Professor of Medicine; Chief, Section of Hepatology, Division of Gastroenterology, Hepatology and Nutrition, Virginia Commonwealth University Health System, Virginia Commonwealth University; Division of Infectious Disease, Virginia Commonwealth University, Richmond, Virginia

CHRISTIAN D. STONE, MD, MPH
Chief, Section of Gastroenterology and Hepatology; Associate Professor of Medicine, University of Nevada School of Medicine, Las Vegas, Nevada

ELLIOT B. TAPPER, MD
Clinical Fellow in Medicine, Liver Center, Beth Israel Deaconess Medical Center, Harvard Medical School, Boston, Massachusetts

MING-MING XU, MD
Fellow, Division of Digestive and Liver Diseases, Department of Medicine, Columbia University College of Physicians & Surgeons, New York, New York

Contents

hepatitis. Presentation can be acute, severe (fulminant), asymptomatic, or chronic. Diagnosis requires multiple findings and exclusion of similar diseases. Treatment with prednisone or prednisolone with azathioprine is recommended. Budesonide with azathioprine has normalized laboratory test with few side effects, but histologic resolution, durability of response, and target population are uncertain. Progressive worsening, incomplete improvement, drug intolerance, and relapse after drug withdrawal are suboptimal outcomes. Calcineurin inhibitors and mycophenolate mofetil are salvage agents in small series and liver transplantation is effective for liver failure.

Overlapping features between autoimmune hepatitis (AIH) and cholestatic disorders (primary biliary cirrhosis (PBC), primary sclerosing cholangitis (PSC), or indeterminate cholestasis), so-called overlap syndromes, usually have a progressive course toward cirrhosis and liver failure without adequate treatment. The diagnosis of overlap syndrome requires the prominent features of classic AIH and secondary objective findings of PBC or PSC. Empiric treatment for patients with AIH-PBC overlap is immunosuppressive therapy plus ursodeoxycholic acid. Empiric treatment for patients with AIH-PSC and AIH-cholestatic overlap is immunosuppressive therapy with or without ursodeoxycholic acid. Liver transplantation is indicated for patients who have end-stage liver disease.

Different imaging modalities including ultrasonography, computed tomography (CT), and MR imaging may be used in the liver depending on the clinical situation. The ability of dedicated contrast-enhanced liver MR imaging or CT to definitively characterize lesions as benign is crucial in avoiding unnecessary biopsy. Liver imaging surveillance in patients with cirrhosis may allow for detection of hepatocellular carcinoma at an earlier stage, and therefore may improve outcome. This article reviews the different imaging modalities used to evaluate the liver and focal benign and malignant hepatic lesions, and the basic surveillance strategy for patients at increased risk for hepatocellular carcinoma.

Newer noninvasive tests have begun to replace liver biopsy for staging purposes. The clinician must evaluate these tools and apply them to individual patients. None of these modalities give the exact same staging of fibrosis as a liver biopsy, but they are excellent tools for risk stratification. Still, it should be recognized that there are disease-specific issues with different utilizations and cutoffs for different clinical diseases. This article provides a framework for incorporating the use of serum biomarkers and elastography-based approaches to stage fibrosis into clinical practice. This review also covers recent developments in this rapidly advancing area.

Portal vein thrombosis (PVT) is a rare event in the general medical setting that commonly complicates cirrhosis with portal hypertension, and can also occur with liver tumors. The diagnosis is often incidental when a thrombus is found in the portal vein on imaging tests. However, PVT may also present with clinical symptoms and can progress to life-threatening complications of ischemic hepatitis, liver failure, and/or small intestinal infarction. This article reviews the pathophysiology of this disorder, with a major focus on PVT in patients with cirrhosis, and presents detailed guidelines on optimal diagnostic and therapeutic strategies.

CLINICS IN LIVER DISEASE

Preface

Consultations in Liver Disease

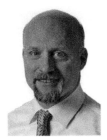

Steven L. Flamm, MD
Editor

Consultations of Gastroenterology practitioners are frequently sought for many complex issues relating to acute and chronic liver disease. Many of the disease entities are uncommon and complicated in scope. Liver disease may occur in the setting of other chronic medical conditions and involve other organ systems, with recommendations for diagnostic strategies and therapeutic approaches somewhat challenging. Serious consequences are often the rule with misdiagnosed or inadequately treated liver disease. A previous issue of *Clinics in Liver Disease* entitled, "Approach to Consultation for Patients with Liver Disease," published in May 2012 dealt with many of these issues to provide a framework for approaching consultation for common liver-related problems for the gastroenterology practitioner. This issue of *Clinics in Liver Disease* is entitled, "Consultations in Liver Disease." Additional timely topics are discussed that will help the practicing gastroenterologist address common but difficult inpatient and outpatient consultations in patients with liver disease.

Liver disease is common in patients with HIV, and there are many unique aspects to diagnosis and therapy. The first article is entitled, "Chronic Liver Disease in the HIV Patient," by Dr Sterling and his colleagues.

One of the rapidly increasing malignancies in incidence in the United States is hepatocellular carcinoma; there have been advances in the diagnosis and therapeutic strategies that Dr Kulik and her co-author outline in their article.

Renal insufficiency is quite common in patients with concomitant liver disease and frequently presents vexing diagnostic and therapeutic dilemmas for the gastroenterology consultant. This topic is covered in detail by Drs Kwo and Bozanich.

Autoimmune liver diseases are not uncommon. Since there are no definitive diagnostic tests for autoimmune disease and therapy can be somewhat complex, consultation can be difficult. Dr Czaja reviews the latest information regarding the approach to diagnosis and management of autoimmune hepatitis, and Drs Reddy and Bunchorntavakul explore the complicated issue of overlap syndromes.

Clin Liver Dis 19 (2015) xiii–xiv
http://dx.doi.org/10.1016/j.cld.2014.10.001
1089-3261/15/$ – see front matter © 2015 Published by Elsevier Inc.

Radiology procedures are often central to the workup of patients with acute and chronic liver disease. In recent years, there have been advances, and new techniques are now available. They may be somewhat confusing for the gastroenterology practitioner. Dr Miller and colleagues carefully discuss the ins and outs of contemporary liver imaging.

The determination of hepatic fibrosis is critical for the management of chronic liver diseases. Dr Afdhal and his co-authors review recent important developments in the noninvasive assessment of hepatic fibrosis.

When patients develop decompensated liver disease, liver transplantation referral may be indicated. Drs Brown and Xu outline the process of liver transplantation evaluation.

One of the more difficult inpatient consultations for the gastroenterologist is for evaluation of jaundice in the hospitalized patient. Drs Ahn and Kathpalia describe how to approach this problem.

On occasion, gastroenterologists are consulted about liver disease in the adolescent. Dr Alonso and her co-author provide insight into the issues of concern in this population.

Finally, two common problems are presented. Drs Brown and Salgia describe contemporary diagnostic and management strategies for genetic hemochromatosis, and Dr Gish and his co-authors review an approach to evaluation and management of portal vein thrombosis.

This issue of *Clinics in Liver Disease* complements the last one and provides guidance on many complex topics that are common challenges to the practicing gastroenterologist.

I would again like to express my gratitude to Dr Norman Gitlin for allowing me to serve as editor of a second issue of *Clinics of Liver Disease* and to Kerry Holland and Casey Jackson for their assistance in preparing the articles for publication.

Steven L. Flamm, MD
Liver Transplantation Program
Professor of Medicine and Surgery
Northwestern Feinberg School of Medicine
676 North St. Clair
Arkes 19-041
Chicago, IL 60611, USA

E-mail address:
s-flamm@northwestern.edu

Chronic Liver Disease in the Human Immunodeficiency Virus Patient

Chathur Acharya, MD[a], Narayan Dharel, MD, PhD[b], Richard K. Sterling, MD, MSc[c,d],*

KEYWORDS

- Highly active antiretroviral therapy • Hepatitis • Fatty liver
- Nonalcoholic fatty liver disease • Nonalcoholic steatohepatitis • Metabolic syndrome
- Drug-induced liver injury • Opportunistic infections

KEY POINTS

- Liver disease in HIV is an emerging etiology of morbidity in HIV. It is the second most common cause of mortality after HIV itself and hence merits vigilance and meticulous work-up.
- Hepatitis C virus is the most common viral hepatitis in HIV. It is hoped that newer all-oral drug regimens soon will allow for improved efficacy and increased compliance in all patients; they are already effective in some.
- Fatty liver in HIV is a multifactorial, potentially reversible etiology for chronic liver disease. No definitive treatment is available yet.
- Drug-induced liver injury is a common etiology of elevated liver functions in HIV, but close monitoring and identification of the culprit drug prevent morbidity.
- Opportunistic infections are on the decline in the age of highly active antiretroviral therapy but should still be considered as clinical situations dictate.

Disclosure: None.

[a] Department of General Medicine, Virginia Commonwealth University, Richmond, VA 23298, USA; [b] Division of Gastroenterology, Hepatology and Nutrition, Virginia Commonwealth University, Richmond, VA 23298, USA; [c] Section of Hepatology, Division of Gastroenterology, Hepatology and Nutrition, Virginia Commonwealth University Health System, Virginia Commonwealth University, Richmond, VA 23298, USA; [d] Division of Infectious Disease, Virginia Commonwealth University, Richmond, VA 23298, USA

* Corresponding author. Section of Hepatology, Division of Gastroenterology, Hepatology and Nutrition, Virginia Commonwealth University Health System, Richmond, VA 23298.

E-mail address: rksterli@vcu.edu

INTRODUCTION

Since the discovery of the human immunodeficiency virus (HIV) 3 decades ago to the initiation of combination highly active antiretroviral therapy (HAART), the epidemiology of HIV and AIDS in the United States has fluctuated. Currently, there are 1.1 million HIV-positive individuals living in the Unites States, with nearly 16% of them being unaware of their infection.

With HIV-infected patients now living longer, liver disease has emerged as a significant cause of morbidity and mortality,[1,2] and liver enzyme elevations are frequently noted in patients with HIV.[3] Due to well-controlled HIV, opportunistic infections (OIs) involving the liver are now rarely seen. Although HIV-infected patients are not protected from having any specific liver disease, most liver diseases now seen in patients with HIV include drug-induced liver injury (DILI), viral hepatitis, and both alcohol and nonalcohol-related steatohepatitis (fatty liver).

This article discusses the common etiologies of increased liver enzymes or otherwise abnormal liver panel and hepatitis in HIV (**Fig. 1**), keeping in mind the pathogenesis for various etiologies. It shall briefly discuss diagnostics and treatment strategies for each condition, with the overall goal of providing the reader a basic framework for the management of liver disease in HIV. In general, the severity of liver enzyme elevations should be assessed using the National Institutes of Health (NIH)-NIAI (National Institute for Allergy and Immunology) guidelines (**Table 1**). In addition, liver synthetic function should be assessed with total and direct bilirubin and prothrombin time (PT) and international normalized ratio (INR). Those with evidence of hepatic decompensation (ascites, jaundice, hepatic encephalopathy), regardless of the etiology, should be considered for referral to a specialized liver center.

HEPATITIS C VIRUS/HUMAN IMMUNODEFICIENCY VIRUS COINFECTION

Globally there are 40 million HIV-infected individuals. The prevalence of hepatitis C virus (HCV) infection by itself was estimated at 4 million in the United States,[4] and HCV has recently overtaken HIV as a cause of mortality.[5] Because of shared routes of transmission, coinfection with hepatitis C and HIV, is common and the incidence of HCV/HIV coinfection ranges from 10% in those who acquired HIV sexually, to over 80% in those who acquired HIV by intravenous drug use.[4] With the mortality of AIDS on the decline because of effective treatment strategies, liver disease caused by hepatitis C coinfection has become the leading cause of mortality in this group.[6]

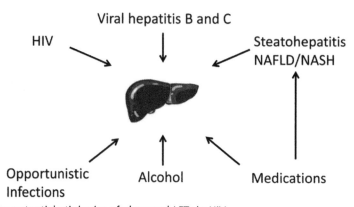

Fig. 1. The potential etiologies of abnormal LFTs in HIV.

Grade	With Normal Baseline AST/ALT	With Elevated Baseline AST/ALT
0	<1.25 × ULN	<1.25 × BL
1	1.25–2.5 × ULN	1.25–2.5 × BL
2	2.6–5.0 × ULN	2.6–3.5 × BL
3	5.1–10 × ULN	3.6–5 × BL
4	>10 × ULN	>5 × BL

Table 1
NIH-NIAI guidelines for grading abnormal liver function tests

Abbreviations: BL, below limit; ULN, upper limit of normal.

The presence of HIV skews the natural history of HCV infection, leading to increased viral load and increased rates of persistence, with an increase in liver-related mortality and morbidity. The risk of progression to chronicity in the presence of HIV increases to 95%, and death from hepatocellular cancer is as high as 13%.[7,8]

Although the risk of progression of liver disease to cirrhosis and end-stage liver disease (ESLD) in HCV/HIV coinfection is double and amplified sixfold, respectively,[8] the presence of HCV does not influence disease progression of HIV to AIDS, even with HAART.[9] This translates to cirrhosis being diagnosed within 12 years[10] and hepatic decompensation by 15 years. Interestingly, HCV foretells a threefold likelihood of hepatotoxicity from older regimens of HAART,[11–13] and close monitoring of liver function is required.

Pathogenesis

The mechanisms by which HCV promotes rapid progression of fibrosis and ESLD are under study and better understood. Apart from HIV causing dysregulation of T cells and increased replication of HCV, there are many other important mechanisms through which HIV accelerates the natural course of HCV (**Fig. 2**).

HIV is associated with intestinal villous effacement and CD4 cell depletion, and this in turn is associated with an increase in intestinal microbial product translocation into

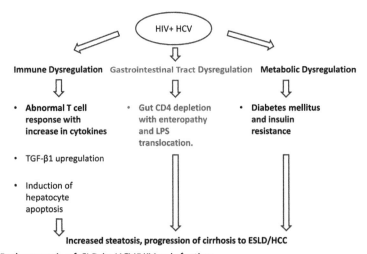

Fig. 2. Pathogenesis of CLD in HCV/HIV coinfection.

the portal venous system. The liver filters the portal venous blood and is exposed to lipopolysaccharide (LPS). Free LPS binds to Kupffer cells via interactions with circulating LPS-binding protein, cell surface CD14 (sCD14), and toll-like receptor 4 (TLR-4), leading to up-regulation of proinflammatory and profibrogenic cytokines, including tumor necrosis factor (TNF)-α, interleukin (IL)-1, IL-6, and IL-12.[14,15]

HCV induced TGF-β1 release from hepatocytes is enhanced by HIV.[16] TGF-β1 is a profibrogenic cytokine that is instrumental in the immunopathogenesis of coinfection through various stimulatory pathways.

There is accelerated hepatocyte apoptosis in coinfection, leading to more inflammation and fibrosis.[17,18] There is also an increase in steatohepatitis, which in turn up-regulates inflammation in the liver and is pro-fibrogenic.[19,20] Finally, there is also evidence that HIV directly infects the stellate cells, and this promotes inflammation and secretion of fibrogenic stroma.[21]

Diagnosis

All HIV patients should be screened for HCV by enzyme-linked immunosorbent assay (ELISA). However, false-negative antibody tests can occur in those with CD4 counts less than 100. In those with a negative antibody, repeat testing is recommended yearly as long as patients have ongoing risks of transmission (high-risk sexual activity, illicit drug use). In addition, the presence of elevated liver enzymes should trigger diagnostic testing for HCV, although moderate elevations in liver enzymes from other etiologies can also be observed.[3] Patients who test negative for HCV Ab should be counseled on risk factors for HCV.

In subjects with a positive HCV antibody, HCV infection must be confirmed by HCV RNA testing (**Fig. 3**). In those with a positive RNA, HCV genotype is required if treatment is contemplated. All HCV RNA-positive patients require assessment of disease severity, and although liver biopsy remains the gold standard for disease staging, it can be associated with complications. As such, noninvasive strategies for assessment of hepatic fibrosis have been developed. These can be divided into biochemical tests (simple and proprietary) and elastography (which measures liver stiffness). Two commonly used noninvasive fibrosis scores are APRI

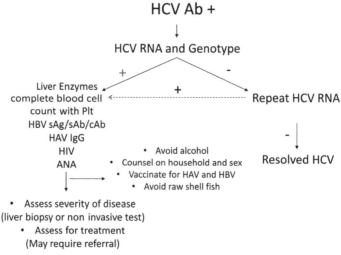

Fig. 3. Evaluation of HCV.

(aspartate aminotransferase to platelet ratio index) and the FIB-4 indices (patient age, aspartate aminotransferase, alanine aminotransferase, and platelets). Each has shown clinical utility in HIV-HCV.[22–24] Noninvasive imaging studies such as transient elastography[25,26] and magnetic resonance elastography are other means for staging but need referral to specialized centers. Those with suspected or proven cirrhosis require screening for esophageal varices and hepatocellular carcinoma (**Fig. 4**).

Management

Treatment of HCV/HIV coinfection is based on similar principles as treatment of HCV without HIV. Given the increased mortality with HCV in HIV, most patients should be considered for treatment. Given the improved response rates and lower adverse effect profiles of interferon-free treatment strategies, the most important determining factor to initiate treatment is the current stage of HCV (mild vs significant fibrosis), presence or absence of comorbidities, the control of HIV, and compliance. In certain individuals, treatment could be deferred if there is no fibrosis and/or if there are contraindications to treatment.

Until recently, the standard US Food and Drug Administration (FDA)-approved therapy for HCV has been pegylated interferon alfa (Peg-IFN) and ribavirin (RBV).[27] The field of HCV treatment is moving fast, and it is anticipated that several interferon-free, all-oral regimens will be available for those with chronic HCV genotype 1, regardless of HIV coinfection, by 2015. All-oral regimens are currently available for HCV genotypes 2 and 3. Overall, sustained virologic response (SVR) rates exceeding 90% for genotypes 1, 2, and 4 are expected. Genotype 3 patients remain a challenge, particularly if patients have cirrhosis and have previously failed Peg-IFN and RBV. While choosing the appropriate drugs, consideration should also be given to the class due to strong drug–drug interactions between HAART and certain classes of HCV direct-acting antiviral agents. For those who develop ESLD and decompensation, liver transplant can be considered. Although overall post-transplant survival is suboptimal, if patients are carefully selected, outcomes approach HCV mono-infected patients.[28] Hopefully, with more effective pre and post-transplant HCV therapy, this will become even less of an issue.

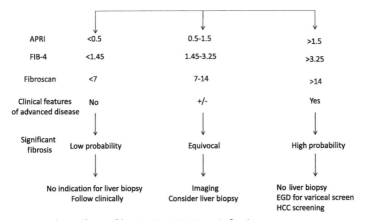

Fig. 4. Diagnosis of significant fibrosis in HCV/HIV coinfection.

HEPATITIS B VIRUS/HUMAN IMMUNODEFICIENCY VIRUS COINFECTION

Similar to HCV/HIV coinfection, HBV coinfection among HIV-positive persons is common because of shared route of transmission.[29,30] Worldwide, an estimated 2 to 4 million people are currently living with HBV/HIV coinfection. In the United States, the prevalence is around 8%, which is approximately 20 times higher than the general US population. Up to two-thirds of HIV-infected individuals have markers of past exposure to HBV,[31] and about 10% of these patients have chronic HBV coinfection.[29,30] HIV coinfection adversely affects the natural history of HBV[32] at every stage, and is associated with increased HBV replication and increased levels of HBV DNA.[33] Coinfected individuals consequently are up to 6 times more likely to progress to chronicity.[34,35] The progression of fibrosis is accelerated; the risk of cirrhosis and hepatocellular carcinoma is subsequently higher,[36] and these patients are more likely to die from liver-related causes than HBV mono-infected individuals.[1,37,38] Chronic HBV infection, however, does not appear to have a significant impact on the natural history or treatment outcome of HIV disease.[39,40]

Pathogenesis

The exact mechanisms by which the disease course in HBV/HIV coinfection is altered have yet to be studied in detail. In general, the immunopathogenesis is similar to HCV/HIV coinfection (see **Fig. 2**), although only increased intrahepatic apoptosis has been documented in HBV/HIV coinfection.[41] Furthermore, antiretroviral therapy (ART) can lead to hepatocellular injury by immune reconstitution and/or direct hepatoxicity,[42,43] accentuating liver dysfunction in coinfected patients.

Diagnosis

Similar to HIV-negative individuals, the diagnosis of HBV coinfection should be suspected when there is presence of elevated serum aminotransferases and the detection of hepatitis B surface antigen (HBsAg) and/or HBV DNA in the serum. Initial screening serology should include HBsAg, hepatitis B surface antibody (HBsAb), and anti-HBc (total or immunoglobulin g [IgG]) as detailed in **Fig. 5**. The hepatitis B e antigen (HBeAg) may or may not be detectable and is not essential for diagnosis.

	Immune tolerant	Immune active	Chronic inactive carrier	Reactivation
ALT[a]	Persistently normal	Persistently high	Normal to minimal elevation	Elevated
Serology	HBsAg + HBsAb - HBeAg + Anti-HBe -	HBsAg + HBsAb - HBeAg +/- Anti-HBe +/-	HBsAg + HBsAb - HBeAg - Anti-HBe +/-	HBsAg + HBsAb - HBeAg - HBcAb +
HBV DNA[b]	High	Moderate to high	Low to undetectable	Elevated
Clinical picture	Asymptomatic Usually young individuals	Symptomatic Clinically diagnosed as chronic hepatitis B	Asymptomatic Inactive histology but can have significant fibrosis	Symptomatic May behave like acute infection

[a] Normal ALT is < 30 IU/mL for males and < 20 IU/mL for females
[b] High HBV DNA is > 20,000 IU/mL and low HBV DNA is < 2000 IU/mL

Fig. 5. Clinical phases of chronic hepatitis B infection and diagnosis.

HBV DNA should be tested as a marker of viral replication, and should also be obtained in all patients with positive isolated core antibody (presence of anti-HBc in the absence of HBsAg or HBsAb) to rule out occult HBV infection.[44] Because spontaneous seroreversion (disappearance of HBsAb and reappearance of HBsAg) is possible among HIV-infected patients, especially those with very low CD4 counts (<200 cells/µL),[45,46] HBV serologic tests should be repeated in the event of unexplained liver enzyme abnormalities to rule out reemergence of HBV infection. Noninvasive studies for diagnosis of fibrosis have been validated in HIV coinfected patients and have been discussed in the HCV/HIV co-infection section. The role of liver biopsy is more defined during follow-up after therapy initiation, but can also be used to aid in decision-making for patients not clearly meeting criteria for treatment.

Management

Management should be initiated in specialized centers with a multidisciplinary approach. The primary goal of anti-HBV therapy among HBV/HIV coinfected patients is to prevent liver-related complications by sustained suppression of HBV replication to the lowest achievable level.[30] Because HBV DNA integrates into the host nuclear material, long-term treatment is usually needed. In most cases, dual therapy for HBV and HIV is started concomitantly; however anti-HBV therapy should be considered for all HBV coinfected individuals irrespective of the need for ART because of the overwhelming liver-related mortality.[47,48]

Three anti-HBV agents, tenofovir (TDF), emtricitabine (FTC), and lamivudine (3TC), have potent antiretroviral activity and are also approved for HIV treatment. Entecavir appears to have weak antiretroviral activity. The preferred regimen is TDF in combination with either FTC or 3TC (which will also act as the nucleoside reverse transcriptase inhibitor backbone of ART) along with a third agent, such as efavirenz (EFV) or raltegravir (aidsinfo.nih.gov, WHO 2013 AIDS guideline). In the event of prior 3TC exposure or resistance, TDF plus FTC should be used. In case TDF cannot be used, (eg, because of bone or renal toxicity) entecavir can be used as a substitute, but only in the context of fully suppressive ART. When there is no indication for ART, then agents without antiretroviral activity such as peginterferon, adefovir, and telbivudine should be used.[30] Agents with antiretroviral activity (TDF, FTC, 3TC, and entecavir) should be avoided in this setting as they can lead to selection of resistant HIV strains. Liver transplant for ESLD could be considered for the appropriate candidate, as long as the patient is maintained on HAART, and HIV is well controlled.[49,50]

HUMAN IMMUNODEFICIENCY VIRUS—FATTY LIVER

Abnormal liver enzymes are common and occur in 40% to 60% of HIV-infected patients on ART, even in the absence of viral hepatitis.[3,13,51] Given its prevalence in the general population, the majority of these subjects may have nonalcoholic fatty liver disease (NAFLD). NAFLD affects one-third of the US population and is the most common cause of elevated aminotransferases in the general population.[52,53] The prevalence of NASH in estimated to be approximately 3% to 5%,[54] and NASH-associated cirrhosis is projected to be the most common etiology for liver transplantation in the future.[55,56] Few studies have looked at the prevalence of NAFLD and NASH in HIV-infected persons, and most of the data on prevalence of steatosis come from studies of HCV/HIV coinfected patients. Not so surprisingly, the prevalence of NAFLD in HCV/HIV coinfected patients is significant, between 40% and 75%,[57–59] while the prevalence of NAFLD in the HIV population without comorbidities such as viral hepatitis is slightly lower, at 31%.[60] NASH is prevalent, at 26%.[61] Similar to

HIV-negative patients, those with NAFLD, and in particular NASH, have increased cardiovascular disease and increased all-cause and cardiovascular mortality as well.[62] With a significantly higher burden of NASH in the coinfected population, it is important to recognize that this population is also at heightened risk for cardiovascular incidents and for the development of progressive liver disease and eventually cirrhosis.

Pathogenesis

NAFLD in the general population is said to be the hepatic manifestation of the metabolic syndrome. The risk factors of obesity, hypertension, insulin resistance, dyslipidemia, and diabetes mellitus are prevalent, even for HIV patients. However, HIV patients also have additional complicating risk factors to make them more prone to NAFLD. In HIV, NAFLD could be caused by HIV itself, secondary to hepatitis viruses (HCV genotype 3), or due to certain HAART medication toxicity acting directly on the liver or via lipodystrophy (**Box 1**). Enumerated are some of the pathogenic mechanisms and risk factors related to NAFLD in HIV:

Presence of ART is an independent risk factor for developing NAFLD in HIV.[13,63–65]
HIV itself is associated with impaired glucose tolerance/insulin resistance.[66]
Presence of HCV genotype 3 may be directly responsible for NAFLD.[67]

Increased intestinal permeability through villous effacement and depletion of CD4 cells increases the amount of bacterial lipopolysaccharide reaching the liver and upregulates inflammation, accelerating NAFLD/NASH. Elevated soluble CD14 (sCD14, a marker of monocyte activation via LPS engagement of TLR-4) and soluble tumor necrosis factor (TNF) receptor II (sTNFRII) have been associated with severity of fibrosis in HCV/HIV coinfection, and have also been noted to be elevated in non-HIV NAFLD subjects.[68,69]

Diagnosis

As with most chronic liver diseases, liver biopsy is the benchmark for diagnosis, but clinicians are implementing other noninvasive means to aid in diagnosis and assessment of hepatic fibrosis. Liver ultrasound or abdominal computed tomography (CT) scan is sensitive in detecting NALFD,[70] but results are not consistent in patients with less than 30% steatosis. A noninvasive test with 84% sensitivity for NALFD is the fatty liver index (FLI). It incorporates body mass index (BMI), waist circumference, triglycerides, and gamma glutamyl transpeptidase (GGT),[71] but has not been independently tested on HIV patients. Other noninvasive means of diagnosis of NAFLD are the

---

Box 1
Pathogenesis of NAFLD in HIV

Insulin resistance and lipodystrophy related to the use of nucleoside inhibitors and other HAART drugs. Presence of ART is an independent risk factor for developing NAFLD in HIV.

HIV is associated with impaired glucose tolerance/insulin resistance. HIV is a direct suppressor of peroxisome proliferator-activated receptor and indirectly alters the signal pathway affecting modulation of TNF.

Presence of HCV genotype 3 may be directly responsible for NAFLD.

Intestinal permeability through villous effacement and depletion of CD4 cells increases the amount of bacterial lipopolysaccharide reaching the liver and upregulates inflammation, accelerating NAFLD/NASH.

liver fat score (LFS) and lipid accumulation product (LAP), which have been assessed in HIV patients.[72]

Management

HIV patients have comorbidities including DM (diabetes mellitus) and obesity, and similar to the rest of the US population, they are increasing in prevalence.[73,74] At present, there are no therapeutic interventions to treat NASH that have been studied in the HIV-infected patient. Once a diagnosis of NAFLD unrelated to HCV/HIV coinfection has been established, a management strategy of conservative measures to control these modifiable risk factors would be beneficial. No studies have been performed, however, in HIV patients to confirm benefit. Although therapy with vitamin E or pioglitazone has been shown to reduce fibrosis in NAFLD,[75] further studies to validate this effect in HIV patients are needed. Once decompensation occurs in the setting of cirrhosis, if there are no contraindications, liver transplantation should be considered. It should be noted that no studies have been performed regarding transplantation for NAFLD in an HIV population.

MISCELLANEOUS
Drug-Induced Liver Injury

Elevated liver enzymes related to drug toxicity (see **Table 1**) have been well documented[3,13,51] and occur frequently, in 40% to 60% of patients on HAART, especially on older regimens. DILI has significant consequences on the health care of HIV individuals. First, it is associated with medication substitution or discontinuation of HAART, which leads to increase in OIs and a direct effect on mortality. Second, it has also been shown to increase the burden on the health care system in terms of office visits and health care costs. The spectrum of DILI in HIV-infected patients ranges from asymptomatic elevations of aminotransferases to hepatic failure and death.[76]

Classically, the NRTIs (nucleoside reverse transcriptase inhibitor) were most studied for association with hepatotoxicity. Compared with protease inhibitors (PIs), NRTIs have shown a greater rise in lactic acid and hepatotoxicity.[77] The incidence of grade 3 or 4 hepatotoxicity in NRTIs is low, approximately 1%, although the presence of symptomatic lactic acidosis is high.[78–80] NRTIs are also known to be associated with a syndrome of hepatic steatosis.[81,82] Comparing NRTIs to NNRTIs (non-nucleoside reverse transcriptase inhibitor), NRTIs are more hepatotoxic. In clinical studies, nevirapine has been shown to have more hepatotoxicity than efavirenz.[64,83] Overall, however, NNRTIs have a low rate of clinically significant hepatotoxicity.[84,85] Among PIs, ritonavir and ritonavir-boosted HAART regimens have been most studied and identified as independent risk factors for the development of hepatotoxicity. Wit and colleagues[86] documented ritonavir (full-dose therapy) as an independent risk factor, with a 5.8-fold increased risk of developing grade 4 liver enzyme elevations. Importantly, although full-dose ritonavir was identified as an independent risk factor for hepatotoxicity,[63,87] Wit and colleagues also showed that low-dose ritonavir (defined as ≤200 mg twice daily) was not independently associated with an increased risk of liver injury.

The presence of chronic infection with HBV and/or HCV is a major risk factor for DILI, as several studies in HIV-infected patients have demonstrated.[12,63,87] In fact, the presence of HCV coinfection increases the risk of severe hepatotoxicity by twofold after adjusting for the type of medication received and baseline liver enzyme levels.

Pathogenesis
Drugs, in particular NRTIs, have been proposed to cause hepatotoxicity primarily by a direct toxic effect on the hepatocyte mitochondria and resultant break in the

generation of adenosine triphosphate (ATP) and accumulation of lactic acid.[88,89] When greater inhibition of mitochondrial DNA polymerase occurs, a higher degree of hepatotoxicity is observed. No exact mechanism for NNRTI and PI (protease inhibitors)-related hepatotoxicity has been clearly identified yet. The various drug categories and their toxic effects are summarized in **Tables 2** and **3**.

Management

The diagnosis of DILI is one of exclusion. In general, the diagnosis should have the key elements of time of onset with relation to initiation of a drug, clinical features, and course and recovery after discontinuation of the drug.[90] Liver panel abnormalities reflect an elevation of ALT greater than aspartate aminotransferase (AST) and elevated alkaline phosphatase, but certain PIs like indinavir and atazanavir are associated with unconjugated hyperbilirubinemia resembling Gilbert syndrome.[91,92] The dilemma of DILI is whether to discontinue the drug, as this impacts the clinical outcome of HIV. A general principle that one should be mindful of in the setting of DILI is that symptomatic hepatitis is more concerning than asymptomatic hepatitis. Symptomatic hepatitis should prompt discontinuation of HAART, as continuation of the offending drug is associated with worse outcomes.[93] There is expert consensus that drugs that elevate ALT or AST levels greater than 10 times the upper limit of normal should be discontinued even if the patient is asymptomatic.[94] When dealing with drug hypersensitivity reactions like fevers and rash, the offending drug should be discontinued immediately, as readministration could be fatal. Any symptoms of mitochondrial toxicity should also prompt discontinuation pending work-up of possible lactic acidosis. Drugs associated with hepatitis and significant direct hyperbilirubinemia are associated with a higher mortality rate and should be discontinued.[95]

Human Immunodeficiency Virus-Associated Noncirrhotic Portal Hypertension or Nodular Regenerative Hyperplasia

Noncirrhotic portal hypertension (NCPH) is now recognized as an uncommon, but serious cause of hepatitis in HIV-infected patients without hepatitis coinfection.[96–99] The most widely cited studies regarding NCPH have reported prevalence ranging from 1% to 8%.[98] Diagnosis of NCPH is one of exclusion, and it is aided with a finding of an abnormal liver panel and portal hypertension in the absence of viral hepatitis, NAFLD, or other causes of portal hypertension. There is no standard diagnostic feature on liver biopsy, but nodular regenerative hyperplasia has been recognized.[98,100,101] Liver biopsies have also revealed the absence of cirrhosis with paucity of and fibrous obliteration of small portal veins.[101,102] Although researchers have not found a single etiology, several studies have noticed an association with older nucleoside inhibitors like didanosine (ddl) and stavudine.[96,103] Studies have shown that cumulative ddl exposure may lead to NCPH, and this led the FDA to issue a warning linking ddl with this serious hepatopathy in 2010. Management is primarily supportive, and studies have shown that substituting ddl prior to development of portal hypertension was associated with slowing of NCPH,[104] and could also result in a decline in mean ALT levels with clinical improvement.[98]

Opportunistic Infections

The common systemic OIs that also affect the liver are *Mycobacteria*, fungi, pneumocystis, Epstein-Barr virus (EBV), cytomegalovirus (CMV), herpes simplex virus (HSV), Kaposi sarcoma and bacillary angiomatosis. OIs affecting AIDS patients with effective HAART are becoming less common in western countries. Management should be directed in conjunction with an infectious disease specialist.

Table 2
Mechanisms of drug-induced liver injury with antiretroviral agents

	Idiosyncratic Reaction or Intrinsic Toxicity	Hypersensitivity Reaction	Mitochondrial Toxicity	Immune Reconstitution	Steatosis
Drug example	NVP	NVP[a]>ABV[a]	ddI>d4T>AZT>ABV = TDF = LAM = FTC	Any	NRTIs PIs
Characteristic	Dose-dependent for intrinsic	Often associated with rash	Lactic acidosis	More common in those with low CD4 and chronic HBV	Metabolic syndrome, lipodystrophy, HCV (especially GT3)
Time of onset	Can vary by agent	Usually within 8 wk	Tends to occur after prolonged exposure	Usually within the first few months	Usually with prolong exposure

Abbreviations: ABV, abacavir; AZT, zidovudine; FTC, emtricitabine; GT, genotype; HBV, hepatitis B virus; LAM, lamividine; NRTI, nucleoside reverse transcriptase inhibitor; NVP, nevirapine; PI, protease inhibitor; TDF, tenofovir.
[a] Increased with certain polymorphisms.

Table 3
Nonhuman immunodeficiency virus drugs associated with drug induced liver injury

Drug	Hepatotoxicity	Example
Anti-PJP agents	Increased AST, ALT, and ALP possible	Trimethoprim-sulfamethoxazole
Antiherpes and CMV agents	Rare elevations in AST and ALT, bilirubin	Acyclovir
Antifungal agents	Increased AST and ALTInhibits cytochrome P450 and may increase PI levels	Ketoconazole
Macrolide antibiotic	Increased ALPInhibits cytochrome P450 and may increase PI levels	Erythromycin
Antituberculosis agents	Increased AST and ALT	Isoniazid, rifampicin, pyrazinamide
Lipid-lowering agents	Increased AST and ALT	Statins
Anabolic steroids	Increased ALP, bilirubin	Nandrolone

Abbreviations: ALP, alkaline phosphatase; ALT, alanine aminotransferase; AST, aspartate amino-transferase; CMV, cytomegalovirus; PI, protease inhibitor; PJP, *Pneumocystis jirovecci.*

AIDS cholangiopathy

AIDS cholangiopathy is a nonfatal cause for hepatitis in HIV patients.[105–107] It has been reported to affect 24% of HIV patients, but this was prior to the advent of HAART.[108] Its incidence now is said to be on the decline.[109]

The exact pathogenesis is still being studied, but there has been a clear association seen with opportunistic infections such as *Cryptosporidium*, CMV, *Microsporidium*, *Giardia*, *Mycobacterium avium* [MAC], *Cyclospora cayetanensis*, and even *isospora*,[106,109–114] suggesting that HIV cholangiopathy is an infectious sclerosing cholangitis. It is typically observed in patients with CD4 counts of less than 100/mm^3.[105] Patients generally present with biliary pain (ie, right upper quadrant [RUQ]) and/or midepigastric abdominal pain, but can also present with nausea, diarrhea,[114–118] weight loss, and jaundice.[105] Blood chemistry studies reveal mild-to-moderate elevation in alkaline phosphatase and gamma-glutamyl transferase levels.[106] Diagnosis is best confirmed by ERCP, which is the most specific diagnostic tool. It has an added advantage of therapeutic intervention with sphincterotomy. Similar to ERCP for diagnosis, but a cheaper initial screening test is a simple biliary ultrasound. Based on a positive or negative screen, further confirmatory diagnostic tests like MRCP or ERCP can be obtained.

Treatment consists of endoscopic retrograde cholangiopancreatography (ERCP) with sphincterotomy. This procedure has been shown to alleviate symptoms, but has no bearing on mortality[105,116,117,119] or improvement in liver enzymes. The only definitive therapy is initiation of HAART, which has the most important effect on survival.[119,120]

Mycobacterial infections

Prior to HAART, mycobacterial infections (tuberculosis and MAC) were the most commonly diagnosed infections on liver biopsy in patients with HIV. In a retrospective study by Lanjewar and colleagues[121] examining liver specimens from 171 patients, the most prevalent infection found was tuberculosis (41%). In another large study in North America, MAC was identified in 17.4% of liver biopsies in HIV-positive patients.[122] Symptoms are systemic and nonspecific, including fever, weight loss, and diarrhea. On biochemical testing, abnormal liver enzyme elevations with jaundice can occur, which can be due to extrahepatic obstruction from porta hepatis and peripancreatic lymphadenopathy. Diagnostic work-up is initiated with an abdominal ultrasound, which in the case of tuberculosis would reveal focal lesions, and in the case of MAC would show hepatosplenomegaly. Confirmation of tuberculosis of the liver is by liver biopsy that reveals granulomas. For MAC, liver biopsy shows microscopic obstruction of small biliary ducts, similar to AIDS cholangiopathy. Treatment of HIV with HAART is of the utmost importance. For tuberculosis, adjunctive treatment with RIPE (Rifampin, Isoniazid, Pyrazinamide, Ethambutol) therapy is necessary. For MAC, adjunctive therapy with macrolide antibiotics is indicated, until there is a CD4 cell response to the HAART.

Fungal infections
The common fungal infections that affect the liver are *Cryptococcus*, *Histoplasma*, *Coccidiomycosis*, and *Candida*. Incidence of opportunistic fungal disease in general, localized or widespread in form has been reported to be 58% to 81%. Fungal involvement of the liver is usually in the context of disseminated disease with a low CD4 count. In 2001, Shibuya and colleagues[123] retrospectively found liver involvement with generalized cryptococcosis in 66.7% of 162 patients with evident fungal infection. Lamps and colleagues[124] found that of 36 patients retrospectively analyzed with histoplasma involving the liver, 47% had enlarged liver, but only 17% had discrete grossly apparent hepatic lesions on pathology. Apart from HAART, rapid initiation of specific antifungals helps reduce mortality.

Pneumocystis jirovecci infection
The liver is a common extrapulmonary site of *Pneumocystis jirovecci* (PJP) involvement in the setting of disseminated disease. PJP has also been reported to be associated with aerosolized pentamidine prophylaxis.[125] The clinical picture resembles hepatitis. Diagnosing PJP of the liver starts with imaging; ultrasound reveals hypoechoic or echogenic foci representing calcifications. CT of the abdomen shows hypodense lesions or calcifications that suggest PJP. Specific treatment is with systemic antibiotics such as sulfamethoxazole/trimethoprim, pentamidine, or dapsone.

Epstein-Barr virus
Hepatic involvement with infectious mononucleosis is estimated in 30% of cases in the elderly and 10% of cases in young adults.[126] It presents with mild elevations of serum aminotransferases and elevated bilirubin in the majority of patients. Fulminant hepatic failure may occur in immunocompetent patients,[127] in those with HIV coinfection,[128] and in patients with complement deficiency, in whom it may be fatal.[129,130] The pathogenesis is likely not direct hepatocyte infection or cytotoxicity, but is more likely related to immune responses to viral antigens expressed on hepatocytes. Diagnosis is primarily by serology with positive antibodies and serum polymerase chain reaction (PCR). EBV has a self-limited course, and initial treatment should be supportive, although several case reports have shown success with ganciclovir in immunocompromised post-liver transplant patients for EBV fulminant hepatitis and immunocompetent patients with severe EBV hepatitis.[131,132]

Cytomegalovirus
CMV is a common OI in HIV, especially in the setting of severe immunosuppression. Liver involvement has been reported in as many as 44% of patients at autopsy in certain studies.[133,134] Most clinically significant infection occurs by reactivation of a previously latent infection. Although liver involvement is generally clinically silent, severe disease can occur in the setting of disseminated/systemic involvement. Serology

and culture are the mainstays of diagnosis. Imaging studies with ultrasound show echogenic liver lesions, and abdominal CT demonstrates multiple low-attenuated lesions. Ganciclovir and related antiviral agents are the mainstays of treatment in setting of the immunocompromised patient, especially with diffuse disease.

Kaposi sarcoma
Once a common presentation of AIDS, the incidence of KS is now on the decline in the HAART era.[135] Previously, prevalence rates of up to 22% were reported in autopsy series. Herpesvirus 8 has classically been associated with Kaposi sarcoma. Liver involvement presents with hepatomegaly and related abdominal pain and is observed in the setting of other manifestations of Kaposi sarcoma. Ultrasound shows multiple hyperechoic periportal bands and nodules, and CT of the abdomen shows periportal involvement. Liver biopsy is confirmatory for diagnosis. Treatment of Kaposi sarcoma is with HAART, in particular ritonavir-boosted therapy, which has antiangiogenic effects and will resolve tumor burden.[136]

Bacillary angiomatosis
Bacillary angiomatosis commonly manifests as a mucocutaneous disease irrespective of HIV status. In HIV, it is considered to be a late-stage infection, and although seropre-valence can be high,[137] clinical prevalence rates have been reported to be low at 1.2 cases per 1000 patients.[138] Bacillary angiomatosis presents with lymphadenopathy and abdominal pain, and manifests as disseminated lesions on the skin, and in the liver and other solid organs.[139–141] In the liver, cystic spaces filled with blood (peliosis hep-atis) are seen. Diagnosis is by radiography, with findings of hepatomegaly and cystic lesions.[142,143] Diagnosis is confirmed by biopsy of cutaneous lesions, which reveal *Bartonella henselae* and *Bartonella quintana* on Warthin-Starry staining. Management is with HAART and antibiotics for 4 to 6 months. The disease is fatal if not treated early.

SUMMARY

Chronic liver disease in the HIV-infected individual is common and poses a challenge to clinicians and scientists. It is an entity that requires management in specialized centers. The more common etiologies that clinicians are now encountering are viral hepatitis coinfection, fatty liver, and DILI. Despite extensive research, much has yet to be elucidated about the underlying pathophysiology. For HCV/HIV coinfection, newer drug therapies that offer better SVR, compliance, and fewer systemic adverse effects are forthcoming. The future era in HIV and chronic liver disease should be a promising one.

REFERENCES

1. Weber R, Sabin CA, Friis-Moller N, et al. Liver-related deaths in persons infected with the human immunodeficiency virus: the D:A:D study. Arch Intern Med 2006; 166(15):1632–41.
2. Bica I, McGovern B, Dhar R, et al. Increasing mortality due to end-stage liver disease in patients with human immunodeficiency virus infection. Clin Infect Dis 2001;32(3):492–7.
3. Sterling RK, Chiu S, Snider K, et al. The prevalence and risk factors for abnormal liver enzymes in HIV-positive patients without hepatitis B or C coinfections. Dig Dis Sci 2008;53(5):1375–82.
4. Sulkowski MS, Thomas DL. Hepatitis C in the HIV-infected person. Ann Intern Med 2003;138(3):197–207.

5. Ly KN, Xing J, Klevens RM, et al. The increasing burden of mortality from viral hepatitis in the United States between 1999 and 2007. Ann Intern Med 2012; 156(4):271–8.
6. Salmon-Ceron D, Lewden C, Morlat P, et al. Liver disease as a major cause of death among HIV infected patients: role of hepatitis C and B viruses and alcohol. J Hepatol 2005;42(6):799–805.
7. Pineda JA, Garcia-Garcia JA, Aguilar-Guisado M, et al. Clinical progression of hepatitis C virus-related chronic liver disease in human immunodeficiency virus-infected patients undergoing highly active antiretroviral therapy. Hepatology 2007;46(3):622–30.
8. Graham CS, Baden LR, Yu E, et al. Influence of human immunodeficiency virus infection on the course of hepatitis C virus infection: a meta-analysis. Clin Infect Dis 2001;33(4):562–9.
9. Rockstroh JK, Mocroft A, Soriano V, et al. Influence of hepatitis C virus infection on HIV-1 disease progression and response to highly active antiretroviral therapy. J Infect Dis 2005;192(6):992–1002.
10. Benhamou Y, Bochet M, Di Martino V, et al. Liver fibrosis progression in human immunodeficiency virus and hepatitis C virus coinfected patients. The Multivirc Group. Hepatology 1999;30(4):1054–8.
11. Sulkowski MS, Benhamou Y. Therapeutic issues in HIV/HCV-coinfected patients. J Viral Hepat 2007;14(6):371–86.
12. den Brinker M, Wit FW, Wertheim-van Dillen PM, et al. Hepatitis B and C virus co-infection and the risk for hepatotoxicity of highly active antiretroviral therapy in HIV-1 infection. AIDS 2000;14(18):2895–902.
13. Sulkowski MS, Thomas DL, Chaisson RE, et al. Elevated liver enzymes following initiation of antiretroviral therapy. JAMA 2000;283(19):2526–7.
14. Jerala R. Structural biology of the LPS recognition. Int J Med Microbiol 2007; 297(5):353–63.
15. Guo J, Friedman SL. Toll-like receptor 4 signaling in liver injury and hepatic fibrogenesis. Fibrogenesis Tissue Repair 2010;3:21. http://dx.doi.org/10.1186/1755-1536-3-21.
16. Lin W, Weinberg EM, Tai AW, et al. HIV increases HCV replication in a TGF-beta1-dependent manner. Gastroenterology 2008;134(3):803–11.
17. Jang JY, Shao RX, Lin W, et al. HIV infection increases HCV-induced hepatocyte apoptosis. J Hepatol 2011;54(4):612–20.
18. Macias J, Japon MA, Saez C, et al. Increased hepatocyte fas expression and apoptosis in HIV and hepatitis C virus coinfection. J Infect Dis 2005;192(9):1566–76.
19. Sterling RK, Contos MJ, Smith PG, et al. Steatohepatitis: risk factors and impact on disease severity in human immunodeficiency virus/hepatitis C virus coinfection. Hepatology 2008;47(4):1118–27.
20. Macias J, Berenguer J, Japon MA, et al. Hepatic steatosis and steatohepatitis in human immunodeficiency virus/hepatitis C virus-coinfected patients. Hepatology 2012;56(4):1261–70.
21. Tuyama AC, Hong F, Saiman Y, et al. Human immunodeficiency virus (HIV)-1 infects human hepatic stellate cells and promotes collagen I and monocyte chemoattractant protein-1 expression: implications for the pathogenesis of HIV/hepatitis C virus-induced liver fibrosis. Hepatology 2010; 52(2):612–22.
22. Smith JO, Sterling RK. Systematic review: non-invasive methods of fibrosis analysis in chronic hepatitis C. Aliment Pharmacol Ther 2009;30(6):557–76.

23. Sterling RK, Lissen E, Clumeck N, et al. Development of a simple noninvasive index to predict significant fibrosis in patients with HIV/HCV coinfection. Hepatology 2006;43(6):1317–25.

24. Shah AG, Smith PG, Sterling RK. Comparison of FIB-4 and APRI in HIV-HCV coinfected patients with normal and elevated ALT. Dig Dis Sci 2011;56(10): 3038–44.

25. Bonder A, Afdhal N. Utilization of FibroScan in clinical practice. Curr Gastroenterol Rep 2014;16(2):372. http://dx.doi.org/10.1007/s11894-014-0372-6.

26. Tapper EB, Castera L, Afdhal NH. FibroScan (vibration controlled transient elastography): where does it stand in the US practice. Clin Gastroenterol Hepatol 2014. [Epub ahead of print].

27. Chung RT, Andersen J, Volberding P, et al. Peginterferon Alfa-2a plus ribavirin versus interferon alfa-2a plus ribavirin for chronic hepatitis C in HIV-coinfected persons. N Engl J Med 2004;351(5):451–9.

28. Terrault NA, Roland ME, Schiano T, et al. Outcomes of liver transplant recipients with hepatitis C and human immunodeficiency virus coinfection. Liver Transpl 2012;18(6):716–26.

29. Alter MJ. Epidemiology of viral hepatitis and HIV co-infection. J Hepatol 2006; 44(Suppl 1):S6–9.

30. Thio CL. Hepatitis B and human immunodeficiency virus coinfection. Hepatology 2009;49(Suppl 5):S138–45.

31. Francisci D, Baldelli F, Papili R, et al. Prevalence of HBV, HDV and HCV hepatitis markers in HIV-positive patients. Eur J Epidemiol 1995;11(2):123–6.

32. McMahon BJ. The natural history of chronic hepatitis B virus infection. Hepatology 2009;49(Suppl 5):S45–55.

33. Colin JF, Cazals-Hatem D, Loriot MA, et al. Influence of human immunodeficiency virus infection on chronic hepatitis B in homosexual men. Hepatology 1999;29(4):1306–10.

34. Bodsworth NJ, Cooper DA, Donovan B. The influence of human immunodeficiency virus type 1 infection on the development of the hepatitis B virus carrier state. J Infect Dis 1991;163(5):1138–40.

35. Gilson RJ, Hawkins AE, Beecham MR, et al. Interactions between HIV and hepatitis B virus in homosexual men: effects on the natural history of infection. AIDS 1997;11(5):597–606.

36. Clifford GM, Rickenbach M, Polesel J, et al. Influence of HIV-related immunodeficiency on the risk of hepatocellular carcinoma. AIDS 2008;22(16):2135–41.

37. Data Collection on Adverse Events of Anti-HIV drugs (D:A:D) Study Group, Smith C, Sabin CA, et al. Factors associated with specific causes of death amongst HIV-positive individuals in the D:A:D Study. AIDS 2010;24(10):1537–48.

38. Hoffmann CJ, Seaberg EC, Young S, et al. Hepatitis B and long-term HIV outcomes in coinfected HAART recipients. AIDS 2009;23(14):1881–9.

39. Konopnicki D, Mocroft A, de Wit S, et al. Hepatitis B and HIV: prevalence, AIDS progression, response to highly active antiretroviral therapy and increased mortality in the EuroSIDA cohort. AIDS 2005;19(6):593–601.

40. Nikolopoulos GK, Paraskevis D, Hatzitheodorou E, et al. Impact of hepatitis B virus infection on the progression of AIDS and mortality in HIV-infected individuals: a cohort study and meta-analysis. Clin Infect Dis 2009;48(12): 1763–71.

41. Iser DM, Avihingsanon A, Wisedopas N, et al. Increased intrahepatic apoptosis but reduced immune activation in HIV-HBV co-infected patients with advanced immunosuppression. AIDS 2011;25(2):197–205.

42. Cooper CL. HIV antiretroviral medications and hepatotoxicity. Curr Opin HIV AIDS 2007;2(6):466–73.
43. Drake A, Mijch A, Sasadeusz J. Immune reconstitution hepatitis in HIV and hepatitis B coinfection, despite lamivudine therapy as part of HAART. Clin Infect Dis 2004;39(1):129–32.
44. Shire NJ, Rouster SD, Stanford SD, et al. The prevalence and significance of occult hepatitis B virus in a prospective cohort of HIV-infected patients. J Acquir Immune Defic Syndr 2007;44(3):309–14.
45. Biggar RJ, Goedert JJ, Hoofnagle J. Accelerated loss of antibody to hepatitis B surface antigen among immunodeficient homosexual men infected with HIV. N Engl J Med 1987;316(10):630–1.
46. Vento S, Di Perri G, Garofano T, et al. Reactivation of hepatitis B in AIDS. Lancet 1989;2(8654):108–9.
47. Lok AS, McMahon BJ. Chronic hepatitis B: update 2009. Hepatology 2009; 50(3):661–2.
48. European Association For The Study Of The Liver. EASL clinical practice guidelines: management of chronic hepatitis B virus infection. J Hepatol 2012;57(1):167–85.
49. Neff GW, Bonham A, Tzakis AG, et al. Orthotopic liver transplantation in patients with human immunodeficiency virus and end-stage liver disease. Liver Transpl 2003;9(3):239–47.
50. Soriano V, Puoti M, Peters M, et al. Care of HIV patients with chronic hepatitis B: updated recommendations from the HIV-Hepatitis B Virus International Panel. AIDS 2008;22(12):1399–410.
51. Meraviglia P, Schiavini M, Castagna A, et al. Lopinavir/ritonavir treatment in HIV antiretroviral-experienced patients: evaluation of risk factors for liver enzyme elevation. HIV Med 2004;5(5):334–43.
52. Williams CD, Stengel J, Asike MI, et al. Prevalence of nonalcoholic fatty liver disease and nonalcoholic steatohepatitis among a largely middle-aged population utilizing ultrasound and liver biopsy: a prospective study. Gastroenterology 2011;140(1):124–31.
53. Vernon G, Baranova A, Younossi ZM. Systematic review: the epidemiology and natural history of non-alcoholic fatty liver disease and non-alcoholic steatohepatitis in adults. Aliment Pharmacol Ther 2011;34(3):274–85.
54. Lazo M, Hernaez R, Eberhardt MS, et al. Prevalence of nonalcoholic fatty liver disease in the United States: the Third National Health and Nutrition Examination Survey, 1988-1994. Am J Epidemiol 2013;178(1):38–45.
55. Agopian VG, Kaldas FM, Hong JC, et al. Liver transplantation for nonalcoholic steatohepatitis: the new epidemic. Ann Surg 2012;256(4):624–33.
56. Charlton MR, Burns JM, Pedersen RA, et al. Frequency and outcomes of liver transplantation for nonalcoholic steatohepatitis in the United States. Gastroenterology 2011;141(4):1249–53.
57. Marks KM, Petrovic LM, Talal AH, et al. Histological findings and clinical characteristics associated with hepatic steatosis in patients coinfected with HIV and hepatitis C virus. J Infect Dis 2005;192(11):1943–9.
58. Monto A, Dove LM, Bostrom A, et al. Hepatic steatosis in HIV/hepatitis C coinfection: prevalence and significance compared with hepatitis C monoinfection. Hepatology 2005;42(2):310–6.
59. Bani-Sadr F, Carrat F, Bedossa P, et al. Hepatic steatosis in HIV-HCV coinfected patients: analysis of risk factors. AIDS 2006;20(4):525–31.
60. Crum-Cianflone N, Dilay A, Collins G, et al. Nonalcoholic fatty liver disease among HIV-infected persons. J Acquir Immune Defic Syndr 2009;50(5):464–73.

61. Sterling RK, Smith PG, Brunt EM. Hepatic steatosis in human immunodeficiency virus: a prospective study in patients without viral hepatitis, diabetes, or alcohol abuse. J Clin Gastroenterol 2013;47(2):182–7.

62. Sanyal AJ, Banas C, Sargeant C, et al. Similarities and differences in outcomes of cirrhosis due to nonalcoholic steatohepatitis and hepatitis C. Hepatology 2006;43(4):682–9.

63. Sulkowski MS, Thomas DL, Chaisson RE, et al. Hepatotoxicity associated with antiretroviral therapy in adults infected with human immunodeficiency virus and the role of hepatitis C or B virus infection. JAMA 2000;283(1):74–80.

64. Sulkowski MS, Thomas DL, Mehta SH, et al. Hepatotoxicity associated with nevirapine or efavirenz-containing antiretroviral therapy: role of hepatitis C and B infections. Hepatology 2002;35(1):182–9.

65. Sulkowski MS, Mehta SH, Chaisson RE, et al. Hepatotoxicity associated with protease inhibitor-based antiretroviral regimens with or without concurrent ritonavir. AIDS 2004;18(17):2277–84.

66. Grunfeld C, Kotler DP, Hamadeh R, et al. Hypertriglyceridemia in the acquired immunodeficiency syndrome. Am J Med 1989;86(1):27–31.

67. Duseja A, Dhiman RK, Chawla Y, et al. Insulin resistance is common in patients with predominantly genotype 3 chronic hepatitis C. Dig Dis Sci 2009;54(8): 1778–82.

68. Harte AL, da Silva NF, Creely SJ, et al. Elevated endotoxin levels in non-alcoholic fatty liver disease. J Inflamm (Lond) 2010;7:15. http://dx.doi.org/10.1186/1476-9255-7-15.

69. Seki E, De Minicis S, Osterreicher CH, et al. TLR4 enhances TGF-beta signaling and hepatic fibrosis. Nat Med 2007;13(11):1324–32.

70. Iwasaki M, Takada Y, Hayashi M, et al. Noninvasive evaluation of graft steatosis in living donor liver transplantation. Transplantation 2004;78(10):1501–5.

71. Bedogni G, Bellentani S, Miglioli L, et al. The Fatty Liver Index: a simple and accurate predictor of hepatic steatosis in the general population. BMC Gastroenterol 2006;6:33.

72. Siddiqui MS, Patidar KR, Boyett S, et al. Validation of non-invasive methods for detecting hepatic steatosis in patients with HIV infection. Clin Gastroenterol Hepatol 2014. [Epub ahead of print].

73. Amorosa V, Synnestvedt M, Gross R, et al. A tale of 2 epidemics: the intersection between obesity and HIV infection in Philadelphia. J Acquir Immune Defic Syndr 2005;39(5):557–61.

74. Crum-Cianflone N, Tejidor R, Medina S, et al. Obesity among patients with HIV: the latest epidemic. AIDS Patient Care STDS 2008;22(12):925–30.

75. Chalasani NP, Sanyal AJ, Kowdley KV, et al. Pioglitazone versus vitamin E versus placebo for the treatment of non-diabetic patients with non-alcoholic steatohepatitis: PIVENS trial design. Contemp Clin Trials 2009; 30(1):88–96.

76. Reisler RB, Han C, Burman WJ, et al. Grade 4 events are as important as AIDS events in the era of HAART. J Acquir Immune Defic Syndr 2003;34(4):379–86.

77. Carr A. HIV protease inhibitor-related lipodystrophy syndrome. Clin Infect Dis 2000;30(Suppl 2):S135–42.

78. Falco V, Rodriguez D, Ribera E, et al. Severe nucleoside-associated lactic acidosis in human immunodeficiency virus-infected patients: report of 12 cases and review of the literature. Clin Infect Dis 2002;34(6):838–46.

79. Boubaker K, Flepp M, Sudre P, et al. Hyperlactatemia and antiretroviral therapy: the Swiss HIV Cohort Study. Clin Infect Dis 2001;33(11):1931–7.

80. John M, Moore CB, James IR, et al. Chronic hyperlactatemia in HIV-infected patients taking antiretroviral therapy. AIDS 2001;15(6):717–23.
81. Brivet FG, Nion I, Megarbane B, et al. Fatal lactic acidosis and liver steatosis associated with didanosine and stavudine treatment: a respiratory chain dysfunction? J Hepatol 2000;32(2):364–5.
82. Miller KD, Cameron M, Wood LV, et al. Lactic acidosis and hepatic steatosis associated with use of stavudine: report of four cases. Ann Intern Med 2000; 133(3):192–6.
83. van Leth F, Phanuphak P, Ruxrungtham K, et al. Comparison of first-line antiretroviral therapy with regimens including nevirapine, efavirenz, or both drugs, plus stavudine and lamivudine: a randomised open-label trial, the 2NN Study. Lancet 2004;363(9417):1253–63.
84. Dieterich DT, Robinson PA, Love J, et al. Drug-induced liver injury associated with the use of nonnucleoside reverse-transcriptase inhibitors. Clin Infect Dis 2004;38(Suppl 2):S80–9.
85. Palmon R, Koo BC, Shoultz DA, et al. Lack of hepatotoxicity associated with nonnucleoside reverse transcriptase inhibitors. J Acquir Immune Defic Syndr 2002;29(4):340–5.
86. Wit FW, Weverling GJ, Weel J, et al. Incidence of and risk factors for severe hepatotoxicity associated with antiretroviral combination therapy. J Infect Dis 2002; 186(1):23–31.
87. Aceti A, Pasquazzi C, Zechini B, et al. Hepatotoxicity development during antiretroviral therapy containing protease inhibitors in patients with HIV: the role of hepatitis B and C virus infection. J Acquir Immune Defic Syndr 2002;29(1):41–8.
88. Brinkman K, ter Hofstede HJ, Burger DM, et al. Adverse effects of reverse transcriptase inhibitors: mitochondrial toxicity as common pathway. AIDS 1998; 12(14):1735–44.
89. Tolomeo M, Mancuso S, Todaro M, et al. Mitochondrial disruption and apoptosis in lymphocytes of an HIV infected patient affected by lactic acidosis after treatment with highly active antiretroviral therapy. J Clin Pathol 2003;56(2):147–51.
90. Fontana RJ, Seeff LB, Andrade RJ, et al. Standardization of nomenclature and causality assessment in drug-induced liver injury: summary of a clinical research workshop. Hepatology 2010;52(2):730–42.
91. Molina JM, Andrade-Villanueva J, Echevarria J, et al. Once-daily atazanavir/ritonavir versus twice-daily lopinavir/ritonavir, each in combination with tenofovir and emtricitabine, for management of antiretroviral-naive HIV-1-infected patients: 48 week efficacy and safety results of the CASTLE study. Lancet 2008;372(9639):646–55.
92. Rotger M, Taffe P, Bleiber G, et al. Gilbert syndrome and the development of antiretroviral therapy-associated hyperbilirubinemia. J Infect Dis 2005;192(8): 1381–6.
93. Soriano V, Puoti M, Garcia-Gasco P, et al. Antiretroviral drugs and liver injury. AIDS 2008;22(1):1–13.
94. Sulkowski MS. Management of hepatic complications in HIV-infected persons. J Infect Dis 2008;197(Suppl 3):S279–93.
95. Bjornsson E. Drug-induced liver injury: Hy's rule revisited. Clin Pharmacol Ther 2006;79(6):521–8.
96. Kovari H, Ledergerber B, Peter U, et al. Association of noncirrhotic portal hypertension in HIV-infected persons and antiretroviral therapy with didanosine: a nested case–control study. Clin Infect Dis 2009;49(4):626–35.

97. Maida I, Nunez M, Rios MJ, et al. Severe liver disease associated with prolonged exposure to antiretroviral drugs. J Acquir Immune Defic Syndr 2006; 42(2):177–82.

98. Mallet V, Blanchard P, Verkarre V, et al. Nodular regenerative hyperplasia is a new cause of chronic liver disease in HIV-infected patients. AIDS 2007;21(2): 187–92.

99. Kovari H, Ledergerber B, Battegay M, et al. Incidence and risk factors for chronic elevation of alanine aminotransferase levels in HIV-infected persons without hepatitis b or c virus co-infection. Clin Infect Dis 2010;50(4):502–11.

100. Podevin P, Spiridon G, Terris B, et al. Nodular regenerative hyperplasia of the liver after IL-2 therapy in an HIV-infected patient. AIDS 2006;20(2):313–5.

101. Vispo E, Moreno A, Maida I, et al. Noncirrhotic portal hypertension in HIV-infected patients: unique clinical and pathological findings. AIDS 2010;24(8): 1171–6.

102. Schiano TD, Kotler DP, Ferran E, et al. Hepatoportal sclerosis as a cause of noncirrhotic portal hypertension in patients with HIV. Am J Gastroenterol 2007; 102(11):2536–40.

103. Schiano TD, Uriel A, Dieterich DT, et al. The development of hepatoportal sclerosis and portal hypertension due to didanosine use in HIV. Virchows Arch 2011; 458(2):231–5.

104. Cachay ER, Peterson MR, Goicoechea M, et al. Didanosine Exposure and Noncirrhotic Portal Hypertension in a HIV Clinic in North America: a Follow-up Study. Br J Med Med Res 2011;1(4):346–55.

105. Bouche H, Housset C, Dumont JL, et al. AIDS-related cholangitis: diagnostic features and course in 15 patients. J Hepatol 1993;17(1):34–9.

106. Ducreux M, Buffet C, Lamy P, et al. Diagnosis and prognosis of AIDS-related cholangitis. AIDS 1995;9(8):875–80.

107. Vakil NB, Schwartz SM, Buggy BP, et al. Biliary cryptosporidiosis in HIV-infected people after the waterborne outbreak of cryptosporidiosis in Milwaukee. N Engl J Med 1996;334(1):19–23.

108. Margulis SJ, Honig CL, Soave R, et al. Biliary tract obstruction in the acquired immunodeficiency syndrome. Ann Intern Med 1986;105(2):207–10.

109. Chen XM, LaRusso NF. Cryptosporidiosis and the pathogenesis of AIDS-cholangiopathy. Semin Liver Dis 2002;22(3):277–89.

110. Enns R. AIDS cholangiopathy: "an endangered disease." Am J Gastroenterol 2003;98(10):2111–2.

111. Pitlik SD, Fainstein V, Rios A, et al. Cryptosporidial cholecystitis. N Engl J Med 1983;308(16):967.

112. Aronson NE, Cheney C, Rholl V, et al. Biliary giardiasis in a patient with human immunodeficiency virus. J Clin Gastroenterol 2001;33(2):167–70.

113. Mahajani RV, Uzer MF. Cholangiopathy in HIV-infected patients. Clin Liver Dis 1999;3(3):669–84.

114. Cello JP. Acquired immunodeficiency syndrome cholangiopathy: spectrum of disease. Am J Med 1989;86(5):539–46.

115. Cello JP, Chan MF. Long-term follow-up of endoscopic retrograde cholangiopancreatography sphincterotomy for patients with acquired immune deficiency syndrome papillary stenosis. Am J Med 1995;99(6):600–3.

116. Forbes A, Blanshard C, Gazzard B. Natural history of AIDS related sclerosing cholangitis: a study of 20 cases. Gut 1993;34(1):116–21.

117. Benhamou Y, Caumes E, Gerosa Y, et al. AIDS-related cholangiopathy. Critical analysis of a prospective series of 26 patients. Dig Dis Sci 1993;38(6):1113–8.

118. Schneiderman DJ, Cello JP, Laing FC. Papillary stenosis and sclerosing cholangitis in the acquired immunodeficiency syndrome. Ann Intern Med 1987;106(4): 546–9.
119. Ko WF, Cello JP, Rogers SJ, et al. Prognostic factors for the survival of patients with AIDS cholangiopathy. Am J Gastroenterol 2003;98(10):2176–81.
120. Devarbhavi H, Dierkhising R, Kremers WK, et al. Single-center experience with drug-induced liver injury from India: causes, outcome, prognosis, and predictors of mortality. Am J Gastroenterol 2010;105(11):2396–404.
121. Lanjewar DN, Rao RJ, Kulkarni SB, et al. Hepatic pathology in AIDS: a pathological study from Mumbai, India. HIV Med 2004;5(4):253–7.
122. Poles MA, Dieterich DT, Schwarz ED, et al. Liver biopsy findings in 501 patients infected with human immunodeficiency virus (HIV). J Acquir Immune Defic Syndr Hum Retrovirol 1996;11(2):170–7.
123. Shibuya K, Coulson WF, Wollman JS, et al. Histopathology of cryptococcosis and other fungal infections in patients with acquired immunodeficiency syndrome. Int J Infect Dis 2001;5(2):78–85.
124. Lamps LW, Molina CP, West AB, et al. The pathologic spectrum of gastrointestinal and hepatic histoplasmosis. Am J Clin Pathol 2000;113(1):64–72.
125. Poblete RB, Rodriguez K, Foust RT, et al. Pneumocystis carinii hepatitis in the acquired immunodeficiency syndrome (AIDS). Ann Intern Med 1989;110(9):737–8.
126. Lawee D. Mild infectious mononucleosis presenting with transient mixed liver disease: case report with a literature review. Can Fam Physician 2007;53(8): 1314–6.
127. Feranchak AP, Tyson RW, Narkewicz MR, et al. Fulminant Epstein-Barr viral hepatitis: orthotopic liver transplantation and review of the literature. Liver Transpl Surg 1998;4(6):469–76.
128. Duffy LF, Daum F, Kahn E, et al. Hepatitis in children with acquired immune deficiency syndrome. Histopathologic and immunocytologic features. Gastroenterology 1986;90(1):173–81.
129. Penman HG. Fatal infectious mononucleosis: a critical review. J Clin Pathol 1970;23(9):765–71.
130. Shaw NJ, Evans JH. Liver failure and Epstein-Barr virus infection. Arch Dis Child 1988;63(4):432–3.
131. Adams LA, Deboer B, Jeffrey G, et al. Ganciclovir and the treatment of Epstein-Barr virus hepatitis. J Gastroenterol Hepatol 2006;21(11):1758–60.
132. Rafailidis PI, Mavros MN, Kapaskelis A, et al. Antiviral treatment for severe EBV infections in apparently immunocompetent patients. J Clin Virol 2010;49(3):151–7.
133. Guarda LA, Luna MA, Smith JL Jr, et al. Acquired immune deficiency syndrome: postmortem findings. Am J Clin Pathol 1984;81(5):549–57.
134. Reichert CM, O'Leary TJ, Levens DL, et al. Autopsy pathology in the acquired immune deficiency syndrome. Am J Pathol 1983;112(3):357–82.
135. Simard EP, Pfeiffer RM, Engels EA. Spectrum of cancer risk late after AIDS onset in the United States. Arch Intern Med 2010;170(15):1337–45.
136. Pati S, Pelser CB, Dufraine J, et al. Antitumorigenic effects of HIV protease inhibitor ritonavir: inhibition of Kaposi sarcoma. Blood 2002;99(10):3771–9.
137. Pons I, Sanfeliu I, Nogueras MM, et al. Seroprevalence of Bartonella spp. infection in HIV patients in Catalonia, Spain. BMC Infect Dis 2008;8:58. http://dx.doi.org/10.1186/1471-2334-8-58.
138. Plettenberg A, Lorenzen T, Burtsche BT, et al. Bacillary angiomatosis in HIV-infected patients–an epidemiological and clinical study. Dermatology 2000; 201(4):326–31.

139. Czapar CA, Weldon-Linne CM, Moore DM, et al. Peliosis hepatis in the acquired immunodeficiency syndrome. Arch Pathol Lab Med 1986;110(7):611–3.
140. Velho PE, Pimentel V, Del Negro GM, et al. Severe anemia, panserositis, and cryptogenic hepatitis in an HIV patient infected with *Bartonella henselae*. Ultrastruct Pathol 2007;31(6):373–7.
141. Mohle-Boetani JC, Koehler JE, Berger TG, et al. Bacillary angiomatosis and bacillary peliosis in patients infected with human immunodeficiency virus: clinical characteristics in a case-control study. Clin Infect Dis 1996;22(5): 794–800.
142. Braden B, Helm B, Fabian T, et al. Bacillary angiomatosis of the liver, a suspected ultrasound diagnosis? Z Gastroenterol 2000;38(9):785–9.
143. Radin DR, Kanel GC. Peliosis hepatis in a patient with human immunodeficiency virus infection. AJR Am J Roentgenol 1991;156(1):91–2.

Evaluation and Management of Hepatocellular Carcinoma

 CrossMark

Laura M. Kulik, MD*, Attasit Chokechanachaisakul, MD

KEYWORDS

- Hepatocellular carcinoma • Evaluation • Management • Diagnosis • Treatment

KEY POINTS

- HCC is increasing in incidence.
- The role of HCC surveillance is to diagnose disease at a curative stage.
- Therapy for HCC is dependent upon the burden of tumor and degree of liver dysfunction.
- Potential curative options for HCC include hepatic resection, transplantation or ablation (in solitary lesion < 3 cm).
- Response to locoregional therapy, both radiographic and AFP decline, can be used to gain insight into tumor biology.

INTRODUCTION

The incidence of hepatocellular carcinoma (HCC) is increasing in the United States and is predicted to continue to increase.[1] Over the last several decades, the escalation in HCC has mirrored the increase in the incidence of hepatitis C virus (HCV)-induced cirrhosis, which carries the highest risk for the development of HCC, at an estimated 2% to 8% per year. The peak incidence of HCV-induced HCC is projected to occur in 2020. Despite an anticipated decline in HCV-induced cirrhosis and hence HCC, HCC related to nonalcoholic fatty liver disease is anticipated to increase.

There have been changing trends in the epidemiology of HCC in the United States, most notably with Hispanic men, who represent the fastest increase in the incidence of HCC, and a shift toward a younger age at diagnosis.[2]

Diagnosis at an incurable stage is associated with a dismal prognosis. Although there have been advancements in the treatment of HCC and a doubling of long-term survival, the overall 5-year survival remains low, at 18%, underscoring the need for novel therapeutic options.[3]

Disclosures: None.
Kovler Organ Transplantation Center, NMH, Arkes Family Pavilion, Suite 1900, 676 North Saint Clair, Chicago, IL 60611, USA
* Corresponding author.
E-mail address: lkulik@nmff.org

Clin Liver Dis 19 (2015) 23–43
http://dx.doi.org/10.1016/j.cld.2014.09.002
1089-3261/15/$ – see front matter © 2015 Elsevier Inc. All rights reserved.

The management of HCC is complicated by the superimposed morbidity/mortality related to cirrhosis, which is present in 80% to 90% of cases of HCC. Treatment of HCC is equally dictated by tumor burden, degree of liver dysfunction (Child-Pugh [CP] class), and the patients' Eastern Cooperative Oncology Group (ECOG) performance status (**Table 1**). The Barcelona Clinic of Liver Cancer (BCLC) encompasses all these factors when making decisions regarding HCC therapy and is endorsed by the American and European associations (**Table 2**).[4] More recently, a staging system from Hong Kong was published.[5]

Given the complexities of caring for a patient with HCC, the vital necessity of a multidisciplinary approach cannot be overstated. Improvement in patient outcome, including more patients receiving curative therapies and prolonged overall survival (OS), has been reported in the setting of a multidisciplinary team.[6]

In this article, the approach to patients at risk for the development of HCC and various treatment options are summarized.

RECOMMENDATIONS FOR HEPATOCELLULAR CARCINOMA SURVEILLANCE

The rationale for HCC surveillance is to diagnose at an early stage, when potential curative options are viable (resection, transplant, ablation). The recommendation for HCC surveillance is limited to a single randomized controlled trial (RCT) from China of 18,816 patients with hepatitis B that reported a 37% decrease in HCC mortality in those undergoing ultrasonography (US) + α-fetoprotein (AFP) every 6 months compared with the control group, despite low compliance in the surveillance group.[7] The decline in mortality among the surveillance group was related to detection of early HCC in 60% compared with 0% in the control group and a resection rate of 47% among those randomized to US + AFP versus 7.5% in the nonsurveillance group. It is not clear if these findings would be applicable to patients with cirrhosis in the United States. Nonetheless, an RCT of HCC surveillance is unlikely because of ethical concerns, and the feasibility of such a study has been reported to be remote, with only 0.5% of patients agreeable to randomization.[8]

A meta-analysis,[9] including more than 15,000 patients with cirrhosis, concluded that HCC surveillance led to earlier stage detection with improved curative treatment rates and OS. The results remained unchanged even after adjusting for lead time bias.

The screening interval is not determined by the risk for the development of HCC but rather the doubling time of HCC, which has been estimated to range from 1 to

Table 1 ECOG performance status	
Grade	ECOG
0	Fully active, able to carry on all predisease performance without restriction
1	Restricted in physically strenuous activity but ambulatory and able to carry out work of a light or sedentary nature (eg, light house work, office work)
2	Ambulatory and capable of all self-care but unable to carry out any work activities. Up and about more than 50% of waking hours
3	Capable of only limited self-care, confined to bed or chair more than 50% of waking hours
4	Completely disabled. Cannot carry on any self-care. Totally confined to bed or chair
5	Dead

From Oken MM, Creech RH, Tormey DC, et al. Toxicity and response criteria of the Eastern Cooperative Oncology Group. Am J Clin Oncol 1982;5:649–55.

Table 2
Effect of tumor number and presence of portal hypertension on 5-year OS and HCC recurrence

OS (%)	5-y
PHT CP A	56
No PHT CP A	71
Multiple HCC CP A	58
Single HCC CP A	68
Recurrence (%)	**5-y**
PHT CP A	75
No PHT CP A	58
Multiple HCC CP A	75
Single HCC CP A	60

Abbreviation: PHT, portal hypertension.

19 months, with a median of 4 to 6 months.[10–12] Semiannual screening has been reported to be superior to annual imaging in detecting HCC at an earlier stage.[13] An RCT[14] found no improvement in the detection of early tumors when screening was performed every 3 months compared with every 6 months.

The American Association for the Study of Liver Disease and European Association for the Study of the Liver (EASL) both advocate US every 6 months for patients with cirrhosis and those with hepatitis B without cirrhosis (men >40 years, women >50 years, Africans >20 years and at time of diagnosis if there is a positive family history).[15,16] The EASL guidelines also recommend surveillance in HCV with stage 3 fibrosis. Surveillance is not recommended in decompensated cirrhotic patients who are not listed for transplantation, because they are unlikely to be candidates for resection or ablation. Similarly, those with substantial comorbidities that prohibit therapy are unlikely to derive a benefit from HCC surveillance. The cost-effectiveness of HCC surveillance has been shown, with curative options available for those with early stage disease.[17]

US has the advantage of being noninvasive, inexpensive, and without radiation. The limitations of US are greatest among those with a more coarsened echotexture and in obese patients. In addition, results are dependent on the experience of the operator. Contrast-enhanced US (used in Europe) can aid in distinguishing regenerative nodules from malignant nodules; however, it is not available in the United State and is not anticipated to be approved by the US Food and Drug Administration, because of concern for cardiac toxicity. Furthermore, the use of contrast-enhanced US is not endorsed by guidelines, because of its inability to distinguish HCC from intrahepatic cholangiocarcinoma.[16]

Since 2000, US technology has improved, allowing for the detection of smaller nodules, median 1.6 ± 0.6 cm.[18] This development is reflected in studies that have reported improved survival among patients undergoing HCC surveillance in cohorts since 2000.[19]

Computed tomography (CT) and MRI have been studied only as diagnostic tests. There are insufficient data to recommend cross-sectional imaging for surveillance purposes. However, a study examining the factors that affect US efficacy[20] identified those with the greatest chance of failure of surveillance with US (HCC diagnosed exceeding Milan criteria or HCC detected after a negative US by CT or MRI performed for inadequate US quality or AFP >50 ng/mL), including those with features suggestive of an aggressive HCC (AFP >200 ng/mL, infiltrating tumor, vascular invasion, or metastases) or patients with more advanced liver disease (leading to a more coarsened echo texture) or who are overweight.

AFP is no longer supported by the current guidelines for surveillance because of high false-negative and false-positive results.[21] AFP levels can be normal in up to 40% of patients with HCC. On the other hand, the presence of viral hepatitis, particularly in HCV, can lead to an increase in AFP levels in the absence of HCC. A persistently increasing AFP or disassociation of aspartate transaminase (AST) and AFP (increasing AFP level with no significant change in AST) is worrisome for underlying HCC.[22] Despite the changes to the guidelines, many physicians continue to use AFP as part of a surveillance regimen. AFP should never be used alone for surveillance.

Other markers to improve the detection of early HCC have not been shown to be of benefit. The largest biomarker study comprising 836 patients failed to show lectin bound AFP (AFP-L3) or des-γ-carboxyprothrombin (DCP) to be more sensitive than AFP.[23] A cutoff AFP level of 10.3 had the highest sensitivity for the diagnosis of very early/early HCC.

Education of physicians who care for patients at risk of HCC is required to improve the less than 20% of cirrhotics who are undergoing appropriate surveillance.[24,25] Davila and colleagues[25] reported that gastroenterologists/hepatologists as well as physicians affiliated with an academic institution are more likely to implement appropriate surveillance. A survey of the attitudes of primary care physicians (PCP) regarding HCC surveillance reported that the responsibility of surveillance is equal between the PCP and specialty physicians.[26] The most common identified barriers to proper surveillance included a lack of knowledge of the current guidelines, difficulty discussing surveillance with patients, and competing clinical issues.

DIAGNOSIS OF HEPATOCELLULAR CARCINOMA

Once a lesion greater than 1 cm is detected on US, 4-phase CT, or contrast-enhanced MRI is required to make a diagnosis of HCC. Because of the difficulty and accuracy of liver biopsy (up to 40% false-negative results in lesions $\leq$2 cm), HCC diagnosis is frequently based on radiographic imaging.[27] The classic descriptions of HCC imaging findings are intense contrast uptake in the arterial phase, followed by washout venous delayed phase. Biopsy is required if radiologic findings are not typical for HCC or cirrhosis is not present.[28] Development of intrahepatic cholangiocarcinoma is also a risk in chronic liver disease and should be distinguished from HCC, because transplant is generally not recommended as a result of reported poor outcomes with high recurrence rates.

TREATMENT OF HEPATOCELLULAR CARCINOMA

The recognized potentially curative options for HCC include hepatic resection, orthotopic liver transplant (OLT), or ablation for a lesion 3 cm or smaller. Selection criteria are critical to achieve the best possible outcomes.

Hepatic Resection

In the last 2 decades, surgical outcomes have significantly improved. This situation has largely been attributed to measures to decrease blood loss (maintaining a low central venous pressure of <5 cm H_2O during hepatic transaction, the Pringle maneuver [cross-clamping of the hilum], and laparoscopic surgery).[29,30] RCTs have shown decreased morbidity with use of total parenteral nutrition and avoidance of drains.[31]

The experience of the surgical team cannot be understated; an inpatient mortality of 10% has been reported in low-volume hospitals performing resection in the United States.[32] The expected clinical outcomes in a CP A patient undergoing hepatic resection include less than 3% perioperative mortality, less than 10% transfusion requirement, and 5-year OS of greater than 50%.[33]

The selection criteria used in the West for candidacy for hepatic resection have been the Barcelona criteria, which take into account clinically relevant portal hypertension and serum bilirubin levels. The 5-year OS status after resection was 74% in patients with a serum bilirubin level less than 1.0 mg/dL and hepatic venous pressure gradient (HVPG) less than 10 mm Hg compared with 25% in those not meeting these criteria.[34] Surrogate markers used to predict an HVPG exceeding 10 mm Hg include the presence of esophageal varices, platelet count less than 100,000, or a spleen size greater than 12 cm on imaging. However, a lack of any of these findings does not necessarily preclude an HVPG greater than 10 mm Hg and therefore its measurement is still recommended. These criteria are for a solitary lesion with no upper limit of size; however, larger lesions (>5 cm) are more likely to have vascular invasion, and outcomes have been reported to be inferior, with 5-year OS of approximately 39%.[35,36] Conversely, others[37] have reported similar OS to smaller lesions.

The Model for End-Stage Liver Disease (MELD) score has also been shown to have prognostic value in potential resection candidates. A MELD of 8 or less predicts the best outcomes in patients with cirrhosis; higher MELD scores were associated with higher morbidity and lower OS.[38,39]

The Makucchi criteria originated in Japan and have been used largely in the East to select appropriate candidates for resection.[40] The extent of resection is based on the serum bilirubin level and a quantitative liver function test known as indocyanine green retention rate at 15 minutes (a normal liver has a retention of <10% at 15 minutes, whereas $\geq$40% at 15 minutes indicates that no resection is feasible, irrespective of how much liver removed). These criteria are not widely used in the United States.

Single institutions have devised their own criteria for resection, such as the University of Texas MD Anderson Cancer Center.[41] A patient is deemed appropriate for a minor resection ($\leq$2 segments) if the patient is a CP A, with a bilirubin level of 2 mg/dL or less, no ascites, and platelet count greater than 100,000. For a major resection ($\geq$3 segments), the bilirubin level must be 1 mg/dL or less as well as meeting the other criteria for a minor resection.

In patients with compensated cirrhosis being considered for resection, CT and MRI volumetry are used to calculate the future liver remnant (FLR). An inadequate FLR is associated with postoperative complications and liver failure. Although there is no strict consensus on what volume constitutes a safe FLR, it is recommended that a remnant of 20% to 30% in normal livers, 30% to 40% in those with fibrosis or steatosis, and 40% to 50% in compensated cirrhosis be present after resection to sustain normal postoperative liver function.[42] In those with a smaller predicted FLR, portal vein (PV) embolization (PVE) to occlude PV flow ipsilateral to the tumor to attempt to hypertrophy the remnant lobe has been used. An FLR hypertrophy of 5% or less after PVE is an indicator of poor regenerative capacity and is associated with higher postoperative complications and therefore a contraindication to resection.[43] There are no RCTs examining the safety and efficacy of PVE before resection. Prospective trials have reported fewer postoperative complications and mortality without increased risk of HCC recurrence in patients undergoing a major resection with preoperative PVE compared with no PVE.[44,45] The EASL guidelines have urged additional data be generated, specifically in the era of laparoscopic resection, before PVE can be endorsed as standard of care.

Others[46] have challenged the notion of resection in patients in more than 1 lesion and in the presence of portal hypertension. The 5-year OS was significantly lower (see **Table 2**) among those with multiple lesions or presence of portal hypertension; however, these factors were not independent predictors of OS. Recurrence risk was significantly higher among those with multiple tumors.

Resection in the setting of macrovascular invasion has been considered a contraindication. However, in patients with branch PV thrombosis (PVT) and preserved liver function, resection may be a consideration after careful evaluation.[47]

The risk of recurrent HCC is estimated to be approximately 70% at 5 years and the leading cause of mortality after resection. Nearly three-quarters of recurrences are caused by intrahepatic spread, with recurrence within 2 years of surgery. The remainder of recurrences occur later and are caused by de novo HCC as a result of the field defect of underlying cirrhosis.[48] Factors that have been associated with a lower 5-year OS after resection include multiple nodules versus single, greater than 5 cm versus less than 5 cm, tumor margin 1 cm versus 2 cm, and higher median intraoperative blood loss.[48–51] A meta-analysis[52] has shown that an anatomic resection results in improved clinical outcomes compared with nonanatomic resection. Although an anatomic resection results in a smaller FLR, it allows for the removal of potential undetected tumor draining into the portal venules.

The National Comprehensive Cancer Network guideline recommends imaging every 3 to 6 months for 2 years, then, annually after surgical resection. In addition, if pretreatment AFP levels were increased, repeat serum AFP is recommended every 3 months for 2 years, then, every 6 months.[53]

There are no proven adjuvant therapies to prevent HCC recurrence after resection. The STORM (Sorafenib as Adjuvant Treatment in the Prevention of Recurrence of Hepatocellular Carcinoma) trial, an international phase 3 trial designed to evaluate efficacy/safety of adjuvant sorafenib (400 twice a day) versus placebo after curative ablation or resection failed to show a benefit among the 1100 patients, of whom approximately 80% underwent hepatic resection (maximal tumor size 3.4 cm; 90% had a solitary lesion).[54] There are data that suggest that the risk of HCC recurrence after resection is associated with HCV. With the advent of direct antiviral agents, this finding could play an important role in diminishing HCC recurrence among those with HCV.[55]

Transplantation

The early experience with OLT for HCC was wrought with high HCC recurrence rates and thus poor OS (5 year <35%), leading to OLT being declared a contraindicated in HCC.[56] The inception of the Milan criteria[57] in 1996 (1 lesion ≤5 cm, 3 lesions with no one >3 cm, no vascular invasion, and no metastasis) revolutionized the role of OLT for in early HCC. Excellent 5-year OS exceeding 70% has been reported in patients meeting the Milan criteria.[58] OLT serves the dual purpose of removal of tumor and the underlying cirrhotic liver that predisposed to the development of HCC. The United Network for Organ Sharing (UNOS)[59] allows a MELD exception for those meeting the Milan criteria starting at 22 points and increasing every 3 months in conjunction with repeat imaging to confirm that the tumor burden has not exceeded Milan criteria. Patients outside the Milan criteria are not granted prioritization, leading to the question of if the Milan criteria are too stringent. The obvious concern for expansion beyond the Milan criteria is the potential for negatively affecting posttransplant outcomes (with higher recurrence rates) and further straining the limited resource of organs available. More patients with HCC awaiting OLT with a MELD upgrade could incur harm to those awaiting OLT without HCC.[60] A consensus statement on OLT for HCC[61] recommended consideration for OLT in patients outside the Milan criteria if the dynamics of the wait list would not be negatively affected among other potential recipients without HCC.

Progression of HCC while awaiting OLT can lead to dropout; the risk at 1 year ranges from 15% to 30%.[62] Recognized factors that increase the risk of dropout include tumor greater than 3 cm, AFP level greater than 200 ng/mL, waiting time exceeding 6 months, and lack of proven response to locoregional therapy (LRT).[63] There are no RCTs that have addressed the role of LRT while awaiting OLT.

However, it is recommended to consider LRT in patients anticipated to wait longer than 6 months in the hopes of decreasing dropout.[61]

Downstaging is defined as a treatment that intends to facilitate or make possible a surgical procedure that otherwise is too risky or unfeasible.[64] There have been multiple reports, mostly limited to single-center experience of downstaging to OLT in patients who have on presentation exceeded the Milan criteria.[64] Successful downstaging has been reported to vary from 40% to 90%. The heterogeneity of these results is caused by differences among these reports in terms of inclusion criteria (initial tumor size/number, AFP, tumor grade), type of LRT used, criteria defining response (ie, within Milan criteria based on total tumor size or taking into account tumor necrosis and only measuring viable tumor, decline in tumor markers; AFP/DCP) and enforcing a mandated period of observation after downstaging (3 or 6 months) before activation on the waiting list with a MELD upgrade to mitigate risk of HCC recurrence after OLT. The University of California, San Francisco group[65] has reported encouraging results of 4-year OS of 92% in an initial cohort of patients enrolled in a downstaging protocol. In an updated analysis of 122 patients, there was no significant difference in posttransplant 5-year OS among those who were successfully downstaged to Milan criteria (N = 68) compared with those who met Milan criteria at time of presentation (80 vs 81%, P = not significant).[66] Identified predictors of failure of downstaging were an initial AFP level greater than 1000 ng/mL and receiving more than 3 treatment sessions with LRT. In aggregate, the data suggest that there is a subgroup of patients who exceed the Milan criteria who have excellent posttransplant outcomes associated with successful downstaging procedures.

Patients with T1 lesions (solitary lesion <2 cm) are not granted a MELD upgrade for HCC. A common practice has been to closely observe solitary lesions less than 2 cm and wait until the lesion is 2 cm or greater before initiation of LRT to qualify for a MELD upgrade. However, this strategy incurs the potential risk of a lesion rapidly growing and exceeding Milan criteria. Mehta and colleagues[67] examined the intention-to-treat outcome of watchful waiting in 114 patients with T1 HCC: 1.0 to 1.9 cm (median initial tumor diameter was 1.4 cm). Patients underwent imaging every 3 months. The median time for tumors to progress from T1 to T2 (1 lesion 2–5 cm or 2–3 lesions ≤3 cm) was 6.8 months, compared with 5.1 months for a tumor to progress from T1 to T3 (N = 6, of which 2 patients developed advanced disease with PVT or metastatic disease). The factors associated with increased risk of tumor progression beyond the Milan criteria included rapid tumor growth (defined as >1 cm growth within 3 months) and an initial AFP level greater than 500 ng/mL. Overall, the risk of progressing beyond T2 in an initial T1 lesion without LRT was less than 10%. However, in those patients with an initial AFP level more than 500 ng/mL or rapid tumor growth, early LRT is recommended, even if the tumor is not yet at a T2 status.

Living donor liver transplant (LDLT) offers a timely transplant and hence would be anticipated to decrease dropout and simultaneously expand the donor pool. The number of LDLT (not limited to HCC) performed in the United States has remained low, with only a few hundred per year.[68] Donor safety is a major concern; donor death has been reported to be approximately 0.5%, morbidity 38%, with most complications not being life threatening or altering.[69] Also fast tracking to transplant with an LDLT has led to concern for an inadequate observational period to gain insight into the biological behavior of the tumor such that a limited waiting time to transplant in an aggressive tumor may lead an increase in HCC recurrence after OLT.[70] No significant difference in HCC recurrence has been found between LDLT and deceased donor liver transplant (DDLT) when the same selection criteria are used.[71] However, in A2ALL (Adult to Adult Living Donor Liver Transplantation Cohort Study), a higher rate of HCC recurrence after transplant was observed after adjusting for tumor characteristics among the entire cohort; however, in the MELD era this difference was no longer statistically significant.[72] The difference in HCC recurrence may be attributed to not only difference in tumor characteristics (LDLT offers an option for OLT in those exceeding the Milan criteria), but also pretransplant HCC therapy and waiting time between LDLT and DDLT.

In a CP A patient with HCC, resection or OLT may both be possible treatment options. Although OLT is generally reserved for nonresectable lesions, this decision is influenced by center experience, cultural attitudes toward OLT, practice patterns, and organ availability. The pros and cons for each approach are highlighted in **Table 3**. Intention-to-treat analysis has shown a lower OS in transplant compared with resection caused by dropout while awaiting OLT.[34] Salvage OLT is a transplant that occurs after resection as a result of either hepatic decompensation or recurrent tumor within the Milan criteria. The benefit of such an approach is it engenders the potential for greater availability of organs in those without HCC and negates the need for immunosuppression (if salvage OLT is never required). It is estimated that up to approximately 40% of patients with HCC recurrence after resection are not candidates for salvage OLT because of recurrence beyond the Milan criteria. Several studies[73–75] have reported no significant difference between a primary OLT for HCC compared with salvage OLT. A meta-analysis[76] that examined primary OLT versus resection followed by salvage OLT found a gain in life expectancy of only 7 months associated with primary OLT in CP A patients within the Milan criteria. Primary OLT was the preferable approach over resection when 5-year OS postprimary OLT exceeded 60%. Sensitivity analysis found a gain in life expectancy in listed patients without HCC with resection followed by salvage OLT when the there is a higher percentage of HCC patients listed for OLT and when waiting times are longer. Because of the shortage of organs available, such dynamics need to be taken into account to maximize outcomes for both those with HCC and non-HCC patients listed for OLT. Resection explant characteristics that have been reported to predict HCC recurrence include presence of microvascular invasion, greater than 3 cm, poorly differentiated tumors, satellite nodules, and cirrhosis.[77] Those with 3 or more of these factors

Table 3			
Comparison between hepatic resection and transplantation for HCC			
Transplantation		Hepatic Resection	
Pro	Con	Pro	Con
Removes cirrhotic liver and treats HCC 5-y OS >70% (within Milan)	Shortage of organs Dropout because of HCC progression Potential recurrence of original disease	No waiting time 5-y OS: 50%–70% (selected patients; CP A with single nodule) Provides histologic information	High recurrence rates; (70% at 5 y) Limited appropriate candidates

were significantly more likely to recur beyond the Milan criteria. Such patients should be considered for transplant before recurrence, known as de principle transplant.[78] The recognized limitation is ability to obtain an organ, because there is no HCC MELD upgrade given after resection. Discussion for LDLT may be the most appropriate in these situations in those who would otherwise be a transplant candidate.

No guidelines are in place for monitoring patients after OLT for HCC recurrence. Recommendations regarding frequency and duration of imaging have been suggested based on explant pathology: low (Milan + well/moderately differentiated, no VI) versus high (>Milan or poorly differentiated or + VI) risk.[79] When possible, HCC recurrence should be treated with resection. LRT, or sorafenib can be used for unresectable lesion(s). The safety and efficacy of sorafenib in high-risk patients is being investigated in an RCT (NCT00997022).

Locoregional Therapy

LRT can be used for multiple purposes. LRT may be appropriate in patients who are not surgical candidates. The other role for LRT is as a bridge to OLT and to downstage a patient to OLT or resection. The various types of LRT are listed in **Box 1**.

The response to LRT (radiographic and AFP decline) has emerged as a selection criteria for OLT. The notion of ablate and wait allows for a period of observation to gain insight into the biological behavior of a tumor.[80] A lack of response to transarterial chemoembolization (TACE), regardless of Milan status, was associated with significantly higher post-OLT HCC recurrence rates.[81] In addition, a lack of response has been reported, with a greater chance of dropout independent of tumor size.[82] AFP level closest to transplant is an independent predictor of OS after OLT.[83–85] However, a decline in AFP level associated with LRT results in no identified increase mortality. These findings indicate that the AFP level should be considered in determining patients' candidacy for OLT regardless of tumor size/number. Although not yet implemented, a UNOS consensus conference[86] recommended that patients listed for OLT with HCC should not be granted an upgrade unless AFP level is less than 500 ng/mL.

Ablative therapies

Percutaneous ethanol injection (PEI) was first used in the 1980s to treat small tumors. Thermal ablative therapies including radiofrequency ablation (RFA) and microwave ablation (MWA) have largely replaced PEI because of superiority, with a need for fewer therapies and better local tumor control in tumors greater than 2 cm. Moreover, OS with thermal ablation were higher in a meta-analysis.[87,88] Both RFA (thermal injury) and MWA (electromagnetic energy) induce coagulative necrosis and can be

---

Box 1
List of LRT

1. Percutaneous ethanol ablation
2. Radiofrequency ablation
3. Microwave ablation
4. Transarterial chemoembolization
5. Drug-eluting beads
6. Radioembolization
7. Stereotactic body radiation therapy

performed via percutaneous, laparoscopic, or open laparotomy approach. General anesthesia is usually required. The size of the tumor is the best predictor of response. Complete response is reported in 90% of tumors less than 2.5 cm, whereas less than 50% achieve complete response when greater than 5 cm.[89] Many factors influence the decision for ablative therapy, including tumor size, number, location (near organs or large blood vessels, which can create heat sink and decrease response). An advantage of MWA is less reported heat sink, and it may be more appropriate for use near large blood vessels.[90] For lesions greater than 3 cm, RFA + TACE may lead to improved OS at 5 years compared with RFA alone, whereas in lesions less than 3 cm there seems to be no significant benefit of combination therapy.[91]

RFA is an alternative to hepatic resection in solitary lesions less than 3 cm. An RCT of hepatic resection versus RFA for patients meeting the Milan criteria[92] showed superior OS at 5 years and less recurrence among those who had resection. A subanalysis in those with a solitary lesion less than 3 cm did not alter these results. However, RFA is less invasive, requires shorter hospitalization, and is associated with less morbidity and cost. A meta-analysis[93] showed RFA to be the treatment of choice in patients older than 75 years, because there was less mortality compared with resection.

Intra-arterial therapies

TACE is the most common LRT used in the treatment of HCC, largely because of an RCT showing improved OS compared with no therapy in patients with preserved liver function with intermediate HCC (BCLC B).[94,95] The hypervascular nature of HCC is the rationale for injection of chemotherapy emulsified in lipiodol (delivery agent) with particles to embolize the feeding hepatic artery supplying the tumor inducing hypoxemia and subsequent tumor necrosis. Postembolization syndrome with symptoms of abdominal pain, fever, nausea, and vomiting is common. Ischemic hepatitis with hepatic decompensation can result in those with compromised blood flow in the PV because of PVT, hepatofugal flow, or presence of a transjugular intrahepatic portosystemic shunt. Although there are reports of TACE being feasible in branch PVT, main PVT is an absolute contraindication for TACE.[96]

Drug-eluting beads (DEBs) offer an advantage over conventional TACE by delivering maximal and sustained intratumoral concentrations of doxorubicin and minimizing toxicity as a result of lower systemic absorption.[97] DEBs also enable standardization (generating a consensus statement), which has been difficult to achieve with conventional TACE.[98] A bead size of 100 to 300 μ is recommended to achieve maximal chemotherapy delivery and embolic effect. There are reports of DEBs in the presence of PVT.[99,100]

PRECISION, an international RCT of DEB versus TACE, failed to meet the primary end point of radiographic response (EASL) at 6 months.[101] However, improved radiographic response with DEBs was observed in those with ECOG 1, bilobar disease, CP B, or recurrent disease, along with significantly less serious side effects/liver toxicity compared with conventional TACE. Encouraging results with DEB from a prospective trial reported an OS of 48 months in CP A patients.[102] DEBS has shown significantly higher rates of necrosis on explants and improved 3-year recurrence-free survival after OLT compared with conventional TACE.[103,104]

Transarterial radioembolization (TARE) is another form of intra-arterial therapy. Microspheres impregnated with yttrium 90 (Y90) are injected into the hepatic artery. Because of the hypervascular nature of HCC and the small size of the microspheres, 25 to 30 μ, Y90 is preferentially delivered to the capillary bed of the tumor, leading to high intralesional radiation and minimization of radiation to nontarget surrounding tissue. Before administration of Y90, a staging angiogram is performed to identify aberrant anatomy that may require coil embolization to prevent nontarget delivery of microspheres, correct catheter position, and determine degree of pulmonary shunting via a technetium 99 macroaggregated albumin scan. The amount of radiation is calculated via dosimetry.[105] If the degree of shunting is too high (>30 Gy with single injection and cumulative dose of >50 Gy), therapy may not be performed or alternatively the dose of radiation can be lowered according to the degree of shunting. Within 7 to 10 days, the patient returns for administration of Y90; both procedures are outpatient. Same day administration is being performed in some centers.

Unlike chemoembolization, Y90 is not macroembolic; and therefore; the patency of the hepatic artery is maintained. The use of Y90 has been shown to be safe in patients with PVT (bland or tumor).[106–109] OS is affected by both the CP class and locations of PVT (branch vs main) (**Table 4**). Another consideration is an emphasis on delivering intra-arterial therapies in a selective/superselective manner to minimize injury to surrounding tissue. It has been suggested that TACE should not be performed if greater than 2 segments are encompassed in the treatment field, generally larger tumors.[110] In such cases, TARE has been advocated.

The other area in which Y90 has shown clinical promise is in downstaging. In a retrospective analysis,[111] Y90 led to downstaging to T2 in 58% versus 31% with TACE ($P = .023$), and disease progression at 1 year was significantly lower among the Y90 cohort, 15% versus 32%, $P \leq .05$. Downstaging to resection has been coined radiation lobectomy. Lobar therapy with Y90 can lead to both treatment of the tumor and simultaneous hypertrophy of the FLR, thereby permitting resection in some patients who may have not otherwise been candidates because of concern for a small liver remnant.[112] Although hypertrophy can be seen within 1 month after Y90, the degree of hypertrophy correlates with the time elapsed since treatment, with a median FLR increase of 45% from baseline at 9 months.

Table 4 Impact of PVT on OS and TTP					
Salem et al	OS Median (95% CI)	TTP Median (95% CI)	Mazzaferro et al	OS Median (95% CI)	TTP Median (95% CI)
CP A: 0 PVT, 0 mets (N = 81)	22.1 (17.2–32.5)	15.5 (10.7–25.9)	CP A: 0 PVT, 0 mets (N = 15)	18 (12–38)	13 (6 NC)
Branch (N = 19)	16.6 (8.8–24)	5.6 (3.7–13.6)	Branch (N = 23)	17 (13–21)	7 (6–12)
Main PVT (N = 16)	7.7 (3.3–13.2)	5.8 (1–7.5)	Main PVT (N = 5)	9 (4 NC)	3 (2 NC)
CP B: 0 PVT, 0 mets (N = 65)	14.8 (11.8–29.1)	13.0 (8.4–18.1)	CP B: 0 PVT, 0 mets (N = 2)	NC	No PD
Branch (N = 27)	6.5 (5–8.5)	5.1 (4.2–8.9)	Branch (N = 6)	6.5 (5–12)	NC
Main PVT (N = 30)	4.5 (2.9–6.6)	6.0 (2.3–10.4)	Main PVT (N = 1)	5	No PD

Abbreviations: mets, metastasis; NC, not calculable; PD, progression of disease; TTP, time to progression.

From Salem R, Lewandowski RJ, Mulcahy MF, et al. Radioembolization for hepatocellular carcinoma using Yttrium-90 microspheres: a comprehensive report of long-term outcomes. Gastroenterology 2010;138(1):52–64; and Mazzaferro V, Sposito C, Bhoori S, et al. Yttrium-90 radioembolization for intermediate-advanced hepatocellular carcinoma: a phase 2 study. Hepatology 2013;57:1826–37.

There are no published RCTs of TACE versus Y90. The comparison between the 2 treatment modalities is limited to retrospective analysis.[113,114] Although OS was similar between TACE and Y90 (overall or in BCLC B), there were noted differences from a patient prospective, which may affect patients' treatment decision. Y90 patients required no hospitalization, less abdominal pain, fewer treatment sessions, and improved quality of life.[115]

Systemic Therapy

Sorafenib, a multityrosine kinase inhibitor, remains the only approved systemic therapy for HCC. Two RCTs (SHARP [Sorafenib Hepatocellular Carcinoma Assessment Randomized Protocol] and the Asian-Pacific group) reported improved OS in CP A advanced HCC compared with placebo.[116,117] An interim analysis of the GIDEON (Global Investigation of Therapeutic Decisions in HCC and of its Treatment with Sorafenib) trial,[118] a prospective observational trial of patients treated with sorafenib, highlighted that OS is influenced by CP status: CP A: 10.3 versus CP B 4.8 months. A survival advantage was reported in a small retrospective study in CP B patients treated with sorafenib compared with best supportive care.[119] The safety and efficacy of sorafenib in CP B patients is being examined in an ongoing RCT, Sorafenib in First-line Treatment of Advanced B Child Hepatocellular Carcinoma or BOOST trial (NCT01405573).

CP A patients with PVT are potential candidates for sorafenib or TARE. The role of combining TARE + sorafenib lacks data; several trials are ongoing.

For those who progress or are intolerant to sorafenib, there is an unmet need. RCTs of other tyrosine kinase inhibitors (sunitinib, brivanib, linifanib) compared with sorafenib have not shown improvement over sorafenib.[120–123] One agent has shown clinical promise. Tivantinib, an oral MET inhibitor, significantly improved time to progression (TTP) (11.7 vs 6.1 mo.; $P = .03$) and OS (7.2 vs 3.8; $P = .01$) in patients with high tumor MET expression on biopsy compared with placebo.[124] The most common grade 3 or higher adverse events in the phase 2 trial were neutropenia and anemia, leading to dose alteration from 360 mg to 240 mg. A phase 3 RCT (NCT01755767) is under way to confirm if this agent is a viable second-line therapy. Several other agents are under investigation alone (SGI-110 NCT01752933) or in combination with sorafenib (everolimus NCT01005199), temsirolimus (NCT01687673), pravastatin (NCT0148729).

The use of sorafenib in the pretransplant setting is limited and has conflicting results.[125,126] A pilot RCT of 20 patients (Y90 ± sorafenib) awaiting OLT found no benefit of sorafenib added to Y90 in terms of explant pathology or clinical outcomes.[127,128] However, there was an increased risk of biliary complications and acute cellular rejection within 30 days in the sorafenib group. These findings suggest that sorafenib before OLT should be used only in the context of a clinical trial.

Combination locoregional therapy with systemic therapy

The rationale for combining sorafenib with LRT is to blunt a flare of angiogenesis and hence lead to slower progression of tumor. Three RCTs of conventional TACE or DEB ± sorafenib have reported conflicted results.[129–131] A meta-analysis of 6 studies (which did not include the unpublished SPACE trial) concluded that the combination of sorafenib + TACE improved OS and TTP.[132] Additional research is warranted to confirm this benefit.

Hepatocellular Carcinoma Prevention

HCC is the number 1 cause of mortality among patients with cirrhosis. Patients should be educated on measures to potentially prevent the development of HCC. All patients should be counseled on alcohol abstinence, smoking cessation, maintaining a normal body mass index, and hepatitis B virus (HBV) vaccination. Data support intake of coffee to prevent HCC; however, decaffeinated coffee and other caffeinated beverages have not been shown to have a protective effect on HCC development.[133] Further research is required to determine the effect of low vitamin D levels on the risk of HCC.[134]

SUMMARY

The incidence of HCC is increasing in the United States. HCV carries the highest risk factor for development of HCC. Diagnosis at an early stage is crucial for survival benefits. Major guidelines recommend US surveillance every 6 months for patients with HCC risk factors. HCC diagnosis is based on typical findings on CT or MRI. Biopsy is required if imaging findings are not typical or noncirrhosis. The Barcelona treatment strategy is widely accepted in the West. Hepatic resection, liver transplant, and ablation are the main curative treatment options for early stage HCC. LRT can be used for patients with HCC who are not surgical candidates, downstaging for surgical treatments, or bridging therapy for OLT. Sorafenib is the only approved systemic therapy for HCC. Although there have been advancements in the treatment of HCC and a doubling of long-term survival, diagnosis in advanced stages has a low 5-year OS, at 18%, underscoring the need for novel therapeutic options.

REFERENCES

1. Altekruse SF, McGlynn KA, Reichman ME. Hepatocellular carcinoma incidence, mortality, and survival trends in the United States from 1975 to 2005. J Clin Oncol 2009;27:1485–91.
2. El-Serag H, Kanwal F. Epidemiology of hepatocellular carcinoma in the United States: where are we? Where do we go? Hepatology 2014. [Epub ahead of print].
3. Altekruse SF, McGlynn KA, Dickie LA, et al. Hepatocellular carcinoma confirmation, treatment, and survival in surveillance, epidemiology, and end results registries, 1992–2008. Hepatology 2012;55:476–82.
4. Llovet JM, Brú C, Bruix J. Prognosis of hepatocellular carcinoma: the BCLC staging classification. Semin Liver Dis 1999;19(3):329–38.
5. Yau T, Tang VY, Yao TJ, et al. Development of Hong Kong liver cancer staging system with treatment stratification for patients with hepatocellular carcinoma. Gastroenterology 2014;146:1697–700.
6. Mazzaferro V, Majno P. Principles for the best multidisciplinary meetings. Lancet Oncol 2011;12(4):323–5.
7. Zhang J, Yang BH, Tang ZY, et al. Randomized controlled trial of screening for hepatocellular carcinoma. J Cancer Res Clin Oncol 2004;130(7):417–22.
8. Poustchi H, Farrell GC, Strasser SI, et al. Feasability of conducting a randomized controlled trial for liver cancer screening: is a randomized controlled trial for liver cancer screening feasible or still needed? Hepatology 2011;54(6):1998–2004.
9. Singal AG, Pillai A, Tiro J. Early detection, curative treatment, and survival rates for hepatocellular carcinoma surveillance in patients with cirrhosis: a meta-analysis. PLoS Med 2014;11(4):e1001624.
10. Sheu JC, Sung JL, Chen DS, et al. Growth rate of asymptomatic hepatocellular carcinoma and its clinical implications. Gastroenterology 1985;89:259–66.
11. Barbara L, Benzi G, Gaiani S, et al. Natural history of small untreated hepatocellular carcinoma in cirrhosis: a multivariate analysis of prognostic factors of tumor growth rate and patient survival. Hepatology 1992;16:132–7.

12. Okazaki N, Yoshino M, Yoshida T, et al. Evaluation of the prognosis for small hepatocellular carcinoma based on tumor volume doubling time. A preliminary report. Cancer 1989;63:2207–10.
13. Santi V, Trevisani F, Gramenzi A, et al. Semiannual surveillance is superior to annual surveillance for the detection of early hepatocellular carcinoma and patient survival. J Hepatol 2010;53:291–7.
14. Trinchet J, Chaffaut C, Bourcier V, et al. Ultrasonographic surveillance of hepatocellular carcinoma in cirrhosis: a randomized trial comparing 3- and 6-month periodicities. Hepatology 2011;54:1987–97.
15. Bruix J, Sherman M. Management of hepatocellular carcinoma. Hepatology 2005;42:1208–36.
16. European Association for the Study of the Liver, European Organisation for Research and Treatment of Cancer. EASL-EORTC clinical practice guidelines: management of hepatocellular carcinoma. J Hepatol 2012;56(4):908–43.
17. Andersson KL, Salomon JA, Goldie SJ, et al. Cost effectiveness of alternative surveillance strategies for hepatocellular carcinoma in patients with cirrhosis. Clin Gastroenterol Hepatol 2008;6:1418–24.
18. Sato T, Tateshi R, Yoshida H, et al. Ultrasound surveillance for early detection of hepatocellular carcinoma among patients with chronic hepatitis C. Hepatol Int 2009;3:544–50.
19. Thompson Coon J, Rogers G, Hewson P, et al. Surveillance of cirrhosis for hepatocellular carcinoma: a cost-utility analysis. Br J Cancer 2008;98:1166–75.
20. Del Poggio P, Olmi S, Ciccarese F, et al. Factors that affect efficacy of ultrasound surveillance for early stage hepatocellular carcinoma in patients with cirrhosis. Clin Gastroenterol Hepatol 2014. [Epub ahead of print].
21. Forner A, Reig M, Bruix J. Alpha-fetoprotein for hepatocellular carcinoma diagnosis: the demise of a brilliant star. Gastroenterology 2009;137:26–9.
22. Di Bisceglie AM, Sterling RK, Chung RT, et al. Serum alpha-fetoprotein levels in patients with advanced hepatitis C: results from the HALT-C Trial. J Hepatol 2005;43(3):434–41.
23. Marrero J, Feng Z, Wang Y, et al. Alpha-fetoprotein, des-gamma carboxyprothrombin, and lectin-bound alpha-fetoprotein in early hepatocellular carcinoma. Gastroenterology 2009;137:110–8.
24. Singal AG, Yopp A, S Skinner C, et al. Utilization of hepatocellular carcinoma surveillance among American patients: a systematic review. J Gen Intern Med 2012;27(7):861–7.
25. Davila JA, Morgan RO, Richardson PA, et al. Use of surveillance for hepatocellular carcinoma among patients with cirrhosis in the United States. Hepatology 2010;52:132–41.
26. Dalton-Fitzgerald E, Tiro J, Kandunoori P, et al. Practice patterns and attitudes of primary care providers and barriers to surveillance of hepatocellular carcinoma in patients with cirrhosis. Clin Gastroenterol Hepatol 2014. [Epub ahead of print].
27. Forner A, Vilana R, Ayuso C, et al. Diagnosis of hepatic nodules 20 mm or smaller in cirrhosis: prospective validation of the noninvasive diagnostic criteria for hepatocellular carcinoma. Hepatology 2008;47:97–104.
28. de Lope CR, Tremosini S, Forner A, et al. Management of HCC. J Hepatol 2012; 56(Suppl 1):S75–87.
29. Jarnagin WR, Gonen M, Fong Y, et al. Improvement in perioperative outcome after hepatic resection: analysis of 1,803 consecutive cases over the past decade. Ann Surg 2002;236(4):397–406.

30. Poon R, Fan ST, Lo CM, et al. Improving perioperative outcome expands the role of hepatectomy in management of benign and malignant hepatobiliary diseases: analysis of 1222 consecutive patients from a prospective database. Ann Surg 2004;240:698–710.

31. Lui CL, Fan ST, Lo CM, et al. Abdominal drainage after hepatic resection is contraindicated in patients with chronic liver diseases. Ann Surg 2004;239:194–201.

32. Dimick JB, Cowan JA Jr, Knol JA, et al. Hepatic resection in the United States: indications, outcomes, and hospital procedural volumes from a nationally representative database. Arch Surg 2003;138:185–91.

33. Llovet JM, Schwartz M, Mazzaferro V. Resection and liver transplantation for hepatocellular carcinoma. Semin Liver Dis 2005;25(2):181–200.

34. Llovet JM, Fuster J, Bruix J. Intention-to-treat analysis of surgical treatment for early hepatocellular carcinoma: resection versus transplantation. Hepatology 1999;30:1434–40.

35. Vauthey JN, Pawlik TM, Lauwers GY, et al. Is hepatic resection for large or multinodular hepatocellular carcinoma justified? Results from a multi-institutional database. Ann Surg Oncol 2005;12(5):364–73.

36. Yang LY, Fang F, Ou DP, et al. Solitary large hepatocellular carcinoma: a specific subtype of hepatocellular carcinoma with good outcome after hepatic resection. Ann Surg 2009;249(1):118–23.

37. Shah SA, Wei AC, Cleary SP, et al. Prognosis and results after resection of very large (>10 cm) hepatocellular carcinoma. J Gastrointest Surg 2007;11: 589–95.

38. Cucchetti A, Ercolani G, Vivarelli M, et al. Impact of model for end-stage liver disease (MELD) score on prognosis after hepatectomy for hepatocellular carcinoma on cirrhosis. Liver Transpl 2006;12:966–71.

39. Teh SH, Sheppard BC, Schwartz J, et al. Model for end-stage liver disease score fails to predict perioperative outcome after hepatic resection for hepatocellular carcinoma in patients without cirrhosis. Am J Surg 2008;195:697–701.

40. Makuuchi M, Kosuge T, Takayama T, et al. Surgery for small liver cancers. Semin Surg Oncol 1993;9:298–304.

41. Truty MJ, Vauthey JN. Surgical resection of high-risk hepatocellular carcinoma: patient selection, preoperative considerations and operative technique. Ann Surg Oncol 2010;17:1219–25.

42. Kubota K, Makuuchi M, Kusaka K, et al. Measurement of liver volume and hepatic functional reserve as a guide to decision-making in resectional surgery for hepatic tumors. Hepatology 1997;26(5):1176–81.

43. Ribero D, Abdalla E, Madoff D, et al. Portal vein embolization before major hepatectomy and its effects on regeneration, resectability and outcome. Br J Surg 2007;94(11):1386–94.

44. Farges O, Belghiti J, Kianmanesh R, et al. Portal vein embolization before right hepatectomy: prospective clinical trial. Ann Surg 2002;237:208–17.

45. Palavencino M, Chun YS, Madoff DC, et al. Major hepatic resection for hepatocellular carcinoma with or without portal vein embolization: perioperative outcome and survival. Surgery 2009;145:399–405.

46. Ishizawa T, Hasegawa K, Aoki T, et al. Neither multiple tumors nor portal hypertension are surgical contraindications for hepatocellular carcinoma. Gastroenterology 2008;134(7):1908–16.

47. Pawlik TM, Poon RT, Abdalla EK, et al. Hepatectomy for hepatocellular carcinoma with major portal or hepatic vein invasion: results of a multicenter study. Surgery 2005;137(4):403–10.

48. Imamura H, Matsuyama Y, Tanaka E, et al. Risk factors contributing to early and late phase intrahepatic recurrence of hepatocellular carcinoma after hepatectomy. J Hepatol 2003;38:200–7.

49. Ikai I, Arii S, Kojiro M, et al. Reevaluation of prognostic factors for survival after liver resection in patients with hepatocellular carcinoma in a Japanese nationwide survey. Cancer 2004;101:796–802.

50. Shi M, Guo RP, Lin XJ, et al. Partial hepatectomy with wide versus narrow resection margin for solitary hepatocellular carcinoma: a prospective randomized trial. Ann Surg 2007;245:36–43.

51. Katz SC, Shia J, Liau KH, et al. Operative blood loss independently predicts recurrence and survival after resection of hepatocellular carcinoma. Ann Surg 2009;249:617–23.

52. Ye JZ, Miao ZG, Wu FX, et al. Recurrence after anatomic resection versus nonanatomic resection for hepatocellular carcinoma: a meta analysis. Asian Pac J Cancer Prev 2012;13:1771–7.

53. NCCN guidelines version 2.2014. Panel members hepatobiliary cancers.

54. Bruix J, Takayama T, Mazzaferro V, et al. STORM: a phase III randomized, double-blind, placebo-controlled trial of adjuvant sorafenib after resection or ablation to prevent recurrent of hepatocellular carcinoma (HCC). J Clin Oncol 2014;32:5s suppl; abstr 4006.

55. Shindoh J, Hasegawa K, Matsuyama Y, et al. Low hepatitis C viral load predicts better long-term outcomes in patients undergoing resection of hepatocellular carcinoma irrespective of serologic eradication of hepatitis C virus. J Clin Oncol 2013;31(6):766–73.

56. Iwatsuki S, Gordon RD, Shaw BW Jr, et al. Role of liver transplantation in cancer therapy. Ann Surg 1985;202(4):401.

57. Mazzaferro V, Regalia E, Doci R, et al. Liver transplantation for the treatment of small hepatocellular carcinomas in patients with cirrhosis. N Engl J Med 1996; 334:693–9.

58. Mazzaferro V, Bhoori S, Sposito C, et al. Milan criteria in liver transplantation for hepatocellular carcinoma: an evidence based analysis of 15 years of experience. Liver Transpl 2011;17:S44–57.

59. Policy 9: allocation of liver and liver-intestines. Organ Procurement and Transplant Network (OPTN) policies. Available at: http://www.unos.org/. Accessed July 01, 2014.

60. Volk ML, Vijan S, Marrero JA. A novel model measuring the harm of transplanting hepatocellular carcinoma exceeding Milan criteria. Am J Transplant 2008;8(4): 839–46.

61. Clavien P, Lesurtel M, Bossuyt PM, et al. Recommendations for liver transplantation for hepatocellular carcinoma: an international consensus conference report. Lancet Oncol 2012;13:e11–22.

62. Yao FY, Bass NM, Nikolai B, et al. Liver transplantation for hepatocellular carcinoma: analysis of survival according to intention-to-treat principle and dropout from the waiting list. Liver Transpl 2002;8:873–83.

63. Yao FY, Bass NM, Nikolai B, et al. A follow up analysis of the pattern and predictors of dropout from the waiting list for liver transplantation in patients with hepatocellular carcinoma: implications for the current organ allocation policy. Liver Transpl 2003;9:684–92.

64. Toso C, Mentha G, Kneteman NM, et al. The place of downstaging for hepatocellular carcinoma. J Hepatol 2010;52:930–6.

65. Yao F, Kerlan RK Jr, Hirose R, et al. Excellent outcome following down-staging of hepatocellular carcinoma prior to liver transplantation: an intention-to-treat analysis. Hepatology 2008;48:819–27.
66. Yao FY, Mehta N, Fix OK, et al. Down-staging of hepatocellular carcinoma to within Milan criteria prior to liver transplantation: comparison of long-term outcome with tumors meeting Milan criteria without requiring down-staging. AASLD. Boston, November 9–13, 2012.
67. Mehta N, Yao FY, Roberts JP, et al. Intention-to-treat outcome of T1 hepatocellular carcinoma. Using the approach of "wait and not ablate" until meeting T2 criteria for liver transplant listing. Presented at AASLD. Washington DC, November 01–05, 2013.
68. SRTR & OPTN annual data report, 2011.
69. Abecassis MM, Fisher RA, Olthoff KM, et al. Complications of living donor hepatic lobectomy–a comprehensive report. Am J Transplant 2012;12(5):1208–17.
70. Kulik L, Abecassis M. Living donor liver transplantation for hepatocellular carcinoma. Gastroenterology 2004;127(5 Suppl 1):S277–82.
71. Bhangui P, Vibert E, Majno P, et al. Intention-to-treat analysis of liver transplantation for hepatocellular carcinoma: living versus decreased donor transplantation. Hepatology 2011;53(5):1570–9.
72. Kulik LM, Fisher RA, Rodrigo DR, et al. Outcomes of living and deceased donor liver transplant recipients with hepatocellular carcinoma: results of the A2ALL cohort. Am J Transplant 2012;12(11):2997–3007.
73. Belghiti J, Cortes A, Abdalla EK, et al. Resection prior to liver transplantation for hepatocellular carcinoma. Ann Surg 2003;238(6):885–92.
74. Hwang S, Lee SG, Moon DB, et al. Salvage living donor liver transplantation after prior liver resection for hepatocellular carcinoma. Liver Transpl 2007;13(5):741–6.
75. Del Gaudio M, Ercolani G, Ravaioli M, et al. Liver transplantation for recurrent hepatocellular carcinoma on cirrhosis after liver resection: University of Bologna experience. Am J Transplant 2008;8(6):1177–85.
76. Cucchetti A, Vitale A, Del Gaudio M, et al. Harm and benefits of primary liver resection and salvage transplantation for hepatocellular carcinoma. Am J Transplant 2010;10:619–27.
77. Fuks D, Dokmak S, Paradis V, et al. Benefit of initial resection of hepatocellular carcinoma followed by transplantation in case of recurrence: an intention-to-treat analysis. Hepatology 2012;55:132–40.
78. Sala M, Forner A, Varela M, et al. Prognostic prediction in patients with hepatocellular carcinoma. Semin Liver Dis 2005;25:171–80.
79. Schwartz M, Roayaie S, Llovet J. How should patients with hepatocellular carcinoma recurrence after liver transplantation be treated? J Hepatol 2005;43(4):584–9.
80. Roberts JP, Venook A, Kerlan R, et al. Hepatocellular carcinoma: ablate and wait versus rapid transplantation. Liver Transpl 2010;16(8):925–9.
81. Otto G, Herber S, Heise M, et al. Response to transarterial chemoembolization as a biological selection criterion for liver transplantation in hepatocellular carcinoma. Liver Transpl 2006;12(8):1260–7.
82. Vitale A, D'Amico F, Frigo AC, et al. Response to therapy as a criterion for awarding priority to patients with hepatocellular carcinoma awaiting liver transplantation. Ann Surg Oncol 2010;17(9):2290–302.
83. Mailey B, Artinyan A, Khalili J, et al. Evaluation of absolute serum alpha-fetoprotein levels in liver transplant for hepatocellular cancer. Arch Surg 2011;146(1):26–33.

84. Berry K, Ioannou GN. Serum alpha-fetoprotein level independently predicts post transplant survival in patients with hepatocellular carcinoma. Liver Transpl 2013; 19(6):634–45.

85. Merani S, Majno P, Kneteman NM, et al. The impact of waiting list alpha-fetoprotein changes on the outcome of liver transplant for hepatocellular carcinoma. J Hepatol 2011;55(4):814–9.

86. Pomfret EA, Washburn K, Wald C, et al. Report of a national conference of liver allocation in patients with hepatocellular carcinoma in the United States. Liver Transpl 2010;16:262–78.

87. Orlando A, Leandro G, Olivo M, et al. Radiofrequency thermal ablation vs. percutaneous ethanol injection for small hepatocellular carcinoma in cirrhosis: meta-analysis of randomized controlled trials. Am J Gastroenterol 2009;104(2):514–24.

88. Cho YK, Kim JK, Kim MY, et al. Systematic review of randomized trials for hepatocellular carcinoma treated with percutaneous ablation therapies. Hepatology 2009;49(2):453–9.

89. Livraghi T, Meloni F, Di Stasi M, et al. Sustained complete response and complications rates after radiofrequency ablation of very early hepatocellular carcinoma in cirrhosis: is resection still the treatment of choice? Hepatology 2008; 47(1):82–9.

90. Huang S, Yu J, Liang P, et al. Percutaneous microwave ablation for hepatocellular carcinoma adjacent to large vessels: a long term follow up. Eur J Radiol 2014;83:552–8.

91. Ni JY, Shan S, Xu LF, et al. Meta-analysis of radiofrequency ablation in combination with transarterial chemoembolization for hepatocellular carcinoma. World J Gastroenterol 2013;19(24):3872–82.

92. Huang J, Yan L, Cheng Z, et al. A randomized trial comparing radiofrequency ablation and surgical resection for HCC conforming to the Milan criteria. Ann Surg 2010;252(6):903–12.

93. Molinari M, Helton S. Hepatic resection versus radiofrequency ablation for hepatocellular carcinoma in cirrhotic individuals not candidates for liver transplantation: a Markov model decision analysis. Am J Surg 2009;198(3): 396–406.

94. Llovet JM, Real MI, Montaña X, et al. Arterial embolisation or chemoembolisation versus symptomatic treatment in patients with unresectable hepatocellular carcinoma: a randomised controlled trial. Lancet 2002;359(9319):1734–9.

95. Lo CM, Ngan H, Tso WK, et al. Randomized controlled trial of transarterial lipiodol chemoembolization for unresectable hepatocellular carcinoma. Hepatology 2002;35(5):1164–71.

96. Georgiades CS, Hong K, D'Angelo M, et al. Safety and efficacy of transarterial chemoembolization in patients with unresectable hepatocellular carcinoma and portal vein thrombosis. J Vasc Interv Radiol 2005;16(12):1653–9.

97. Varela M, Real MI, Burrel M, et al. Chemoembolization of hepatocellular carcinoma with drug eluting beads: efficacy and doxorubicin pharmacokinetics. J Hepatol 2007;46(3):474–81.

98. Lencioni R, De Baere T, Burrel M, et al. Transcatheter treatment of hepatocellular carcinoma with doxorubicin DC beads (DEBDOX): technical recommendations. Cardiovasc Intervent Radiol 2012;35(5):980–5.

99. Pawlik TM, Reyes D, Cosgrove D, et al. Phase II trial of sorafenib combined with concurrent transarterial chemoembolization with drug-eluting beads for hepatocellular carcinoma. J Clin Oncol 2011;29(30):3960–7.

100. Kalva S, Pectasides M, Liu R, et al. Safety and effectiveness of chemoemboliza-tion with drug-eluting beads for advanced-stage hepatocellular carcinoma. Cardiovasc Intervent Radiol 2014;37(2):381–7.
101. Lammer J, Malagari K, Vogl T, et al. Prospective randomized study of doxorubicin-eluting-bead embolization in the treatment of hepatocellular carcinoma: results of the PRECISION V study. Cardiovasc Intervent Radiol 2010;33(1):41–52.
102. Burrel M, Reig M, Forner A, et al. Survival of patients with hepatocellular carci-noma treated by transarterial chemoembolisation (TACE) using drug eluting beads. Implications for clinical practice and trial design. J Hepatol 2012; 56(6):1330–5.
103. Nicolini A, Martinetti L, Crespi S, et al. Transarterial chemoembolization with epirubicin-eluting beads versus transarterial embolization before liver transplan-tation for hepatocellular carcinoma. J Vasc Interv Radiol 2010;21(3):327–32.
104. Nicolini D, Svegliati-Baroni G, Candelari R, et al. Doxorubicin-eluting bead vs conventional transcatheter arterial chemoembolization for hepatocellular carci-noma before liver transplantation. World J Gastroenterol 2013;19(34):5622–32.
105. Salem R, Thurston KG. Radioembolization with 90Yttrium microspheres: a state of the art brachytherapy treatment for primary and secondary malignancies: part 1: technical and methodologic considerations. J Vasc Interv Radiol 2006; 17:1251–78.
106. Salem R, Lewandowski RJ, Mulcahy MF, et al. Radioembolization for hepatocel-lular carcinoma using Yttrium-90 microspheres: a comprehensive report of long-term outcomes. Gastroenterology 2010;138(1):52–64.
107. Hilgard P, Hamami M, Fouly AE, et al. Radioembolization with yttrium-90 glass microspheres in hepatocellular carcinoma: European experience on safety and long-term survival. Hepatology 2010;52(5):1741–9.
108. Sangro B, Carpanese L, Cianni R, et al. Survival after yttrium-90 resin micro-sphere radioembolization of hepatocellular carcinoma across Barcelona Clinic Liver Cancer stages: a European evaluation. Hepatology 2011;54:868–78.
109. Mazzaferro V, Sposito C, Bhoori S, et al. Yttrium-90 radioembolization for inter-mediate- advanced hepatocellular carcinoma: a phase 2 study. Hepatology 2013;57:1826–37.
110. Golfieri R, Renzulli M, Mosconi C, et al. Hepatocellular carcinoma responding to superselective transarterial chemoembolization: an issue of nodule dimension? J Vasc Interv Radiol 2013;24(4):509–17.
111. Lewandowski RJ, Kulik LM, Riaz A, et al. A comparative analysis of transarterial downstaging for hepatocellular carcinoma: chemoembolization versus radioem-bolization. Am J Transplant 2009;9(8):1920–8.
112. Vouche M, Lewandowski RJ, Atassi R, et al. Radiation lobectomy: time-dependent analysis of future liver remnant volume in unresectable liver cancer as a bridge to resection. J Hepatol 2013;59(5):1029–36.
113. Salem R, Lewandowski RJ, Kulik L, et al. Radioembolization results in longer time-to-progression and reduced toxicity compared with chemoembolization in patients with hepatocellular carcinoma. Gastroenterology 2011;140(2): 497–507.e2.
114. Moreno-Luna LE, Yang JD, Sanchez W, et al. Efficacy and safety of transarterial radioembolization versus chemoembolization in patients with hepatocellular car-cinoma. Cardiovasc Intervent Radiol 2013;36(3):714–23.
115. Salem R, Gilbertsen M, Butt Z, et al. Increased quality of life among hepatocel-lular carcinoma patients treated with radioembolization, compared with chemo-embolization. Clin Gastroenterol Hepatol 2013;11(10):1358–65.

116. Llovet JM, Ricci S, Mazzaferro V, et al. Sorafenib in advanced hepatocellular carcinoma. N Engl J Med 2008;359(4):378–90.
117. Cheng AL, Kang YK, Chen Z, et al. Efficacy and safety of sorafenib in patients in the Asia-Pacific region with advanced hepatocellular carcinoma: a phase III randomised, double-blind, placebo-controlled trial. Lancet Oncol 2009;10(1):25–34.
118. Lencioni R, Venook A, Marrero J, et al. Second interim results of the GIDEON (Global Investigation of Therapeutic Decisions in HCC and of its Treatment with Sorafenib) study: Barcelona-Clinic Liver Cancer (BCLC) Stage Subgroup Analysis. In European Multidisciplinary Cancer Congress (ECCO-ESMO). Stockholm, Sweden, September 23–27, 2011.
119. Pinter M, Sieghart W, Hucke F, et al. Prognostic factors in patients with advanced hepatocellular carcinoma treated with sorafenib. Aliment Pharmacol Ther 2011;34(8):949–59.
120. Cheng A, Kang D, Lin J, et al. Phase III trial of sunitib (Su) versus sorafenib (So) in advanced hepatocellular carcinoma (HCC). J Clin Oncol 2011;29. supp; abstract 4000.
121. Johnson P, Qin S, Park JW, et al. Brivanib versus sorafenib as first-line therapy in patients with unresectable, advanced hepatocellular carcinoma: results from the phase 3 BRISK-FL study. Presented at AASLD. Boston, September 11–13, 2012; Abstract LB-6.
122. Llovet JM, Decaens T, Raoul J, et al. Brivanib versus placebo in patients with advanced hepatocellular carcinoma (HCC) who failed or were intolerant to sorafenib: results from the BRISK-PS trial. EASL. Barcelona, Spain, April 18–22, 2012; Abstract 1398.
123. Cainap C, Qin S, Huang WT, et al. Phase III trial of linifanib versus sorafenib in patients with advanced hepatocellular carcinoma (HCC). J Clin Oncol 2013; 31(Suppl 4):249.
124. Santoro A, Rimassa L, Borbath I, et al. Tivantinib for second-line treatment of advanced hepatocellular carcinoma: a randomised, placebo-controlled phase 2 study. Lancet Oncol 2013;14(1):55–63.
125. Truesdale AE, Caldwell SH, Shah NL, et al. Sorafenib therapy for hepatocellular carcinoma prior to liver transplant is associated with increased complications after transplant. Transpl Int 2011;24(10):991–8.
126. Frenette CT, Boktour M, Burroughs SG, et al. Pre-transplant utilization of sorafenib is not associated with increased complications after liver transplantation. Transpl Int 2013;26(7):734–9.
127. Vouche M, Kulik L, Atassi R, et al. Radiological-pathological analysis of WHO, RECIST, EASL, mRECIST and DWI: imaging analysis from a prospective randomized trial of Y90 +/− sorafenib. Hepatology 2013;58(5):1655–66.
128. Kulik L, Vouche M, Koppe S, et al. Prospective randomized pilot study of Y90+/− sorafenib as bridge to transplantation in hepatocellular carcinoma. J Hepatol 2014;61(2):309–17.
129. Kudo M, Imanaka K, Chida N, et al. Phase III study of sorafenib after transarterial chemoembolisation in Japanese and Korean patients with unresectable hepatocellular carcinoma. Eur J Cancer 2011;47(14):2117–27.
130. Sansonno D, Lauletta G, Russi S, et al. Transarterial chemoembolization plus sorafenib: a sequential therapeutic scheme for HCV-related intermediate-stage hepatocellular carcinoma: a randomized clinical trial. Oncologist 2012;17(3): 359–66.
131. Lencioni R, Llovet JM, Han G, et al. Sorafenib or placebo in combination with transarterial chemoembolization (TACE) with doxorubicin-eluting beads

(DEBDOX) for intermediate-stage hepatocellular carcinoma (HCC): phase II, randomized, double-blind SPACE trial. J Clin Oncol 2012;30(Suppl 4) [abstract: LBA154].

132. Zhang L, Hu P, Chen X, Bie P. Transarterial chemoembolization (TACE) plus sorafenib versus TACE for intermediate or advanced stage hepatocellular carcinoma: a meta-analysis. PLoS One 2014;9(6):e100305.

133. Bravi F, Bosetti C, Tavani A, et al. Coffee reduces risk for hepatocellular carcinoma: an updated meta-analysis. Clin Gastroenterol Hepatol 2013;11(11):1413–21.

134. Finkelmeier F, Kronenberger B, Köberle V, et al. Severe 25-hydroxyvitamin D deficiency identifies a poor prognosis in patients with hepatocellular carcinoma–a prospective cohort study. Aliment Pharmacol Ther 2014;39(10):1204–12.

Renal Insufficiency in the Patient with Chronic Liver Disease

Nadia K. Bozanich, MD, Paul Y. Kwo, MD*

KEYWORDS

- Hepatorenal syndrome • Chronic liver disease • Acute kidney injury • Hyponatremia

KEY POINTS

- Acute kidney injury has replaced the previous term acute renal failure and is defined as an abrupt loss of kidney function with retention of urea and electrolyte and fluid imbalances.
- The pathophysiology of renal disease in the setting of chronic liver disease and cirrhosis explains why those with cirrhosis are at risk for kidney injury.
- Hyponatremia is another complication of cirrhosis that may lead to renal injury and disease.

Patients with chronic liver disease frequently develop renal insufficiency, with an estimated prevalence of 20% to 25%.[1] It is essential to determine whether a chronic liver disease patient with renal insufficiency has a single etiology that is affecting liver and kidneys, a kidney disease whose cause is different than the liver disease, or kidney disease as the result of chronic liver disease. Kidney disease from liver disease may be acute or chronic, and may lead to dialysis or kidney transplantation with or without liver transplantation. Finally, kidney disease may affect candidacy for liver transplant and long-term outcomes after transplant.[2–4] Moreover, it is essential that this evaluation occur in a timely manner, as the overall survival of patients with cirrhosis who develop renal failure (from all causes) is poor, at 50% at 1 month and 20% at 6 months.[5] This article will discuss the revised nomenclature of acute and chronic kidney injury, the differential diagnosis of those with renal insufficiency with chronic liver disease, and specific therapies and strategies to reduce the risk of developing renal insufficiency.

DEFINITIONS OF ACUTE KIDNEY AND CHRONIC KIDNEY INJURY

Acute kidney injury (AKI) has replaced the previous term acute renal failure and is defined as an abrupt loss of kidney function with retention of urea and electrolyte

Disclosures: None.
Medicine, Indiana University School of Medicine, 975 West Walnut, IB 327, Indianapolis, IN 46202, USA
* Corresponding author.
E-mail address: pkwo@iu.edu

Clin Liver Dis 19 (2015) 45–56
http://dx.doi.org/10.1016/j.cld.2014.09.003
1089-3261/15/$ – see front matter © 2015 Elsevier Inc. All rights reserved.

liver.theclinics.com

and fluid imbalances. In 2004, a consensus group proposed a set of definitions (RIFLE criteria [Risk, Injury, Failure, Loss, ESRD]) that described 3 levels of renal dysfunction (risk, injury, and failure) along with 2 outcome measures (loss and end-stage renal disease).[6] However, the definition of AKI has been recently modified in the liver disease population. This is because serum creatinine is not a reliable marker in assessing kidney function in patients with liver disease due to the low production of creatinine and decreased muscle mass in those with cirrhosis.[7,8] Thus equations including the Cockcroft-Gault and Modification of Diet in Renal Disease, which include serum creatinine, typically overestimate glumerular filtration rate (GFR) in patients with cirrhosis.[9] In addition, creatinine clearance by urine collection may also overestimate GFR cirrhotic patients, and it is sometimes difficult to collect urine accurately in a cirrhotic patient, making this approach somewhat less practical.[10] The gold standard of assessing GFR in the general population relies on clearance of iohexol or iothalamate, although ascites limits the use of these tests in cirrhotic patients.[1]

For these reasons, the International Ascites Club and the Acute Dialysis Quality Initiative have advocated using the more recent Acute Kidney Injury Network (AKIN) definition of AKI for patients with cirrhosis.[11] The AKIN criteria are classified into 3 stages. Stage 1 is an increase in serum creatinine of at least 0.3 mg/dL or an increase of 150% to 200% from baseline; stage 2 is an increase in serum creatinine greater than 200% to 300%, and stage 3 is a serum creatinine greater than 300%, or at least 0.5 mg/dL in patients with baseline serum creatinine of at least 4 mg/dL or renal replacement therapy (RRT).[12,13] This classification has important prognostic value, as 1 study demonstrated a mortality rate of 2% in stage 1, 15% in stage 2, and 44% in stage 3, although patients with stage 1 AKI with a serum of no more than 1.5 mg/dL had a comparable mortality rate at 3 months as the same population without AKI.[14] A recent report noted that the AKIN definition predicted 30-day mortality, length of hospital stay, and organ failure with a tenfold higher risk of mortality in those with irreversible AKI.[15] Thus clinicians should be aware that even small changes in measured creatinine warrant evaluation and intervention.

THE PATHOPHYSIOLOGY OF THE RENAL CIRCULATION IN CHRONIC LIVER DISEASE

The pathophysiology of renal disease in the setting of chronic liver disease and cirrhosis explains why those with cirrhosis are at risk for kidney injury. The presence of portal hypertension disrupts the normal circulatory system by leading to increased production of vasodilators including nitrous oxide, carbon monoxide, and endogenous cannabinoids in the splanchnic system, and this vasodilatation leads to a reduction in systemic vascular resistance.[16–19] In those with early stage cirrhosis, portal hypertension is not as prominent, and the heart is able to increase cardiac output to compensate for the decrease in vascular resistance, maintaining an effective blood volume.[5,16] As cirrhosis progresses with increased portal hypertension, the decrease in vascular resistance becomes more predominant, and there is no longer cardiovascular compensation; a decrease in cardiac output may be observed.[20] This leads to renin–angiotensin system activation to raise arterial pressures.[18] Although this helps maintain arterial pressures, there are deleterious effects on the kidneys, including sodium and water retention, as well as increased renal vasoconstriction, leading to hypoperfusion of the kidneys. Finally, angiotensin 2-mediated efferent glomerular arteriole vasoconstriction also helps maintain renal perfusion, and all of these mechanisms may lead to or exacerbate edema and ascites.[16,21]

In those with cirrhosis, bacterial translocation (from intestine to extraintestinal sites) plays an important role in leading to kidney injury and disease.[22,23] Bacterial translocation may trigger inflammation, leading to cytokine production and endogenous vasodilators that in turn exacerbate the vasodilated state that exists in those with cirrhosis and portal hypertension. Indeed, patients with evidence of bacterial translocation (circulating bacterial DNA or lipopolysaccharide-binding protein) have higher levels of cytokines, reduced vascular resistance, and increased cardiac output compared with patients who have cirrhosis without evidence of bacterial translocation.[24,25] Additionally, studies have demonstrated that the administration of the antibiotic norfloxacin, which decreases gut bacteria, ameliorates many of the deleterious effects on the vascular system.[26,27]

Hyponatremia is another complication of cirrhosis that may lead to renal injury and disease. Approximately half of the patients with advanced cirrhosis have a serum sodium measurement of less than 135 mEq/L, and the severity of hyponatremia correlates with more advanced disease.[1] Hyponatremia occurs because of the nonosmotic release of vasopressin, which leads to renal tubular reduction in excreting solute-free water and is typically managed by free water restriction, which may be difficult for patients to tolerate. Vasopressin 2 receptor blockers (such as tolvaptan) have been used in this type of hyponatremia, although tolvaptan has been associated with hepatotoxicity in polycystic kidney disease and is contraindicated in those with advanced liver disease.[28,29]

PREVALENCE AND TYPES OF ACUTE KIDNEY INJURY

AKI is common in patients with liver disease.[14] As cirrhosis advances, likelihood of AKI has been reported in up to 19% of hospitalized patients with cirrhosis.[30] AKI has also been shown to be an independent risk factor for mortality in the setting of variceal bleeding and spontaneous bacterial peritonitis (SBP), and in patients admitted for variceal bleeding, the severity of cirrhosis correlates with the development of acute renal failure.[31,32] As in noncirrhotic patients, AKI occurs from prerenal, renal, and postrenal causes.[33] The most common etiologies of AKI this cirrhotic population, which account for 80% to 90% of all cases, include volume depletion, acute tubular necrosis (ATN), and hepatorenal syndrome (HRS).[1] Postrenal causes are rare and are due to the obstruction of the urinary tract.[33]

Prerenal AKI is caused by hypoperfusion to the kidneys without damage of renal structure. Volume depletion typically leads to prerenal AKI and occurs from diuretic use, diarrhea from lactulose use, large volume paracentesis without albumin replacement, and general malaise leading to poor intake. Gastrointestinal (GI) bleeding, typically from varices, also leads to volume depletion, but may also be associated with ATN because of ischemic injury of the renal tubular cells.[34] Intra-abdominal pressure from tense ascites may lead to abdominal compartment syndrome, increasing renin and aldosterone levels, activating the renin angiotensin–aldosterone system and causing AKI. Prerenal AKI usually occurs in patients with ascites due to the low arterial pressure, renal vasoconstriction, and low renal blood flow.[35]

SPONTANEOUS BACTERIAL PERITONITIS AND ACUTE KIDNEY INJURY

Spontaneous bacterial peritonitis is the most common infection in cirrhotic patients and has been known to lead to renal failure with poor outcome.[36–41] Circulatory changes with increase in including tumor necrosis factor alpha (TNF-α) lead to increased systemic vasodilation, which subsequently initiates the compensatory process of renal vasoconstriction and renal hypoperfusion.[36,38,42] One study demonstrated a 10% incidence of renal failure in patients with SBP, and an additional 20% to 40% of SBP patients developed AKI.[36,38] In patients with SBP, the severity of cirrhosis, and, independently, an increased serum creatinine level, correlated with the development of type 1 HRS.[1]

Infections other than SBP also are associated with significant renal disease. One study examined renal failure as a result of sepsis from other infectious causes besides SBP. This study found that 27% of patients with cirrhosis developed AKI after documented sepsis hospitalization as compared with 8% of patients who were hospitalized without sepsis. The type of renal failure correlated with mortality. At 3 months, 100% mortality was seen in those with nonreversible renal failure; 55% mortality was seen in those with reversible renal failure, and 13% mortality was seen in those with no renal failure. Model for End Stage Liver Disease (MELD) score was the only factor that independently predicted prognosis and increased mortality.[43] Another study suggested 70% of patients with cirrhosis hospitalized without known hepatic complication (such as SBP) and with AKI had infection (pneumonia, a urinary tract infection, or bacteremia), with an additional 20% of cirrhotic patients having a GI bleed; thus, a careful evaluation for these etiologies is required in hospitalized cirrhotic patients with AKI.[43]

RENAL CAUSES OF RENAL INSUFFICIENCY

Renal causes of renal insufficiency, also termed intrinsic renal failure or parenchymal renal disease, include acute tubular necrosis (ischemia or toxic injury), glomerulonephritis, or interstitial nephritis.[33] Intrinsic renal failure is usually suspected when there is proteinuria and/or hematuria.[17,33] Ideally, renal causes would be confirmed by renal biopsy, but renal biopsy is seldom done because of the coagulopathy associated with cirrhosis. Nonsteroidal anti-inflammatory drugs (NSAIDs) may cause ATN in patients with cirrhosis, as renal perfusion depends on COX-derived prostaglandin synthesis and may be seen when clinicians give cirrhotic patients NSAIDs for pain relief, rather than acetaminophen, believing that they are sparing hepatotoxicity.[17,44] Aminoglycoside antibiotics are another cause of ATN in patients with cirrhosis.[17]

Acute glomerulonephritis may be seen in patients with cirrhosis and is sometimes caused by pharyngitis, cellulitis, or endocarditis with staphylococci and gram-negative strains, not streptococci as the predominant species.[45] Cryoglobinemic membranoproliferative glomerulonephritis may occur in patients with hepatitis B or hepatitis C with or without cirrhosis.[46,47] The diagnosis of glomerulonephritis is suggested when arterial hypertension is found and can present with the red cell casts and proteinuria in the urine.[12,33,46,48] Renal biopsy will show glomerulonephritis or membranoproliferative glomerulonephritis. For those with chronic hepatitis B infection and documented glomerular disease, treatment with entecavir or tenofovir is warranted in adults. In those with hepatitis C infection, treatment historically has been with pegylated interferon and ribavirin, although it is likely that direct-acting antiviral agents will be the preferred therapy once renal dosing becomes available for these agents.

HEPATORENAL SYNDROME

HRS is a type of prerenal AKI that has no apparent structural kidney damage that occurs from severe renal vasoconstriction and is associated with a high mortality rate.[5] The 5-year risk of developing HRS in patients with cirrhosis has been estimated at 11%, which is a reduction in risk likely due to improved care for cirrhotic patients, particularly administration of albumin and antibiotics for patients with SBP.[1] The underlying pathophysiology is due to the splanchnic vasodilation and renal vasoconstriction with cardiac output unable to compensate for the vasodilation. Indeed, cardiac output in cirrhotic patients with SBP who experience renal failure has been shown to be lower than cardiac output in patients with SBP and no renal failure, even with treated SBB.[39] Low cardiac output and high plasma renin activity have been shown to independently increase the risk of HRS.[20] The exact mechanism of low cardiac output is unknown, but it has been suggested that a shortened systolic and diastolic response to stimuli, repolarization change, and hypertrophy of the myocardium may lead to a cirrhotic cardiomyopathy, thereby reducing cardiac output.[49] The decrease in cardiac preload due to a lower venous return is another potential explanation and could partially explain why intravenous albumin infusion improves renal function.[20]

HRS is classified into types 1 and 2. The definition of type 1 HRS is a doubling of serum creatinine to a level greater than 2.5 mg/dL within 2 weeks, while in type 2 HRS, there is a slower increase in serum creatinine to at least 1.5 mg/dL, with no improvement by administering albumin (1 g/kg of body weight) after at least 2 days off diuretics.[5] Type 2 HRS may be difficult to distinguish from CKD, defined as having a GFR of less than 60 mL/min for at least 3 months.[1] HRS is a diagnosis of exclusion, and it should be suspected in the absence of shock, treatment with nephrotoxic drugs, or any findings of structural renal disease including proteinuria or hematuria. Because of the reduced cardiac output, HRS patients typically have low blood pressures, and if a patient has systemic hypertension, this suggests that the cause of renal failure is not related to HRS. Type 1 HRS may have an abrupt onset, often with multiorgan failure, and it carries a worse prognosis than type 2 HRS. Type 2 HRS progresses more slowly in correlation with the decline of liver function and is typically associated with refractory ascites.[50] For clinicians, it is often challenging to distinguish HRS from other causes of renal failure, particularly ATN, where renal function may not improve after appropriate intravascular volume repletion. However, improvement in renal function with vasoconstrictive therapy can help differentiate HRS from ATN, and there is evidence suggesting that HRS may lead to ATN.[51]

The precipitating factors for HRS include infection (most common etiology is SBP), bleeding, and large-volume paracentesis without albumin replacement.[31,37,43] Not surprisingly, cirrhotic patients with SBP who present with elevated serum creatinine levels, hyponatremia, or high cytokine levels are more likely to develop HRS, with 20% to 30% of patients with SBP progressing to type 1 HRS. For this reason, SBP prophylaxis is important in patients with low-protein ascites (<1.5 g/L), with norfloxacin administration reducing the risk of HRS and mortality by reducing bacterial translocation or creating an anti-inflammatory state by decreasing cytokines and improving renal perfusion.[24–27,52] Hepatorenal syndrome occurs commonly in many of the cirrhosis complications, and clinicians should have a high index of suspicion in decompensated cirrhotic patients who are admitted with renal insufficiency. In cirrhotic patients with GI bleeding, 5% may develop type 1 HRS.[31] Ten percent of patients admitted with ascites treated by large-volume paracentesis, and 25% of patients with acute alcoholic hepatitis, will develop HRS, and HRS is the primary cause of death in patients with cirrhosis admitted to the hospital with severe alcohol-induced hepatitis.[42,53]

USE OF VASOCONSTRICTORS FOR HEPATORENAL SYNDROME

The current treatment of HRS is meant to increase intravascular volume by increasing total plasma volume, typically with albumin to improve renal perfusion, and to reduce the intense peripheral vasodilatation with selected vasoconstrictors.[54–60] Multiple studies have shown that treatment with vasopressin analogues (like terlipressin) is effective in 40% to 50% of patients with type 1 HRS, and terlipressin is to date the most studied vasoconstrictor, although not yet available in the United States or Canada. Terlipressin is typically administered at doses of 1 to 2 mg every 4–6 hours along with albumin at 25 to 50 g/d. Terlipressin binds to the vasopressin (V1) receptor predominantly on vascular smooth muscle cells in the splanchnic circulatory system.[1] This means it can be used as a bolus injection, but continuous administration of the drug is linked with a higher reversal rate of HRS. The mechanism of GFR improvement is not fully understood, but is likely related to improved blood pressure and reductions in plasma renin activity. One theory is that vasopressin analogues constrict the splanchnic system to allow additional blood volume to perfuse other organs including the kidneys and the central compartment, inhibiting the sympathetic and renin–angiotensin systems.[61,62] Studies have shown that treatment of HRS type 1 with renal vasodilators including dopamine or prostaglandins is not effective.[63]

Despite its widespread use in the United States, there are few studies supporting the use of midodrine and norepinephrine for type 1 HRS. In nonrandomized trials, midodrine was combined with octreotide to increase splanchnic vasoconstriction using varying doses and routes of administration.[64,65] One small study noted improvement in 3 of 5 patients who received subcutaneous octreotide 100 μg three times daily and midodrine at a starting dose of 7.5 mg three times daily, titrating to increase in mean arterial pressure (MAP) of 15 mm Hg with daily albumin 20 to 40 g/d that allowed discharge from the hospital. Another retrospective review of 60 patients who received midodrine up to 15 mg three times daily with octreotide 200 μg three times daily subcutaneously with albumin noted improved survival and improved resolution of type 1 HRS compared with those receiving albumin alone.[66] It is the authors' preference to use intravenous octreotide 50 μg/h for inpatients with type 1 HRS with doses of midodrine starting at 7.5 mg three times daily and titrating to 15 mg three times daily. Importantly, octreotide monotherapy has not been shown to improve GFR.[67] The midodrine/octreotide combination may also be administered as an outpatient.[1] Finally, a pilot study of norepinephrine 0.5 to 3 mg/h plus 20 g/L albumin and intravenous furosemide 120 mg as needed reversed type 1 HRS in 10 of 12 cases with decreased plasma renin activity (PRA) and improved urinary sodium excretion, with responses noted in those who failed to improve on terlipressin.[68] Caution must be used with norepinephrine, as there is a higher rate of cardiac arrhythmias than with terlipressin.

Albumin infusion is essential in the therapy of HRS as well as in patients with SBP to prevent development of HRS, and the effect of vasoconstrictors is likely enhanced by albumin.[1] The mechanism of action of albumin is not clear, but it has been postulated to be related to improving renal perfusion by increasing colloidal oncotic pressure and possibly also binding to vasodilators to reduce their deleterious effects on the circulatory system.[69,70] In those with SBP, one randomized controlled trial with albumin administration demonstrated a 66% reduction in incidence of HRS as well as reduction of in-hospital (10% vs 29%) and 3-month mortality rates (22% vs 41%).[71] Another randomized controlled trial allocated patients with SBP to cefotaxime alone or cefotaxime plus intravenous albumin, with the patients who received albumin with cefotaxime developing HRS less frequently at 3 months (22% vs 40%, respectively).[1]

Other therapies to treat HRS include RRT, including hemodialysis or continuous venovenous hemofiltration, especially when a patient is awaiting a transplant or in patients with the expectation of improved hepatic function though RRT is not without risks, including hypotension, infection, and bleeding.[72,73] Transjugular intrahepatic portosystemic shunts (TIPS) have also been used, but limited data are available on their effectiveness in HRS, as most patients with HRS are too decompensated to undergo TIPS placement.[74] Nevertheless, there are reports that have suggested TIPS may benefit a small subset of HRS patients and can be considered as a salvage option in selected patients. Encephalopathy, renal failure, and infection are all risks with TIPS placement. Regardless of the therapy, HRS may recur after vasoconstrictors are stopped.[58] Type 1 HRS recurs after discontinuation of treatment in about 20% of patients, but retreatment may be successful.[62,75] If the HRS only partially responds to treatment (defined as a decrease in serum creatinine >50% of pretreatment value without decreasing <1.5 mg/dL), renal failure will likely return in a severe and irreversible fashion.[61]

The prognosis of HRS is the poorest of all the renal diseases associated with liver disease unless patients are able to undergo orthotopic liver transplant.[5] The 2-week mortality rate in type 1 HRS is 80% without therapy.[1] Therapy for HRS may improve the prognosis, with 1 multicenter study demonstrating improved 3-month survival of 20% and 40% for type 1 and type 2 HRS respectively when given both vasoconstrictive and albumin therapy. However, other studies have not shown the same benefit (**Fig. 1**).

Assessment of the etiology of renal insufficiency in the setting of liver disease is essential. Patients should be queried regarding fluid losses including diarrhea, vomiting, excess diuresis, and poor oral intake and GI bleeding. Infectious etiologies should be investigated, especially SBP, and a history of fever, cough, abdominal pain and dysuria can point to an infectious contribution to the renal insufficiency. Even if infection is not apparent by history, blood, and urine cultures, chest radiograph, as well as a diagnostic paracentesis for SBP should be done. If acute GI bleeding is suspected in the setting of renal insufficiency, then the patient should be managed in the intensive care unit (ICU) to optimize fluid and blood resuscitation to maintain renal perfusion while arranging urgent endoscopy. The patient's medications should be thoroughly surveyed with special attention nephrotoxic agents,

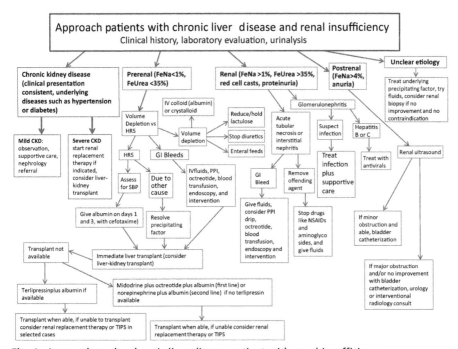

Fig. 1. Approach to the chronic liver disease patient with renal insufficiency.

especially NSAIDs and aminoglycosides, as well as radiocontrast exposure, and these agents should discontinued. The evaluation should include urinalysis for protein, casts, and cells in addition to sodium and osmolality. Urine osmolality, concentration of sodium in the urine, and the fractional excretion of sodium (FeNa) can help determine if the renal failure is due to prerenal causes (including HRS) or ATN.[5,61,63] Prerenal insufficiency due to excess diuresis readily responds to volume expansion with crystalloid and/or albumin. Distinguishing between ATN and HRS may be difficult, as both conditions can cause granular casts in the urine, but usually the finding of renal tubular epithelial cells suggests a diagnosis of ATN.[63] In ATN, the FeNa is usually greater than 1%, and in prerenal failure (HRS), the FeNa is usually less than 1% in patients not receiving diuretics.[5,33] Of note, the urine sodium level is not a reliable marker of the etiology of renal disease, and can be low in ATN or elevated in HRS, and it is no longer required for the diagnosis of HRS.[1] A renal ultrasound will assess for structural renal abnormalities, evidence of chronic kidney disease, and evidence of obstruction.[5] If urinary obstruction is suspected, aggressive intervention is required to prevent further damage to the kidneys. Bladder catheterization should be done if the patient is not able to produce urine, although it is preferable to not initially not leave an indwelling catheter because of infection risk.[63] Renal biopsy is typically not needed but may be helpful in selected cases in which a diagnosis cannot be made clinically, such as cryoglobulinemia.[1]

The management of patients with chronic liver disease and renal disease is dependent upon the etiology of renal disease. It is important that renal failure is identified and treated as early as possible to avoid complications. Patients with severe sepsis and renal failure may have an element of relative adrenal insufficiency and benefit from stress doses of hydrocortisone therapy.[76] Although maintaining euvolemia important is important, especially in ATN, excessive intravenous fluid administration in renal failure in the setting of cirrhosis may lead to fluid overload and increased hyponatremia, ascites, and/or edema because of the solute-free water retention.[5] Infections or bleeding should be treated urgently. Potassium-sparing diuretics (like spironolactone) are contraindicated because of the danger of hyperkalemia, and loop diuretics may contribute to prerenal or intrinsic renal failure and should be prescribed carefully in patients with suboptimal renal function and in patients without peripheral edema.[61,77] Large-volume paracentesis should always be followed by the administration of albumin 8 g/L of ascitic fluid removed.[78] Cirrhosis has not been identified as a significant risk factor for contrast-induced nephropathy; however, important predictive factors for the risk of contrast-induced nephropathy include patients with decreased effective arterial blood volume, diabetes, and chronic renal disease, which often exist in the liver disease patient population.[77] Chronic liver disease patients undergoing imaging requiring contrast medium should be pretreated by standard hydration measures, and creatinine should be monitored after imaging.[79]

Pharmacologic therapy for hepatorenal syndrome consists of vasoconstrictors, including terlipressin or midodrine with octereototide in addition to intravenous albumin. Renal support such as dialysis should be offered as a bridge to transplantation. Finally, liver transplantation should be considered urgently in all patients with cirrhosis experiencing renal disease if appropriate, as renal failure has been shown to lead to worse outcomes after liver transplantation.[2,3]

REFERENCES

1. Gonwa TA, Wadei HM. Kidney disease in the setting of liver failure: core curriculum 2013. Am J Kidney Dis 2013;62:1198–212.

2. Nair S, Verma S, Thuluvath PJ. Pretransplant renal function predicts survival in patients undergoing orthotopic liver transplantation. Hepatology 2002;35:1179–85.

3. Gonwa TA, Klintmalm GB, Levy M, et al. Impact of pretransplant renal function on survival after liver transplantation. Transplantation 1995;59:361–5.

4. Gonwa TA, McBride MA, Anderson K, et al. Continued influence of preoperative renal function on outcome of orthotopic liver transplant (OLTX) in the US: where will MELD lead us? Am J Transpl 2006;6:2651–9.

5. Gines P, Schrier RW. Renal failure in cirrhosis. N Engl J Med 2009;361:1279–90.

6. Bellomo R, Ronco C, Kellum J, et al, Acute Dialysis Quality Initiative workgroup. Acute renal failure—definition, outcome measures, animal models, fluid therapy and information technology needs: the Second International Consensus Conference of the Acute Dialysis Quality Initiative (ADQI) Group. Crit Care 2004;8: R204–12.

7. Francoz C, Nadim MK, Baron A, et al. Glomerular filtration rate equations for liver–kidney transplantation in patients with cirrhosis: validation of current recommendations. Hepatology 2014;59:1514–21.

8. Liangpunsakul S, Agarwal R. Renal failure in cirrhosis: is it time to change the diagnosis and classification? Am J Nephrol 2013;38:342–4.

9. Belcher JM, Parikh CR, Garcia-Tsao G. Acute kidney injury in patients with cirrhosis: perils and promise. Clin Gastroenterol Hepatol 2013;11:1550–8.

10. Proulx NL, Akbari A, Garg AX, et al. Measured creatinine clearance from timed urine collections substantially overestimates glomerular filtration rate in patients with liver cirrhosis: a systematic review and individual patient meta-analysis. Nephrol Dial Transpl 2005;20:1617–22.

11. Wong F, Nadim MK, Kellum JA, et al. Working party proposal for a revised classification system of renal dysfunction in patients with cirrhosis. Gut 2011;60: 702–9.

12. Arroyo V. Acute kidney injury (AKI) in cirrhosis: should we change current definition and diagnostic criteria of renal failure in cirrhosis? J Hepatol 2013;59:415–7.

13. Kellum J, Lameire N. Diagnosis, evaluation, and management of acute kidney injury: a KDIGO summary (part 1). Crit Care 2013;17:1–15.

14. Belcher JM, Garcia-Tsao G, Sanyal AJ, et al. Association of AKI with mortality and complications in hospitalized patients with cirrhosis. Hepatology 2013;57: 753–62.

15. Wong F, O'Leary JG, Reddy KR, et al. New consensus definition of acute kidney injury accurately predicts 30-day mortality in patients with cirrhosis and infection. Gastroenterology 2013;145:1280–8.e1.

16. Schrier RW, Arroyo V, Bernardi M, et al. Peripheral arterial vasodilation hypothesis: a proposal for the initiation of renal sodium and water retention in cirrhosis. Hepatology 1988;8:1151–7.

17. Arroyo V, Gines P, Gerbes AL, et al. Definition and diagnostic criteria of refractory ascites and hepatorenal syndrome in cirrhosis. International Ascites Club. Hepatology 1996;23:164–76.

18. Martin PY, Ginès P, Schrier RW. Nitric oxide as a mediator of hemodynamic abnormalities and sodium and water retention in cirrhosis. N Engl J Med 1998;339: 533–41.

19. Ros J, Claria J, To-Figueras J, et al. Endogenous cannabinoids: a new system involved in the homeostasis of arterial pressure in experimental cirrhosis in the rat. Gastroenterology 2002;122:85–93.

20. Ruiz-del-Arbol L, Monescillo A, Arocena C, et al. Circulatory function and hepatorenal syndrome in cirrhosis. Hepatology 2005;42:439–47.

21. Kew MC, Varma RR, Williams HS, et al. Renal and intrarenal blood-flow in cirrhosis of the liver. Lancet 1971;298:504–10.
22. Wiest R, Das S, Cadelina G, et al. Bacterial translocation in cirrhotic rats stimulates eNOS-derived NO production and impairs mesenteric vascular contractility. J Clin Invest 1999;104:1223–33.
23. Wiest R, Garcia-Tsao G. Bacterial translocation (BT) in cirrhosis. Hepatology 2005;41:422–33.
24. Albillos A, de la Hera A, Gonzalez M, et al. Increased lipopolysaccharide binding protein in cirrhotic patients with marked immune and hemodynamic derangement. Hepatology 2003;37:208–17.
25. Frances R, Zapater P, Gonzalez-Navajas JM, et al. Bacterial DNA in patients with cirrhosis and noninfected ascites mimics the soluble immune response established in patients with spontaneous bacterial peritonitis. Hepatology 2008;47:978–85.
26. Chin-Dusting JP, Rasaratnam B, Jennings GL, et al. Effect of fluoroquinolone on the enhanced nitric oxide-induced peripheral vasodilation seen in cirrhosis. Ann Intern Med 1997;127:985–8.
27. Rasaratnam B, Kaye D, Jennings G, et al. The effect of selective intestinal decontamination on the hyperdynamic circulatory state in cirrhosis. A randomized trial. Ann Intern Med 2003;139:186–93.
28. Okita K, Kawazoe S, Hasebe C, et al. Dose-finding trial of tolvaptan in liver cirrhosis patients with hepatic edema: a randomized, double-blind, placebo-controlled trial. Hepatol Res 2014;44:83–91.
29. Torres VE, Chapman AB, Devuyst O, et al. Tolvaptan in patients with autosomal dominant polycystic kidney disease. N Engl J Med 2012;367:2407–18.
30. Garcia-Tsao G, Parikh CR, Viola A. Acute kidney injury in cirrhosis. Hepatology 2008;48:2064–77.
31. Cardenas A, Gines P, Uriz J, et al. Renal failure after upper gastrointestinal bleeding in cirrhosis: incidence, clinical course, predictive factors, and short-term prognosis. Hepatology 2001;34:671–6.
32. Tandon P, Garcia-Tsao G. Renal dysfunction is the most important independent predictor of mortality in cirrhotic patients with spontaneous bacterial peritonitis. Clin Gastroenterol Hepatol 2011;9:260–5.
33. Thadhani R, Pascual M, Bonventre JV. Acute renal failure. N Engl J Med 1996;334:1448–60.
34. Grewal P, Martin P. Pretransplant management of the cirrhotic patient. Clin Liver Dis 2007;11:431–49.
35. Moreau R, Gaudin C, Hadengue A, et al. Renal hemodynamics in patients with cirrhosis: relationship with ascites and liver failure. Nephron 1993;65:359–63.
36. Sort P, Navasa M, Arroyo V, et al. Effect of intravenous albumin on renal impairment and mortality in patients with cirrhosis and spontaneous bacterial peritonitis. N Engl J Med 1999;341:403–9.
37. Follo A, Llovet JM, Navasa M, et al. Renal impairment after spontaneous bacterial peritonitis in cirrhosis: incidence, clinical course, predictive factors and prognosis. Hepatology 1994;20:1495–501.
38. Navasa M, Follo A, Filella X, et al. Tumor necrosis factor and interleukin-6 in spontaneous bacterial peritonitis in cirrhosis: relationship with the development of renal impairment and mortality. Hepatology 1998;27:1227–32.
39. Ruiz-del-Arbol L, Urman J, Fernández J, et al. Systemic, renal, and hepatic hemodynamic derangement in cirrhotic patients with spontaneous bacterial peritonitis. Hepatology 2003;38:1210–8.

40. Perdomo Coral G, Alves de Mattos A. Renal impairment after spontaneous bacterial peritonitis: incidence and prognosis. Can J Gastroenterol 2003;17:187–90.
41. Such J, Hillebrand DJ, Guarner C, et al. Nitric oxide in ascitic fluid is an independent predictor of the development of renal impairment in patients with cirrhosis and spontaneous bacterial peritonitis. Eur J Gastroenterol Hepatol 2004;16:571–7.
42. Gines A, Escorsell A, Gines P, et al. Incidence, predictive factors, and prognosis of the hepatorenal syndrome in cirrhosis with ascites. Gastroenterology 1993; 105:229–36.
43. Terra C, Guevara M, Torre A, et al. Renal failure in patients with cirrhosis and sepsis unrelated to spontaneous bacterial peritonitis: value of MELD score. Gastroenterology 2005;129:1944–53.
44. Laffi G, La Villa G, Pinzani M, et al. Arachidonic acid derivatives and renal function in liver cirrhosis. Semin Nephrol 1997;1997:530–48.
45. Montseny JJ, Meyrier A, Kleinknecht D, et al. The current spectrum of infectious glomerulonephritis. Experience with 76 patients and review of the literature. Medicine (Baltimore) 1995;74:63–73.
46. Meyers CM, Seeff LB, Stehman-Breen CO, et al. Hepatitis C and renal disease: an update. Am J Kidney Dis 2003;42:631–57.
47. Martin P, Fabrizi F. Hepatitis C virus and kidney disease. J Hepatol 2008;49: 613–24.
48. Navarro J, García-Nieto V, Bihari D, et al. Acute renal failure. Lancet 1996;347: 478–9.
49. Jeyarajah DR, Gonwa TA, McBride M, et al. Hepatorenal syndrome: combined liver kidney transplants versus isolated liver transplant. Transplantation 1997; 64:1760–5.
50. Angeli P, Merkel C. Pathogenesis and management of hepatorenal syndrome in patients with cirrhosis. J Hepatol 2008;48(Suppl 1):S93–103.
51. Abuelo JG. Diagnosing vascular causes of renal failure. Ann Intern Med 1995; 123:601–14.
52. Fernandez J, Navasa M, Planas R, et al. Primary prophylaxis of spontaneous bacterial peritonitis delays hepatorenal syndrome and improves survival in cirrhosis. Gastroenterology 2007;133:818–24.
53. Akriviadis E, Botla R, Briggs W, et al. Pentoxifylline improves short-term survival in severe acute alcoholic hepatitis: a double-blind, placebo-controlled trial. Gastroenterology 2000;119:1637–48.
54. Guevara M, Gines P, Fernandez-Esparrach G, et al. Reversibility of hepatorenal syndrome by prolonged administration of ornipressin and plasma volume expansion. Hepatology 1998;27:35–41.
55. Gulberg V, Bilzer M, Gerbes AL. Long-term therapy and retreatment of hepatorenal syndrome type 1 with ornipressin and dopamine. Hepatology 1999;30:870–5.
56. Kiser TH, Fish DN, Obritsch MD, et al. Vasopressin, not octeotide, may be beneficial in the treatment of hepatorenal syndrome: a retrospective study. Nephrol Dial Transplant 2005;20:1813–20.
57. Moreau R, Durand F, Poynard T, et al. Terlipressin in patients with cirrhosis and type 1 hepatorenal syndrome: a retrospective multicenter study. Gastroenterology 2002;122:923–30.
58. Gluud LL, Christensen K, Christensen E, et al. Terlipressin for hepatorenal syndrome. Cochrane Database Syst Rev 2012;(9):CD005162.
59. Sanyal AJ, Boyer T, Garcia-Tsao G, et al. A randomized, prospective, double-blind, placebo-controlled trial of terlipressin for type 1 hepatorenal syndrome. Gastroenterology 2008;134:1360–8.

60. Martin-Llahi M, Pepin MN, Guevara M, et al. Terlipressin and albumin vs albumin in patients with cirrhosis and hepatorenal syndrome: a randomized study. Gastroenterology 2008;134:1352–9.

61. Salerno F, Gerbes A, Gines P, et al. Diagnosis, prevention and treatment of hepatorenal syndrome in cirrhosis. Postgrad Med J 2008;84:662–70.

62. Ortega R, Gines P, Uriz J, et al. Terlipressin therapy with and without albumin for patients with hepatorenal syndrome: results of a prospective, nonrandomized study. Hepatology 2002;36:941–8.

63. Moreau R, Lebrec D. Acute renal failure in patients with cirrhosis: perspectives in the age of MELD. Hepatology 2003;37:233–43.

64. Angeli P, Volpin R, Gerunda G, et al. Reversal of type 1 hepatorenal syndrome with the administration of midodrine and octreotide. Hepatology 1999;29:1690–7.

65. Wong F, Pantea L, Sniderman K. Midodrine, octreotide, albumin, and TIPS in selected patients with cirrhosis and type 1 hepatorenal syndrome. Hepatology 2004;40:55–64.

66. Esrailian E, Pantangco ER, Kyulo NL, et al. Octreotide/Midodrine therapy significantly improves renal function and 30-day survival in patients with type 1 hepatorenal syndrome. Dig Dis Sci 2007;52:742–8.

67. Pomier-Layrargues G, Paquin SC, Hassoun Z, et al. Octreotide in hepatorenal syndrome: a randomized, double-blind, placebo-controlled, crossover study. Hepatology 2003;38:238–43.

68. Duvoux C, Zanditenas D, Hézode C, et al. Effects of noradrenalin and albumin in patients with type I hepatorenal syndrome: a pilot study. Hepatology 2002;36: 374–80.

69. Fernandez J, Navasa M, Garcia-Pagan JC, et al. Effect of intravenous albumin on systemic and hepatic hemodynamics and vasoactive neurohormonal systems in patients with cirrhosis and spontaneous bacterial peritonitis. J Hepatol 2004;41:384–90.

70. Quinlan GJ, Martin GS, Evans TW. Albumin: biochemical properties and therapeutic potential. Hepatology 2005;41:1211–9.

71. Brinch K, Moller S, Bendtsen F, et al. Plasma volume expansion by albumin in cirrhosis. Relation to blood volume distribution, arterial compliance and severity of disease. J Hepatol 2003;39:24–31.

72. Keller F, Heinze H, Jochimsen F, et al. Risk factors and outcome of 107 patients with decompensated liver disease and acute renal failure (including 26 patients with hepatorenal syndrome): the role of hemodialysis. Ren Fail 1995;17:135–46.

73. Capling RK, Bastani B. The clinical course of patients with type 1 hepatorenal syndrome maintained on hemodialysis. Ren Fail 2004;26:563–8.

74. Boyer TD. Transjugular intrahepatic portosystemic shunt: current status. Gastroenterology 2003;124:1700–10.

75. Uriz J, Gines P, Cardenas A, et al. Terlipressin plus albumin infusion: an effective and safe therapy of hepatorenal syndrome. J Hepatol 2000;33:43–8.

76. Tsai MH, Peng YS, Chen YC, et al. Adrenal insufficiency in patients with cirrhosis, severe sepsis and septic shock. Hepatology 2006;43:673–81.

77. Moore KP, Wong F, Gines P, et al. The management of ascites in cirrhosis: report on the consensus conference of the International Ascites Club. Hepatology 2003; 38:258–66.

78. Garcia-Tsao G. Current management of the complications of cirrhosis and portal hypertension: variceal hemorrhage, ascites, and spontaneous bacterial peritonitis. Gastroenterology 2001;120:726–48.

79. McCullough PA. Contrast-induced acute kidney injury. J Am Coll Cardiol 2008;51: 1419–28.

Diagnosis and Management of Autoimmune Hepatitis

Albert J. Czaja, MD

KEYWORDS

- Autoimmune • Hepatitis • Diagnosis • Steroids • Suboptimal responses
- Salvage therapies

KEY POINTS

- Autoimmune hepatitis has diverse presentations, and the diagnosis must be considered in all patients with acute or chronic liver disease or graft dysfunction after liver transplantation.
- Diagnostic criteria have been codified and scoring systems can aid in the diagnosis.
- Prednisone or prednisolone in combination with azathioprine is the mainstay therapy.
- Budesonide in combination with azathioprine is associated with a higher frequency of laboratory resolution with fewer side effects than conventional therapy after 6 months of frontline treatment.
- Corticosteroid-related side effects can develop in budesonide-treated patients with cirrhosis. The frequency of histologic resolution, durability of response, and target population for off-label frontline therapy with budesonide is uncertain.
- Calcineurin inhibitors (cyclosporine and tacrolimus) have been effective as off-label salvage agents in multiple small observational studies and they can be considered in steroid-refractory disease.
- Mycophenolate mofetil can be used off-label as a salvage agent and it is more effective as a treatment of patients with azathioprine intolerance than with refractory liver disease.
- Liver transplantation is the ultimate rescue therapy for patients with autoimmune hepatitis and liver failure.

INTRODUCTION

Autoimmune hepatitis is characterized by abnormal serum aspartate (AST) and alanine (ALT) aminotransferase levels, autoantibodies, increased serum IgG concentration, and

Disclosures: This article did not receive financial support from a funding agency or institution, and A.J. Czaja has no conflict of interests to declare.
Division of Gastroenterology and Hepatology, Mayo Clinic College of Medicine, 200 First Street Southwest, Rochester, MN 55905, USA
E-mail address: czaja.albert@mayo.edu

Clin Liver Dis 19 (2015) 57–79
http://dx.doi.org/10.1016/j.cld.2014.09.004   **liver.theclinics.com**

interface hepatitis on histologic examination.[1,2] It is primarily a disease of young women; however, it affects all ages and genders.[3,4] Autoimmune hepatitis has been described in diverse ethnic populations and geographic regions,[5] and its clinical presentation can vary from mild asymptomatic disease[6,7] to acute severe (fulminant) liver failure.[8] Disease activity can fluctuate spontaneously from none to severe[9]; progression to cirrhosis can be indolent and unsuspected[10]; and the histologic manifestations can include centrilobular zone 3 necrosis,[8] multilobular collapse,[11] and bile duct injury.[12] Autoimmune hepatitis can also recur or develop de novo after liver transplantation.[13]

- The mean annual incidence of autoimmune hepatitis in white northern Europeans is 0.85 to 1.9 per 100,000 persons, and its point prevalence is 10.7 to 16.9 per 100,000 persons.[14,15]
- The frequencies of autoimmune hepatitis in acute liver failure (2%–16%),[16,17] cryptogenic cirrhosis (10%–54%),[18] and recurrent (8%–12% at 1 year and 36%–68% at 5 years) or de novo (1%–7%) autoimmune hepatitis after liver transplantation[13] compel its consideration in all patients with acute and chronic hepatitis of uncertain cause.

DIAGNOSIS

Autoimmune hepatitis is diagnosed by suspecting the disease in all clinical settings and by applying codified diagnostic criteria (**Table 1**).[19,20] The diagnostic features can be typical and render a definite diagnosis, or they can be less pronounced or associated with other confounders (drug or alcohol exposure, alpha-1 anti-trypsin deficiency, steatosis, or iron excess) and render a probable diagnosis.[21] The diagnosis is suspect without hypergammaglobulinemia, especially an increased serum IgG concentration.[21] Normal serum IgG levels are present in only 3% of patients.[22]

- Chronic viral hepatitis, drug-induced chronic liver disease (most commonly associated with minocycline or nitrofurantoin therapy), Wilson disease, and the immune-mediated cholangiopathies (primary biliary cirrhosis [PBC] and primary sclerosing cholangitis [PSC]) must be excluded.[21]
- The diagnosis is especially difficult in patients with acute severe (fulminant) presentations because laboratory (low titer or absent autoantibodies, normal or near-normal serum IgG levels), and histologic (centrilobular zone 3 necrosis) findings can dissuade its consideration.[17]
- Celiac disease must not be overlooked because it can be associated with an acute or chronic liver disease and improve with gluten restriction.[1,23]

Diagnostic Scoring Systems

A comprehensive diagnostic scoring system was developed originally as a research tool to ensure the homogeneity of study populations, but it has evolved into a clinical tool that ensures the systematic assessment of the key features of autoimmune hepatitis (**Table 2**).[21] The comprehensive scoring system can be applied before and after conventional corticosteroid therapy, and the treatment response can upgrade or downgrade the diagnosis. A simplified scoring system has been developed to facilitate its clinical application, and it does not score treatment response (**Table 3**).[24]

- The comprehensive scoring system has greater sensitivity for the diagnosis of autoimmune hepatitis than the simplified scoring system (100% vs 95%), and the simplified scoring system has greater specificity (90% vs 73%) and accuracy (92% vs 82%).[25]

Table 1
Codified international criteria for the diagnosis of autoimmune hepatitis

Features	Definite Autoimmune Hepatitis	Probable Autoimmune Hepatitis
Abnormal serum AST, ALT, and AP levels	Abnormal serum AST and ALT levels of any degree with less pronounced serum AP abnormality	Abnormal serum AST and ALT levels of any degree with less pronounced serum AP abnormality
Serum α_1-antitrypsin, copper, and ceruloplasmin levels	Normal serum levels	Any abnormal serum level provided Wilson disease excluded
Abnormal serum globulin, γ-globulin, or IgG level	Serum globulin or γ-globulin, or IgG level >1.5-fold ULN	Serum globulin or γ-globulin or IgG level >ULN
ANA, SMA, anti-LKM1 one or more positive	Serum titers >1:80 by IIF or levels strongly positive by ELISA	Serum titers or levels weakly positive or negative and supplemented by positivity for other nonstandard antibodies
AMA titer or level	AMA negative	AMA negative
IgM anti-HAV, HBsAg, anti-HCV	All markers negative for active viral infection	All markers negative for active viral infection
Interface hepatitis on histologic examination	Moderate-to-severe interface hepatitis without destructive biliary changes, granulomas, or other prominent features that suggest alternative diagnosis	Moderate-to-severe interface hepatitis without destructive biliary changes, granulomas, or other prominent features that suggest alternative diagnosis
No other causal factors	Alcohol <25 g/d No recent exposure to hepatotoxic drugs No celiac disease	Alcohol <50 g/d Some drug or alcohol exposure Celiac disease concurrent but unlikely primary cause of liver injury

Abbreviations: AMA, antimitochondrial antibodies; ANA, antinuclear antibodies; AP, alkaline phosphatase; AST, aspartate aminotransferase; HAV, hepatitis A virus; HBsAg, hepatitis B surface antigen; HBV, hepatitis B virus; HCV, hepatitis C virus; IgM, immunoglobulin M; IIF, indirect immunofluorescence; ULN, upper limit of normal range.

Adapted from Alvarez F, Berg PA, Bianchi FB, et al. International Autoimmune Hepatitis Group Report: review of criteria for diagnosis of autoimmune hepatitis. J Hepatol 1999;31:933; with permission of Elsevier BV and the European Association for the Study of the Liver.

- Patients with absent or atypical features are best evaluated by the comprehensive scoring system to ensure that every component of the disease is assessed and graded.[25]
- Patients with typical features of autoimmune hepatitis or other diseases that must be excluded from autoimmune hepatitis are best evaluated by the simplified scoring system.[25]
- Neither scoring system has been validated by prospective studies nor can they be used as discriminative diagnostic indices or as instruments for defining syndromes with mixed or overlapping features of autoimmune hepatitis.[26]

Table 2
Comprehensive diagnostic scoring system of the international autoimmune hepatitis group

Clinical Features	Points
Female	+2
AP:AST (or ALT) ratio	
<1.5	+2
1.5–3.0	0
>3.0	−2
Serum globulin or IgG level above ULN	
>2.0	+3
1.5–2.0	+2
1.0–1.5	+1
<1.0	0
ANA, SMA, or anti-LKM1	
>1:80	+3
1:80	+2
1:40	+1
<1:40	0
AMA positive	−4
Hepatitis markers	
Positive	−3
Negative	+3
Hepatotoxic drug exposure	
Positive	−4
Negative	+1
Average alcohol intake	
<25 g/d	+2
>60 g/d	−2
Histologic findings	
Interface hepatitis	+3
Lymphoplasmacytic infiltrate	+1
Rosette formation	+1
Biliary changes	−3
Other atypical changes	−3
None of above	−5
Concurrent immune disease	+2
Other autoantibodies	+2
HLA DRB1*03 or DRB1*04	+1
Response to corticosteroids	
Complete	+2
Relapse after drug withdrawal	+3
Aggregate score pretreatment	
Definite autoimmune hepatitis	>15
Probable autoimmune hepatitis	10–15

(continued on next page)

Table 2 (continued)	
Clinical Features	**Points**
Aggregate score posttreatment	
Definite autoimmune hepatitis	>17
Probable autoimmune hepatitis	12–17

Abbreviations: AMA, antimitochondrial antibodies; ANA, antinuclear antibodies; AP, alkaline phosphatase; AST, aspartate aminotransferase; LKM1, liver/kidney microsome type 1; SMA, smooth muscle antibodies; ULN, upper limit of the normal range.

Adapted from Alvarez F, Berg PA, Bianchi FB, et al. International Autoimmune Hepatitis Group Report: review of criteria for diagnosis of autoimmune hepatitis. J Hepatol 1999;31:934; with permission of Elsevier BV and the European Association for the Study of the Liver.

- The performance parameters of the scoring systems have been based on clinical judgment, and the results of the scoring systems can never supersede the diagnosis based on clinical judgment.[25]

Autoantibodies

Autoantibodies are the serologic manifestations of autoimmune hepatitis, and their occurrence in a patient with an acute or chronic liver disease compels consideration of this diagnosis (**Fig. 1**).[1,2] Autoantibodies do not establish the presence of autoimmune hepatitis, and the diagnostic effort must extend beyond their detection.[19]

Standard autoantibodies

The standard serologic battery for diagnosing autoimmune hepatitis includes antinuclear antibodies (ANA), smooth muscle antibodies (SMA), and antibodies to liver kidney microsome type 1 (anti-LKM1) (**Table 4**).[1,21]

Table 3 Simplified diagnostic scoring system of the international autoimmune hepatitis group			
Category	**Scoring Elements**	**Results**	**Points**
Autoantibodies	ANA or SMA	1:40 by IIF	+1
	ANA or SMA	≥1:80 by IIF	+2
	Anti-LKM1 (alternative to ANA and SMA)	≥1:40 by IIF	+2
	Anti-SLA (alternative to ANA, SMA and LKM1)	Positive	+2
Immunoglobulins	IgG level	>ULN	+1
		>1.1 times ULN	+2
Histologic findings	Interface hepatitis	Compatible features	+1
		Typical features	+2
Viral markers	IgM anti-HAV, HBsAg, HBV DNA, HCV RNA	No viral markers	+2
		Probable diagnosis	≥6
		Definite diagnosis	≥7

Abbreviations: ANA, antinuclear antibodies; HAV, hepatitis A virus; HBsAg, hepatitis B surface antigen; HBV, hepatitis B virus; HCV, hepatitis C virus; IIF, indirect immunofluorescence; LKM1, liver microsome type 1; SLA, soluble liver antigen; SMA, smooth muscle antibodies; ULN, upper limit of the normal range.

Adapted from Hennes EM, Zeniya M, Czaja AJ, et al. Simplified criteria for the diagnosis of autoimmune hepatitis. Hepatology 2008;48:171; with permission of John Wiley & Sons, Inc. and the American Association for the Study of Liver Disease.

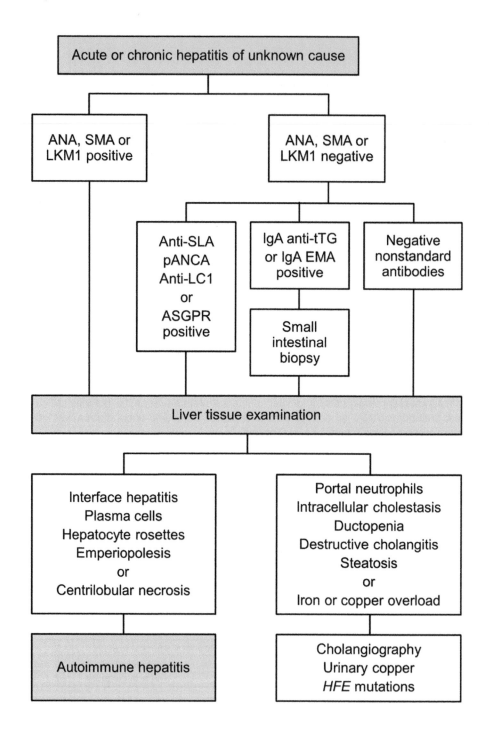

- ANA are the classical markers of autoimmune hepatitis, but they lack organ-specificity and disease-specificity. They are present in 80% of patients with auto-immune hepatitis, but they also occur in chronic alcoholic liver disease (21%), nonalcoholic fatty liver disease (32%), chronic viral hepatitis (28%), and the chol-angiopathies of PBC and PSC (39%).[27]
- SMA also lack organ-specificity and disease-specificity, but they occur less frequently than ANA in autoimmune hepatitis (63% vs 80%) and other chronic liver diseases such as chronic hepatitis C (7%), alcoholic liver disease (4%), PBC (6%), and PSC (16%).[27]
- The concurrence of ANA and SMA has a sensitivity (43%), specificity (99%), and diagnostic accuracy (74%) for autoimmune hepatitis that exceeds the perfor-mance parameters of either antibody alone.[27]
- Anti-LKM1 occur in only 3% to 4% of adults with autoimmune hepatitis in the United States, but they have high specificity for the diagnosis (99%).[27]
- Anti-LKM1 are most common in European children with autoimmune hepatitis (occurrence, 14%–38% in the United Kingdom).[3,28]
- Anti-LKM1 coexist with ANA or SMA in only 1% to 3% of instances, and the sep-aration of these markers has justified the designation of 2 types of autoimmune hepatitis.[27] Type 1 autoimmune hepatitis is characterized by ANA and/or SMA, and type 2 autoimmune hepatitis is characterized by anti-LKM1.[29]
- The designations of type 1 and type 2 autoimmune hepatitis are mainly clinical descriptors, and they have not been endorsed by the International Autoimmune Hepatitis Group.[21]

Nonstandard autoantibodies

Nonstandard autoantibodies have been incorporated into the codified diagnostic criteria and scoring systems for autoimmune hepatitis (see **Fig. 1**),[21] and they are typi-cally assessed as supplemental markers when the standard serologic battery is nega-tive or nondiagnostic (see **Table 4**).[30,31]

- Atypical perinuclear antineutrophil cytoplasmic antibodies (pANCA) react to the nuclear membrane of human neutrophils, and they have been detected in 50% to 92% of patients with type 1 autoimmune hepatitis.[30] These antibodies are ab-sent in type 2 autoimmune hepatitis, but they are common in chronic ulcerative colitis and PSC.[30,32] Atypical pANCA have been used to evaluate patients with liver disease of undetermined nature.[30]

Fig. 1. Diagnostic algorithm for acute or chronic hepatitis of unknown cause. All patients are evaluated and negative for viral markers, drug, alcohol or toxic exposures, decreased ceruloplasmin level, transferrin saturation greater than 45%, antimitochondrial antibodies, and family history of liver disease. Antinuclear antibodies (ANA), smooth muscle antibodies (SMA), and antibodies to liver kidney microsome type 1 (LKM1) constitute the standard sero-logic battery, and atypical perinuclear antineutrophil cytoplasmic antibodies (pANCA), IgA antibodies to tissue transglutaminase (IgA anti-tTG) or endomysium (EMA), and antibodies to soluble liver antigen (SLA), liver cytosol type 1 (LC1), asialoglycoprotein receptor (ASGPR) constitute the nonstandard serologic battery. The absence of serologic markers and the presence of histologic findings atypical of autoimmune hepatitis justify additional diag-nostic studies based on the clinical findings. These may include cholangiography, urinary copper excretion, and determinations of the *High iron FE (HFE) gene* mutations for hemochromatosis.

Table 4
Standard and nonstandard autoantibodies in the diagnosis of autoimmune hepatitis

Diagnostic Battery	Autoantibody Type	Antigenic Target	Clinical Attributes
Standard	ANA	Ribonucleoproteins Centromere	Overall occurrence, 80%[27] Combined with SMA, 43%[27] Helps define type 1 AIH[29,30] Frequent in other liver diseases[27]
	SMA	Actin Tubulin Intermediate filaments	Diagnostic accuracy with ANA, 74%[27] Helps define type 1 AIH[29] Occurs in other liver diseases[27]
	anti-LKM1	CYP2D6	Defines type 2 AIH[29] Mainly in European children, 14%–38%[3] Rare in North American adults, 3%–4%[30] Can occur in chronic hepatitis C, 0%–10%[30]
Nonstandard	pANCA	Neutrophilic nuclear lamins	High occurrence in type 1 AIH, 50%–92%[30] Absent in type 2 AIH[30] Frequent in CUC and PSC[30,32] May reclassify cryptogenic hepatitis[30]
	Soluble liver antigen (anti-SLA)	Transfer ribonucleoprotein complex	Occurrence in US, 15%[33] Diagnostic specificity, >90%[33] Associated with severity and relapse[36,37] May be sole marker of AIH[33]
	Actin (anti-actin)	Polymerized F-actin	Occurrence with SMA, 99%[30] Absent when SMA positive, 14%[30] Assay-dependent prognostic implications[39]
	Liver cytosol type 1 (anti-LC1)	Formiminotransferase cyclodeaminase	Associated with anti-LKM1[30] Rare in USA[31]
	Asialoglycoprotein receptor	Transmembrane glycoprotein	Occurrence, 88%[30] Associated with relapse[30]
	IgM tissue transglutaminase	Enzyme interacting with gliadin	Celiac disease in AIH, 4%[40] Liver disease can be due to celiac disease[23]

Abbreviations: AIH, autoimmune hepatitis; CUC, chronic ulcerative colitis; CYP2D6, cytochrome monooxygenase; pANCA, atypical perinuclear antineutrophil cytoplasmic antibodies; US, United States.

- Antibodies to soluble liver antigen (anti-SLA) have high specificity (>90%) but low sensitivity (15%) for autoimmune hepatitis.[33] They have been closely associated with antibodies to ribonucleoprotein or Sjögren syndrome A antigen (anti-Ro/SSA) (96% concurrence),[34,35] and they may identify individuals with severe disease and long-term treatment dependence.[36,37] They may also reclassify 26% of patients with cryptogenic hepatitis as autoimmune hepatitis.[30,33]
- Antibodies to actin (anti-actin) have been proposed as a replacement for SMA, but not all patients with SMA have anti-actin.[38] Anti-actin have characterized patients with severe disease and limited treatment response, especially if they coexist with antibodies to α-actinin.[39] The assay for anti-actin has not been standardized, and tests for anti-actin remain outside the standard repertoire for autoimmune hepatitis.[20]
- Antibodies to asialoglycoprotein receptor (anti-ASGPR) and antibodies to liver cytosol type 1 (anti-LC1) are other nonstandard autoantibodies that may strengthen the diagnosis of autoimmune hepatitis or clarify the nature of cryptogenic liver disease.[20,30]
- IgM antibodies to tissue transglutaminase or endomysium can suggest the diagnosis of celiac disease and help identify a concurrent disease associated with autoimmune hepatitis (4% concurrence)[40] or a cause of acute and chronic liver injury that may respond to gluten restriction.[23]

Histologic Assessment

Interface hepatitis is the principal histologic pattern associated with autoimmune hepatitis, and it is characterized by a lymphoplasmacytic infiltrate of the portal tract, disruption of the limiting plate, and extension of mononuclear cells into the hepatic lobule (**Fig. 2**).[1] Plasma cells are prominent in 66% of cases, hepatocyte rosettes and emperiopolesis (penetration of one cell into and through a larger cell) can be present, and lymphoid and pleomorphic cholangitis are evident in 7% to 9% of cases.[12,41–43]

- The histologic features of autoimmune hepatitis are not disease-specific, and they can occur in acute and chronic viral hepatitis, drug-induced liver injury, PBC, and PSC.[41]

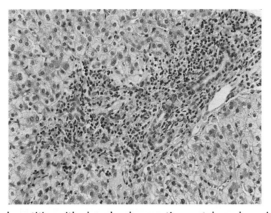

Fig. 2. Interface hepatitis with lymphoplasmacytic portal and periportal infiltrates. Hematoxylin-eosin, original magnification, ×200. (*From* Gonzalez-Koch A, Czaja AJ, Carpenter HA, et al. Recurrent autoimmune hepatitis after orthotopic liver transplantation. Liver Transpl 2001;7:306; with permission from John Wiley & Sons, Inc and the American Association for the Study of the Liver.)

- Histologic assessment at presentation is essential to establish the diagnosis and to identify concurrent features (steatosis, destructive cholangitis, ductopenia, and viral inclusions) that might suggest an alternative diagnosis (infectious, metabolic, hereditary, toxic, cholestatic, or overlap syndrome) or modify the management strategy.[1,44,45]
- Studies suggesting that the liver biopsy is unnecessary to establish the diagnosis have failed to examine the frequency that patients with compatible clinical findings have been excluded from the diagnosis because of the liver tissue examination.[46]
- Centrilobular zone 3 necrosis can be a feature of early-stage severe disease or acute injury on chronic disease.[8,47] Centrilobular zone 3 necrosis coexists with interface hepatitis in 78% of instances, and it can be present in cirrhosis.[47]
- Bile duct injury, including isolated and transient destructive cholangitis, can present in 24% of patients with classic histologic features of autoimmune hepatitis,[12,42] and they should not dissuade the diagnosis or alter therapy in the absence of other features of cholestatic liver disease.[42,48]

Concurrent Immune-Mediated Diseases

Immune-mediated diseases are present in 38% of patients with autoimmune hepatitis, and they may mask the presence of liver disease, especially in elderly patients.[4,49]

- Autoimmune thyroiditis, Graves disease, synovitis, and ulcerative colitis are the most common concurrent immune-mediated diseases.[49]
- Patients aged 60 years or older have autoimmune thyroid diseases (30% vs 13%) and rheumatic diseases (13% vs 0%), including rheumatoid arthritis, Sjögren syndrome, and systemic lupus erythematosus, more commonly than adults 30 years and younger.[4,49]
- Adults aged 30 years or younger with autoimmune hepatitis have ulcerative colitis more frequently (10% vs 0%) than patients aged 60 years or older.[4]
- Concurrent immune-mediated diseases must be managed independently of the liver disease, and only ulcerative colitis can affect the course of autoimmune hepatitis if associated with cholangiographic changes of PSC.[50]

Cholangiography

Sixteen percent of adults with autoimmune hepatitis and ulcerative colitis have focal bile duct strictures and dilations by cholangiography that suggest PSC, and these patients can respond poorly to conventional corticosteroid regimens.[50] Endoscopic cholangiography (ERC) or magnetic resonance cholangiography (MRC) is warranted in all patients with autoimmune hepatitis and ulcerative colitis to identify these potentially problematic individuals.

- Biliary changes suggestive of PSC have been described in 10% of adults with autoimmune hepatitis who undergo MRC,[51] but these changes may reflect biliary distortions associated with hepatic fibrosis.[52]
- Cholangiographic features of PSC (autoimmune sclerosing cholangitis) have also been described in 50% of European children with autoimmune hepatitis, including patients without inflammatory bowel disease, and these individuals tend to improve on conventional corticosteroid therapy.[28]
- ERC or MRC should also be considered in all adults with autoimmune hepatitis who have histologic changes of bile duct injury or loss, marked cholestatic laboratory findings, or corticosteroid-refractory liver disease.[50]

MANAGEMENT

Autoimmune hepatitis is managed by instituting corticosteroid therapy promptly, monitoring the treatment response closely, and individualizing the schedule by adjusting doses of medication, supplementing the original regimen, or supplanting it with other agents (**Fig. 3**).[20,53] All patients with active liver inflammation, evidenced by

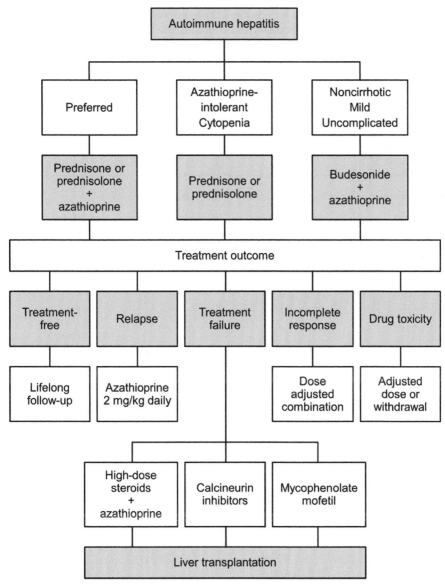

Fig. 3. Management algorithm for autoimmune hepatitis. Three regimens can be considered for treatment-naïve patients. The regimen of budesonide and azathioprine is the least established. The outcomes of initial therapy determine the next management strategy. Progressive disease with features of liver failure warrant evaluation for liver transplantation at any step.

abnormal serum AST, ALT, or IgG levels and histologic features of interface hepatitis, are candidates for treatment.[1,54] Mild asymptomatic disease at presentation becomes symptomatic in 26% to 70% of instances,[6,7] and untreated patients with mild autoimmune hepatitis have a lower 10-year survival than treated patients with severe disease (67% vs 98%).[55] The asymptomatic state or the presence of mild laboratory changes does not preclude the need for treatment.

The supplemental or replacement medications used in frontline and salvage therapies for autoimmune hepatitis include the calcineurin inhibitors (cyclosporine, tacrolimus), next generation glucocorticoid (budesonide), and purine antagonist (mycophenolate mofetil). All are unlicensed in the United States for use in autoimmune hepatitis, and their administration has been for off-label indications.

Corticosteroid Regimens and Ancillary Treatments

The preferred treatment schedule of autoimmune hepatitis is prednisone or prednisolone in combination with azathioprine (**Table 5**).[1,2] A 4-week induction phase is followed by a maintenance phase using lower doses of the same medications that is continued until disease resolution, treatment failure, or drug intolerance. Prednisone

Table 5
Corticosteroid regimens for treatment-naïve autoimmune hepatitis

Regimens	Induction Phase	Maintenance Phase	Side Effects
Prednisone or prednisolone and azathioprine (Combination therapy)[1]	Prednisone or prednisolone: 30 mg/d × 1 wk 20 mg/d × 1 wk 15 mg/d × 2 wk Azathioprine: 50 mg/d	Prednisone or prednisolone: 10 mg/d Azathioprine: 50 mg/d	Prednisone or prednisolone: Cosmetic, 80%[64] Osteopenia, 7%[64] Treatment ending, 12%–29%[55,64] More common in cirrhosis, 25%[58] Azathioprine: Cytopenia, 6%[64] Bone marrow failure, rare[64] Malignancy SIR, 2.7[67] Treatment ending, 5%–10%[64,65]
Prednisone or prednisolone (Monotherapy)[1]	Prednisone or prednisolone: 60 mg/d × 1 wk 40 mg/d × 1 wk 30 mg/d × 2 wk	Prednisone or prednisolone: 20 mg/d	Same as lower dose in combination regimen but more frequent (44% vs 10%)[56]
European Preference[1,2]	Prednisolone: Equivalent dose or 1 mg/kg/d Azathioprine 1–2 mg/kg/d	Prednisolone: Adjusted to response Azathioprine 1–2 mg/kg/d	Same as in other regimens[2]
Budesonide in combination with azathioprine[57]	Budesonide: 6–9 mg/d Azathioprine: 1–2 mg/kg/d	—	Same as with prednisone or prednisolone but mainly in cirrhosis[59–61]

Abbreviation: SIR, standardized incidence ratio.

or prednisolone can be as effective as the combination regimen, and it is preferred in patients with severe cytopenia (leukocyte count, <2.5 × 10^9/l; platelet count, <50 × 10^9/l), absent thiopurine methyltransferase (TPMT) activity, or concerns about the effects of azathioprine on active malignancy or pregnancy.[1,54] Prednisone or prednisolone must be administered in higher dose during the induction and maintenance phases than in the combination regimen, and monotherapy is associated with a higher risk of corticosteroid-induced complications (44% vs 10%).[56]

- Prednisolone is preferred over prednisone in Europe, and the doses of prednisolone (1 mg/kg/d) and azathioprine (1–2 mg/kg/d) are weight-based.[1,2] Clinical experiences have indicated comparable efficacies and safety between the American and European regimens.
- Patients taking budesonide (6–9 mg/d) in combination with azathioprine (1–2 mg/kg body weight/d) had normalized serum AST and ALT levels more frequently (47% vs 18%) and had fewer side effects (28% vs 53%) than patients randomized to prednisone (40 mg/d tapered to 10 mg/d) in combination with azathioprine (1–2 mg/kg body weight/d) during a treatment trial lasting 6 months in treatment-naïve patients.[57]
- Budesonide in combination with azathioprine has been proposed as an alternative frontline therapy despite the uncertain frequency that the regimen induces histologic resolution or a durable response.[58]
- Caveats to treatment with budesonide include the emergence of typical corticosteroid-related side effects in patients with cirrhosis,[59,60] the failure of the drug to salvage refractory disease,[61] and the uncertain identity of its target population. Budesonide therapy may be most appropriate for treatment-naïve, noncirrhotic patients with mild inflammatory activity and uncomplicated autoimmune hepatitis.[58]
- Mycophenolate mofetil (1.5–2 g/d) has also been used as a frontline therapy in combination with prednisolone. This combination has normalized serum ALT and γ-globulin levels in 87%, allowed corticosteroid withdrawal in 58%, and been well tolerated in 97% after 3 to 92 months of treatment (mean duration, 26 months).[62] A preference for this regimen has not been established.
- Ancillary management strategies include pretreatment vaccination of all patients susceptible to infection with the hepatitis A and hepatitis B viruses[1,63]; pretreatment determination of bone density in postmenopausal women[1]; and institution of a bone maintenance regimen in all adults, including calcium and vitamin D supplementation and a regular exercise regimen.[1] Bisphosphonates can be added as indicated by the clinical status or bone density assessment.[1]

Treatment-Related Side Effects

Corticosteroid therapy is complicated by side effects (intolerable cosmetic changes, obesity, hypertension, diabetes, mental instability, and vertebral compression) that compel dose reduction or drug withdrawal in 12% to 29% of patients (see **Table 5**).[55,64] Patients with cirrhosis have a higher frequency of complications than patients without cirrhosis (25% vs 8%), probably because of increased serum levels of unbound prednisolone associated with protracted hypoalbuminemia or hyperbilirubinemia.[58] Patients with cirrhosis are also at risk to develop typical corticosteroid-induced complications when they are treated with budesonide, probably because of decreased hepatic clearance of the drug and increased systemic bioavailability.[58–60]

Nausea, vomiting, rash, liver toxicity, pancreatitis, and cytopenia can complicate chronic azathioprine therapy, and these side effects warrant dose reduction or withdrawal in 5% to 10% of patients.[64–66] Bone marrow failure is a rare complication,[64] and the standardized incidence ratio for extrahepatic malignancy is 2.7 (95% confidence interval 1.8–3.9).[67] Extensive clinical experiences with the use of azathioprine during pregnancy have not indicated an increased risk to the fetus[68,69]; however, azathioprine is listed as a category D drug. Patients with cirrhosis and pretreatment cytopenia are especially difficult to manage with azathioprine, and they must be monitored by frequent assessments of the leukocyte and platelet counts.[64]

- Determinations of TPMT activity by phenotyping or genotyping have not been closely associated with the occurrence of azathioprine-induced side effects.[70–73]
- Routine pretreatment screening for TPMT activity has not been supported by strong clinical evidence,[1,2] but this determination can be useful in identifying the 0.3% of patients with absent enzyme activity.[71,74]

Treatment Outcomes

Corticosteroid therapy ameliorates symptoms, improves liver tests, and reduces histologic activity in 80% of patients.[75] Treatment also prevents or reverses hepatic fibrosis in 79%[76,77] and improves 5-year survival from 40% to greater than 90%.[78,79] Sixty-seven percent of patients improve to normal or near-normal liver tests and liver tissue,[75] 7% worsen despite compliance with therapy (treatment failure),[80] 14% have an incomplete response,[81,82] and at least 12% have treatment-ending side effects (see **Fig. 3**).[55,64] The average duration of treatment until normal or near-normal laboratory tests and liver tissue is 22 months in the United States[81,82] and at least 24 months in Europe.[2,83]

Treatment Withdrawal

Corticosteroid withdrawal is the preferred management strategy after resolution of the disease.[1,2] Normalization of liver tests (serum aminotransferase, γ-globulin, and IgG levels) and liver tissue are requisites before drug withdrawal.[1,2] Patients with cirrhosis are unlikely to normalize their liver tissue, and treatment withdrawal can be considered after 6 to 12 months of persistently normal laboratory indices and histologic demonstration of inactive cirrhosis.[78]

- Histologic resolution is achieved in only 22% of patients who are treated for 56 ± 5 months (range, 9–120 months),[81] and most patients who resolve their liver tests have mild residual histologic manifestations or hepatic fibrosis.[81,84]
- Histologic resolution can reduce the frequency of relapse after drug withdrawal to 28%,[81] and it should be documented by liver tissue examination before drug withdrawal.[1,54]
- Histologic improvement lags behind laboratory resolution by 3 to 8 months, and the liver biopsy assessment should be deferred for this interval.[85]
- Combination therapy should be discontinued in a slowly tapered, well-monitored fashion. The dose of prednisone can be reduced from the maintenance level of 10 mg/d to 7.5 mg/d for 2 weeks, then 5 mg/d for 2 weeks, and then 2.5 mg/d for 2 weeks, before complete withdrawal. The dose of azathioprine can be maintained at 50 mg/d for the first 3 weeks of the withdrawal program and then reduced to 25 mg/d for the final 3 weeks.[86]
- Corticosteroid monotherapy is also discontinued in a slow, gradual fashion. The dose of prednisone or prednisolone can be decreased from 20 mg/d to 15 mg/d for 1 week, then 10 mg/d for 1 week, then 5 mg/d for 2 weeks, and then 2.5 mg/d for 2 weeks, before complete withdrawal.[86]

- Arthralgias and myalgias associated with corticosteroid withdrawal may affect the rapidity of the withdrawal or necessitate a temporary increase in the dose of corticosteroids.[58]
- Serum AST, ALT, and γ-globulin levels should be performed at 3-week intervals during the withdrawal process and for at least 3 months after discontinuation to monitor for relapse. Thereafter, monitoring intervals can be increased to every 3 to 6 months and then to every 12 months depending on clinical stability.[1,87]

Consequences of Treatment Withdrawal

Drug withdrawal can result in the emergence of a treatment-free state or the exacerbation of inflammatory activity (relapse). A stable treatment-free state of at least 3 years duration can be achieved in 19% to 40% of patients who are withdrawn from treatment[81,86,88] and 36% may remain treatment-free for at least 5 years (mean, 130 ± 7 months; range, 68–198 months).[89,90] Relapse can terminate the treatment-free state at any time (longest interval to relapse, 22 years), and patients who achieve a treatment-free state require annual laboratory assessments indefinitely to ensure the continued quiescence of their liver disease.[87] Relapse usually occurs within the first 3 months after drug withdrawal, and its frequency decreases to an average of 3% per year after the first year.[87]

Relapse eventuates in 28% to 87% of patients, and its occurrence relates in part to the degree of histologic improvement before drug withdrawal.[81,86,91,92] Relapse has been associated with progression to cirrhosis during treatment,[91,93] persistent plasma cell infiltration,[84,93] and residual portal or periportal hepatitis.[84,94] Its frequency can be reduced to 28% in patients treated to normal liver tissue, but the risk can never be eliminated.[81]

Management of Suboptimal Responses

The suboptimal responses to conventional corticosteroid treatment are relapse after drug withdrawal, treatment failure, incomplete response, and drug intolerance (see **Fig. 3**). Therapies have been derived mainly from single-center clinical experiences, and they have not been subjected to rigorous clinical trial.

Relapse after drug withdrawal

Serum AST or ALT levels that increase to more than threefold the upper limit of the normal range after drug withdrawal are invariably associated with histologic evidence of interface hepatitis (**Table 6**).[85] These laboratory findings do not require confirmation by liver tissue examination unless other confounding clinical factors or findings are present.

- Relapse is managed by restarting the original corticosteroid regimen until laboratory resolution is again achieved. The dose of azathioprine is then increased to 2 mg/kg body weight/d while the dose of prednisone or prednisolone is gradually withdrawn.[1] Indefinite azathioprine therapy can suppress clinical and histologic activity and be well tolerated in 80% of patients followed for 10 years.[95]
- Low-dose prednisone or prednisolone (<10 mg/d; median dose 7.5 mg/d) can achieve similar results in azathioprine-intolerant patients. Seventy-two percent maintain a stable clinical course (mean treatment duration, 44 ± 7 months), and liver failure resulting in death or liver transplantation occurs in 18%.[96]

Table 6
Management of suboptimal responses

Response	Clinical Features	Management Options
Relapse	Serum AST, ALT or γ-globulin level ≥3-fold ULN Interface hepatitis (biopsy not necessary unless other concerns)	Restart original regimen and continue until laboratory resolution, then adjust dose Azathioprine tolerance[95]: Increase azathioprine to 2 mg/kg/d as prednisone or prednisolone withdrawn Azathioprine intolerance[96]: Steroids at lowest dose for normal tests (median, 7.5 mg/d)
Treatment Failure	Increasing serum AST, ALT or γ-globulin level on original regimen Intensified histologic activity Liver-related symptoms	High-dose prednisone or prednisolone in combination with azathioprine[1]: Prednisone or prednisolone, 30 mg/d, and azathioprine, 150 mg/d × 1 mo Dose reductions of prednisone or prednisolone by 10 mg and azathioprine by 50 mg each month of improvement High-dose prednisone or prednisolone[1]: 60 mg/d × 1 mo 10 mg dose reduction each month Calcineurin inhibitors[66]: Cyclosporine A, 2–5 mg/kg/d (trough levels, 100–300 ng/mL) Tacrolimus, 1–3 mg bid (serum level, 3 ng/ml; range, 1.7–10.7 ng/ml) Mycophenolate mofetil[66]: 1.5–2 g/d Liver transplantation[1]
Incomplete Response	Improved but not fully corrected laboratory tests after 36 mo	Individualized dose reductions to maintain stable mild liver test abnormalities[1]
Drug Intolerance	Drug-specific side effects	Reduce dose or discontinue implicated drug[1] Continue tolerated drug in adjusted dose[1] Consider mycophenolate mofetil for azathioprine intolerance[66]

Abbreviation: ULN, upper limit of normal range.

Treatment failure

Treatment failure can be managed by increasing the doses of prednisone (or prednisolone) and azathioprine, supplanting the corticosteroid regimen with calcineurin inhibitors, or by replacing azathioprine with mycophenolate mofetil (see **Table 6**).[97,98]

- The dose of prednisone or prednisolone is increased to 30 mg/d and the dose of azathioprine is increased to 150 mg/d for at least 1 month.[1] The dose of prednisone or prednisolone is then reduced by 10 mg and the dose of azathioprine is reduced by 50 mg after each month of laboratory improvement until conventional maintenance doses are achieved (prednisone or prednisolone, 10 mg/d, and azathioprine, 50 mg/d).[1]
- Prednisone or prednisolone, 60 mg/d, can be administered alone for at least 1 month in azathioprine intolerant patients.[1] The dose reductions are then reduced by 10 mg after each month of laboratory improvement until a maintenance dose of 20 mg/d is achieved.[1]

- Therapy with high-dose corticosteroids induces clinical and laboratory resolution in greater than 70% of patients within 2 years. Histologic improvement to normal or near-normal liver tissue is achieved in 14% to 20%, treatment must be continued indefinitely, side effects are possible, cirrhosis develops in 82%, and the 5-year survival is 41%.[80,97]
- Therapy with cyclosporine induces laboratory improvement in 93% and a negative response, defined as no response, drug intolerance, and noncompliance, in 7%.[99] The composite experience consists of 32 subjects in 11 studies published during the past 29 years.[99]
- Therapy with tacrolimus induces laboratory improvement in 87% and negative responses in 13%.[99] The composite experience consists of 23 subjects in 4 reports during the past 19 years.[99]
- The limited experience with the calcineurin inhibitors must be counterbalanced against the expense, possible side effects, and uncertain dosing and monitoring schedule of these drugs in autoimmune hepatitis.
- Therapy with mycophenolate mofetil induces laboratory improvement in less than 50% of patients treated for corticosteroid-refractory liver disease or azathioprine intolerance.[66,99] Patients who are treated for azathioprine intolerance improve more commonly than patients who are treated for refractory liver disease (58% vs 12%).[66,99]
- The low frequency of salvage with mycophenolate mofetil must be counterbalanced against its expense, frequency of side effects (3%–34%), indefinite duration, and well-documented teratogenicity.[66,99]
- Liver transplantation for autoimmune hepatitis has a 5-year survival of 75% to 79%, and it should be considered in all patients with a score greater than 16 points by the model of end-stage liver disease (MELD), acute decompensation, intractable symptoms, treatment intolerance, or detection of liver cancer.[100] Autoimmune hepatitis recurs in 8% to 68%, depending on the duration of observation after transplantation, but the actuarial 5-year survival for recurrent disease ranges from 89% to 100%. Graft failure may require retransplantation in 13% to 23%.[100]

Incomplete response

The inability to induce laboratory resolution and normal or near normal histologic findings within 3 years connotes an incomplete response. Further improvement with additional conventional therapy is unlikely.[82] The goals of management must be redirected from disease resolution and treatment withdrawal to long-term suppression of inflammatory activity, prevention of disease progression, and tolerance of the therapeutic regimen (see **Table 6**).

- The dose of prednisone or prednisolone can be reduced to the lowest level possible to maintain stable, albeit often abnormal, laboratory indices while the dose of azathioprine is increased to 2 mg/kg body weight/d.
- The inflammatory activity may diminish or even disappear during long-term observation, and these patients may become eligible for treatment withdrawal.[86]

Drug intolerance

Drug intolerance is managed by reducing the dose of the incriminated medication or discontinuing it, depending on the severity of the presentation (see **Table 6**).[1,64] The inflammatory manifestations can usually be managed by increasing the dose of the tolerated medication. Mycophenolate mofetil has been used as an alternative drug for patients with azathioprine-intolerance, but it does have side effects that may resemble those of azathioprine, including cytopenia.[66]

SUMMARY

- Autoimmune hepatitis must be considered in all patients with acute or chronic liver disease and graft dysfunction after liver transplantation.
- Diagnostic criteria have been codified, and scoring systems can aid in the diagnosis.
- Prednisone or prednisolone in combination with azathioprine is the mainstay therapy.
- Budesonide is an alternative off-label frontline therapy, but it has major uncertainties.
- Cyclosporine or tacrolimus is an off-label salvage therapy for steroid-refractory disease.
- Mycophenolate mofetil can be used off-label as a salvage agent, especially for selected patients with azathioprine intolerance.
- Liver transplantation is the preferred treatment of liver failure.

REFERENCES

1. Manns MP, Czaja AJ, Gorham JD, et al. Diagnosis and management of autoimmune hepatitis. Hepatology 2010;51:2193–213.
2. Gleeson D, Heneghan MA. British Society of Gastroenterology (BSG) guidelines for management of autoimmune hepatitis. Gut 2011;60:1611–29.
3. Gregorio GV, Portmann B, Reid F, et al. Autoimmune hepatitis in childhood: a 20-year experience. Hepatology 1997;25:541–7.
4. Czaja AJ, Carpenter HA. Distinctive clinical phenotype and treatment outcome of type 1 autoimmune hepatitis in the elderly. Hepatology 2006;43:532–8.
5. Czaja AJ. Autoimmune hepatitis in diverse ethnic populations and geographical regions. Expert Rev Gastroenterol Hepatol 2013;7:365–85.
6. Kogan J, Safadi R, Ashur Y, et al. Prognosis of symptomatic versus asymptomatic autoimmune hepatitis: a study of 68 patients. J Clin Gastroenterol 2002;35:75–81.
7. Feld JJ, Dinh H, Arenovich T, et al. Autoimmune hepatitis: effect of symptoms and cirrhosis on natural history and outcome. Hepatology 2005;42:53–62.
8. Kessler WR, Cummings OW, Eckert G, et al. Fulminant hepatic failure as the initial presentation of acute autoimmune hepatitis. Clin Gastroenterol Hepatol 2004;2:625–31.
9. Burgart LJ, Batts KP, Ludwig J, et al. Recent-onset autoimmune hepatitis. Biopsy findings and clinical correlations. Am J Surg Pathol 1995;19:699–708.
10. Davis GL, Czaja AJ, Ludwig J. Development and prognosis of histologic cirrhosis in corticosteroid-treated hepatitis B surface antigen-negative chronic active hepatitis. Gastroenterology 1984;87:1222–7.
11. Czaja AJ, Rakela J, Ludwig J. Features reflective of early prognosis in corticosteroid-treated severe autoimmune chronic active hepatitis. Gastroenterology 1988;95:448–53.
12. Ludwig J, Czaja AJ, Dickson ER, et al. Manifestations of nonsuppurative cholangitis in chronic hepatobiliary diseases: morphologic spectrum, clinical correlations and terminology. Liver 1984;4:105–16.
13. Czaja AJ. Diagnosis, pathogenesis, and treatment of autoimmune hepatitis after liver transplantation. Dig Dis Sci 2012;57:2248–66.

14. Boberg KM, Aadland E, Jahnsen J, et al. Incidence and prevalence of primary biliary cirrhosis, primary sclerosing cholangitis, and autoimmune hepatitis in a Norwegian population. Scand J Gastroenterol 1998;33:99–103.

15. Werner M, Prytz H, Ohlsson B, et al. Epidemiology and the initial presentation of autoimmune hepatitis in Sweden: a nationwide study. Scand J Gastroenterol 2008;43:1232–40.

16. Stravitz RT, Lefkowitch JH, Fontana RJ, et al. Autoimmune acute liver failure: proposed clinical and histological criteria. Hepatology 2011;53:517–26.

17. Czaja AJ. Acute and acute severe (fulminant) autoimmune hepatitis. Dig Dis Sci 2013;58:897–914.

18. Czaja AJ. Cryptogenic chronic hepatitis and its changing guise in adults. Dig Dis Sci 2011;56:3421–38.

19. Czaja AJ. Autoimmune hepatitis. Part B: diagnosis. Expert Rev Gastroenterol Hepatol 2007;1:129–43.

20. Czaja AJ, Manns MP. Advances in the diagnosis, pathogenesis and management of autoimmune hepatitis. Gastroenterology 2010;139:58–72.

21. Alvarez F, Berg PA, Bianchi FB, et al. International Autoimmune Hepatitis Group Report: review of criteria for diagnosis of autoimmune hepatitis. J Hepatol 1999; 31:929–38.

22. Czaja AJ, Carpenter HA. Validation of scoring system for diagnosis of autoimmune hepatitis. Dig Dis Sci 1996;41:305–14.

23. Kaukinen K, Halme L, Collin P, et al. Celiac disease in patients with severe liver disease: gluten-free diet may reverse hepatic failure. Gastroenterology 2002; 122:881–8.

24. Hennes EM, Zeniya M, Czaja AJ, et al. Simplified criteria for the diagnosis of autoimmune hepatitis. Hepatology 2008;48:169–76.

25. Czaja AJ. Performance parameters of the diagnostic scoring systems for autoimmune hepatitis. Hepatology 2008;48:1540–8.

26. Boberg KM, Chapman RW, Hirschfield GM, et al. Overlap syndromes: the International Autoimmune Hepatitis Group (IAIHG) position statement on a controversial issue. J Hepatol 2011;54:374–85.

27. Czaja AJ. Performance parameters of the conventional serological markers for autoimmune hepatitis. Dig Dis Sci 2011;56:545–54.

28. Gregorio GV, Portmann B, Karani J, et al. Autoimmune hepatitis/sclerosing cholangitis overlap syndrome in childhood: a 16-year prospective study. Hepatology 2001;33:544–53.

29. Czaja AJ, Manns MP. The validity and importance of subtypes in autoimmune hepatitis: a point of view. Am J Gastroenterol 1995;90:1206–11.

30. Czaja AJ, Norman GL. Autoantibodies in the diagnosis and management of liver disease. J Clin Gastroenterol 2003;37:315–29.

31. Czaja AJ, Shums Z, Norman GL. Nonstandard antibodies as prognostic markers in autoimmune hepatitis. Autoimmunity 2004;37:195–201.

32. Bansi D, Chapman R, Fleming K. Antineutrophil cytoplasmic antibodies in chronic liver diseases: prevalence, titre, specificity and IgG subclass. J Hepatol 1996;24:581–6.

33. Baeres M, Herkel J, Czaja AJ, et al. Establishment of standardised SLA/LP immunoassays: specificity for autoimmune hepatitis, worldwide occurrence, and clinical characteristics. Gut 2002;51:259–64.

34. Eyraud V, Chazouilleres O, Ballot E, et al. Significance of antibodies to soluble liver antigen/liver pancreas: a large French study. Liver Int 2009;29: 857–64.

35. Montano-Loza AJ, Shums Z, Norman GL, et al. Prognostic implications of anti-bodies to Ro/SSA and soluble liver antigen in type 1 autoimmune hepatitis. Liver Int 2012;32:85–92.

36. Czaja AJ, Donaldson PT, Lohse AW. Antibodies to soluble liver antigen/liver pancreas and HLA risk factors for type 1 autoimmune hepatitis. Am J Gastroenterol 2002;97:413–9.

37. Ma Y, Okamoto M, Thomas MG, et al. Antibodies to conformational epitopes of soluble liver antigen define a severe form of autoimmune liver disease. Hepatology 2002;35:658–64.

38. Frenzel C, Herkel J, Luth S, et al. Evaluation of F-actin ELISA for the diagnosis of autoimmune hepatitis. Am J Gastroenterol 2006;101:2731–6.

39. Gueguen P, Dalekos G, Nousbaum JB, et al. Double reactivity against actin and alpha-actinin defines a severe form of autoimmune hepatitis type 1. J Clin Immunol 2006;26:495–505.

40. Volta U, De Franceschi L, Molinaro N, et al. Frequency and significance of anti-gliadin and anti-endomysial antibodies in autoimmune hepatitis. Dig Dis Sci 1998;43:2190–5.

41. Czaja AJ, Carpenter HA. Sensitivity, specificity, and predictability of biopsy interpretations in chronic hepatitis. Gastroenterology 1993;105:1824–32.

42. Czaja AJ, Carpenter HA. Autoimmune hepatitis with incidental histologic features of bile duct injury. Hepatology 2001;34:659–65.

43. Suzuki A, Brunt EM, Kleiner DE, et al. The use of liver biopsy evaluation in discrimination of idiopathic autoimmune hepatitis versus drug-induced liver injury. Hepatology 2011;54:931–9.

44. Carpenter HA, Czaja AJ. The role of histologic evaluation in the diagnosis and management of autoimmune hepatitis and its variants. Clin Liver Dis 2002;6:685–705.

45. Czaja AJ, Carpenter HA. Optimizing diagnosis from the medical liver biopsy. Clin Gastroenterol Hepatol 2007;5:898–907.

46. Bjornsson E, Talwalkar J, Treeprasertsuk S, et al. Patients with typical laboratory features of autoimmune hepatitis rarely need a liver biopsy for diagnosis. Clin Gastroenterol Hepatol 2011;9:57–63.

47. Miyake Y, Iwasaki Y, Terada R, et al. Clinical features of Japanese type 1 autoimmune hepatitis patients with zone III necrosis. Hepatol Res 2007;37:801–5.

48. Czaja AJ, Muratori P, Muratori L, et al. Diagnostic and therapeutic implications of bile duct injury in autoimmune hepatitis. Liver Int 2004;24:322–9.

49. Czaja AJ. Clinical features, differential diagnosis and treatment of autoimmune hepatitis in the elderly. Drugs Aging 2008;25:219–39.

50. Czaja AJ. Cholestatic phenotypes of autoimmune hepatitis. Clin Gastroenterol Hepatol 2014;12:1430–8.

51. Abdalian R, Dhar P, Jhaveri K, et al. Prevalence of sclerosing cholangitis in adults with autoimmune hepatitis: evaluating the role of routine magnetic resonance imaging. Hepatology 2008;47:949–57.

52. Lewin M, Vilgrain V, Ozenne V, et al. Prevalence of sclerosing cholangitis in adults with autoimmune hepatitis: a prospective magnetic resonance imaging and histological study. Hepatology 2009;50:528–37.

53. Czaja AJ. Advances in the current treatment of autoimmune hepatitis. Dig Dis Sci 2012;57:1996–2010.

54. Czaja AJ. Review article: the management of autoimmune hepatitis beyond consensus guidelines. Aliment Pharmacol Ther 2013;38:343–64.

55. Czaja AJ. Features and consequences of untreated type 1 autoimmune hepatitis. Liver Int 2009;29:816–23.

56. Summerskill WH, Korman MG, Ammon HV, et al. Prednisone for chronic active liver disease: dose titration, standard dose, and combination with azathioprine compared. Gut 1975;16:876–83.
57. Manns MP, Woynarowski M, Kreisel W, et al. Budesonide induces remission more effectively than prednisone in a controlled trial of patients with autoimmune hepatitis. Gastroenterology 2010;139:1198–206.
58. Czaja AJ. Drug choices in autoimmune hepatitis: part A—steroids. Expert Rev Gastroenterol Hepatol 2012;6:603–15.
59. Geier A, Gartung C, Dietrich CG, et al. Side effects of budesonide in liver cirrhosis due to chronic autoimmune hepatitis: influence of hepatic metabolism versus portosystemic shunts on a patient complicated with HCC. World J Gastroenterol 2003;9:2681–5.
60. Efe C, Ozaslan E, Kav T, et al. Liver fibrosis may reduce the efficacy of budesonide in the treatment of autoimmune hepatitis and overlap syndrome. Autoimmun Rev 2012;11:330–4.
61. Czaja AJ, Lindor KD. Failure of budesonide in a pilot study of treatment-dependent autoimmune hepatitis. Gastroenterology 2000;119:1312–6.
62. Zachou K, Gatselis N, Papadamou G, et al. Mycophenolate for the treatment of autoimmune hepatitis: prospective assessment of its efficacy and safety for induction and maintenance of remission in a large cohort of treatment-naive patients. J Hepatol 2011;55:636–46.
63. Worns MA, Teufel A, Kanzler S, et al. Incidence of HAV and HBV infections and vaccination rates in patients with autoimmune liver diseases. Am J Gastroenterol 2008;103:138–46.
64. Czaja AJ. Safety issues in the management of autoimmune hepatitis. Expert Opin Drug Saf 2008;7:319–33.
65. Bajaj JS, Saeian K, Varma RR, et al. Increased rates of early adverse reaction to azathioprine in patients with Crohn's disease compared to autoimmune hepatitis: a tertiary referral center experience. Am J Gastroenterol 2005;100:1121–5.
66. Czaja AJ. Drug choices in autoimmune hepatitis: part B—nonsteroids. Expert Rev Gastroenterol Hepatol 2012;6:617–35.
67. Ngu JH, Gearry RB, Frampton CM, et al. Mortality and the risk of malignancy in autoimmune liver diseases: a population-based study in Canterbury, New Zealand. Hepatology 2012;55:522–9.
68. Francella A, Dyan A, Bodian C, et al. The safety of 6-mercaptopurine for childbearing patients with inflammatory bowel disease: a retrospective cohort study. Gastroenterology 2003;124:9–17.
69. Casanova MJ, Chaparro M, Domenech E, et al. Safety of thiopurines and anti-TNF-alpha drugs during pregnancy in patients with inflammatory bowel disease. Am J Gastroenterol 2013;108:433–40.
70. Langley PG, Underhill J, Tredger JM, et al. Thiopurine methyltransferase phenotype and genotype in relation to azathioprine therapy in autoimmune hepatitis. J Hepatol 2002;37:441–7.
71. Czaja AJ, Carpenter HA. Thiopurine methyltransferase deficiency and azathioprine intolerance in autoimmune hepatitis. Dig Dis Sci 2006;51:968–75.
72. Heneghan MA, Allan ML, Bornstein JD, et al. Utility of thiopurine methyltransferase genotyping and phenotyping, and measurement of azathioprine metabolites in the management of patients with autoimmune hepatitis. J Hepatol 2006;45:584–91.

73. Ferucci ED, Hurlburt KJ, Mayo MJ, et al. Azathioprine metabolite measurements are not useful in following treatment of autoimmune hepatitis in Alaska Native and other non-Caucasian people. Can J Gastroenterol 2011;25:21–7.

74. Stocco G, Londero M, Campanozzi A, et al. Usefulness of the measurement of azathioprine metabolites in the assessment of non-adherence. J Crohns Colitis 2010;4:599–602.

75. Soloway RD, Summerskill WH, Baggenstoss AH, et al. Clinical, biochemical, and histological remission of severe chronic active liver disease: a controlled study of treatments and early prognosis. Gastroenterology 1972;63:820–33.

76. Czaja AJ, Carpenter HA. Decreased fibrosis during corticosteroid therapy of autoimmune hepatitis. J Hepatol 2004;40:646–52.

77. Czaja AJ. Review article: prevention and reversal of hepatic fibrosis in autoimmune hepatitis. Aliment Pharmacol Ther 2014;39:385–406.

78. Roberts SK, Therneau TM, Czaja AJ. Prognosis of histological cirrhosis in type 1 autoimmune hepatitis. Gastroenterology 1996;110:848–57.

79. Delgado JS, Vodonos A, Malnick S, et al. Autoimmune hepatitis in southern Israel: a 15-year multicenter study. J Dig Dis 2013;14:611–8.

80. Montano-Loza AJ, Carpenter HA, Czaja AJ. Features associated with treatment failure in type 1 autoimmune hepatitis and predictive value of the model of end-stage liver disease. Hepatology 2007;46:1138–45.

81. Czaja AJ, Davis GL, Ludwig J, et al. Complete resolution of inflammatory activity following corticosteroid treatment of HBsAg-negative chronic active hepatitis. Hepatology 1984;4:622–7.

82. Czaja AJ. Rapidity of treatment response and outcome in type 1 autoimmune hepatitis. J Hepatol 2009;51:161–7.

83. Kanzler S, Gerken G, Lohr H, et al. Duration of immunosuppressive therapy in autoimmune hepatitis. J Hepatol 2001;34:354–5.

84. Czaja AJ, Carpenter HA. Histological features associated with relapse after corticosteroid withdrawal in type 1 autoimmune hepatitis. Liver Int 2003;23:116–23.

85. Czaja AJ, Wolf AM, Baggenstoss AH. Laboratory assessment of severe chronic active liver disease during and after corticosteroid therapy: correlation of serum transaminase and gamma globulin levels with histologic features. Gastroenterology 1981;80:687–92.

86. Czaja AJ, Menon KV, Carpenter HA. Sustained remission after corticosteroid therapy for type 1 autoimmune hepatitis: a retrospective analysis. Hepatology 2002;35:890–7.

87. Czaja AJ. Late relapse of type 1 autoimmune hepatitis after corticosteroid withdrawal. Dig Dis Sci 2010;55:1761–9.

88. Seo S, Toutounjian R, Conrad A, et al. Favorable outcomes of autoimmune hepatitis in a community clinic setting. J Gastroenterol Hepatol 2008;23:1410–4.

89. Czaja AJ, Beaver SJ, Shiels MT. Sustained remission after corticosteroid therapy of severe hepatitis B surface antigen-negative chronic active hepatitis. Gastroenterology 1987;92:215–9.

90. Czaja AJ. Review article: permanent drug withdrawal is desirable and achievable for autoimmune hepatitis. Aliment Pharmacol Ther 2014;39:1043–58.

91. Czaja AJ, Ammon HV, Summerskill WH. Clinical features and prognosis of severe chronic active liver disease (CALD) after corticosteroid-induced remission. Gastroenterology 1980;78:518–23.

92. Hegarty JE, Nouri Aria KT, Portmann B, et al. Relapse following treatment withdrawal in patients with autoimmune chronic active hepatitis. Hepatology 1983;3:685–9.

93. Verma S, Gunuwan B, Mendler M, et al. Factors predicting relapse and poor outcome in type I autoimmune hepatitis: role of cirrhosis development, patterns of transaminases during remission and plasma cell activity in the liver biopsy. Am J Gastroenterol 2004;99:1510–6.
94. Czaja AJ, Ludwig J, Baggenstoss AH, et al. Corticosteroid-treated chronic active hepatitis in remission: uncertain prognosis of chronic persistent hepatitis. N Engl J Med 1981;304:5–9.
95. Johnson PJ, McFarlane IG, Williams R. Azathioprine for long-term maintenance of remission in autoimmune hepatitis. N Engl J Med 1995;333:958–63.
96. Czaja AJ. Low-dose corticosteroid therapy after multiple relapses of severe HBsAg-negative chronic active hepatitis. Hepatology 1990;11:1044–9.
97. Czaja AJ, Carpenter HA. Empiric therapy of autoimmune hepatitis with mycophenolate mofetil: comparison with conventional treatment for refractory disease. J Clin Gastroenterol 2005;39:819–25.
98. Czaja AJ. Challenges in the diagnosis and management of autoimmune hepatitis. Can J Gastroenterol 2013;27:531–9.
99. Czaja AJ. Autoimmune hepatitis: focusing on treatments other than steroids. Can J Gastroenterol 2012;26:615–20.
100. Czaja AJ. Management of recalcitrant autoimmune hepatitis. Curr Hepat Rep 2013;12:66–77.

Diagnosis and Management of Overlap Syndromes

Chalermrat Bunchorntavakul, MD[a,b], K. Rajender Reddy, MD[a,*]

KEYWORDS

- Overlap syndrome • Autoimmune liver disease • Autoimmune hepatitis
- Primary biliary cirrhosis • Primary sclerosing cholangitis • Autoimmune cholangitis
- Management

KEY POINTS

- Overlapping features between autoimmune hepatitis and cholestatic disorders (primary biliary cirrhosis, primary sclerosing cholangitis, or indeterminate cholestasis), so-called overlap syndromes, are not uncommon and usually show a progressive course toward cirrhosis and liver failure without adequate treatment.

- Overlap syndromes should be considered in the differential diagnosis when a patient with autoimmune liver disease deviates from the normal clinical course, classical biochemical and serologic findings, and expected response to therapy. Autoimmune hepatitis–primary sclerosing cholangitis overlap is increasingly common in patients with young age and inflammatory bowel disease.

- The diagnosis of overlap syndrome requires the prominent features of classical autoimmune hepatitis (positive antinuclear antibody or antismooth muscle antibody findings, elevated immunoglobulin G levels, and interface hepatitis) and secondary objective findings of primary biliary cirrhosis (positive antinuclear antibody findings, elevated immunoglobulin M, and florid duct lesion) or primary sclerosing cholangitis (abnormal cholangiography). The possibility for immunoglobulin G4–associated cholangitis and drug-induced liver injury should also be excluded in patients with possible autoimmune hepatitis–primary sclerosing cholangitis and autoimmune hepatitis–primary biliary cirrhosis overlap, respectively.

Continued

Conflict of Interest: The authors have nothing to disclose.
[a] Division of Gastroenterology and Hepatology, Department of Medicine, University of Pennsylvania, 2 Dulles, 3400 Spruce Street, Philadelphia, PA 19104, USA; [b] Division of Gastroenterology and Hepatology, Department of Medicine, Rajavithi Hospital, College of Medicine, Rangsit University, Rajavithi Road, Ratchathewi, Bangkok 10400, Thailand
* Corresponding author.
E-mail address: rajender.reddy@uphs.upenn.edu

Continued

- Empiric treatment for patients with autoimmune hepatitis–primary biliary cirrhosis overlap is immunosuppressive therapy plus ursodeoxycholic acid, and the response is nearly similar to that of classic autoimmune hepatitis.
- Empiric treatment for patients with autoimmune hepatitis–primary sclerosing cholangitis and autoimmune hepatitis–cholestatic overlap is immunosuppressive therapy with or without ursodeoxycholic acid. However, the clinical responses are highly variable, and disease in most patients eventually progresses to cirrhosis.
- Liver transplantation is indicated for patients with overlap syndrome who have end-stage liver disease. After liver transplantation, such patients tend to have a higher rate and aggressive disease recurrence when compared with patients with single autoimmune liver disorders, but the overall survival seems comparable.

INTRODUCTION

Autoimmune liver diseases encompass a spectrum of immune-mediated disorders targeting the hepatocytes and bile ducts, which are generally defined by a combination of clinical, biochemical, serologic, histologic, radiologic, and liver histology findings. They comprise 2 broad categories: those with a predominance of hepatocellular injury, such as, autoimmune hepatitis (AIH), and those with a predominance of cholestatic features including primary biliary cirrhosis (PBC) and primary sclerosing cholangitis (PSC). Although the exact mechanism is unclear, broadly similar pathogenic themes of injury have been postulated for AIH, PBC, and PSC, and these comprise environmental triggers, genetic predisposition, and failure of immune tolerance mechanisms, which, in turn, collaborate to induce an antibody- and T cell–mediated immune attack against liver-specific targets, leading to a progressive necroinflammatory and fibrotic process in the liver (**Fig. 1**).[1–4] In AIH, immune-mediated liver injury is most pronounced in the portal/periportal areas, although a few patients can have antimitochondrial antibodies (AMA) and coincidental bile duct injury or loss (2%–13%), focal biliary strictures and dilations based on cholangiography (2%–11%), or histologic changes of bile duct injury or loss in the absence of other features (5%–11%).[5] In PBC and PSC, the pattern of liver injury is predominantly directed toward biliary epithelial cells, although a degree of parenchymal damage can be observed.

Conditions exhibiting features of 2 different autoimmune liver diseases occur in a small subgroup of patients and are commonly designated as overlap syndromes. With regard to the pathogenesis of overlapping features between hepatocyte-predominant and bile duct–predominant immune-mediated liver injuries, there remains debate as to whether this syndrome forms a distinct entity or is a variant of AIH. Several clinical presentations and pathophysiologic mechanisms of the overlap syndromes have been suggested: (1) a pure coincidence of 2 independent autoimmune diseases; (2) a different genetic background that determines the clinical, biochemical, and histologic appearance of one autoimmune disease entity; and (3) a representation of the middle of a continuous spectrum of 2 autoimmune diseases.[6,7] The prevalence of overlap features is difficult to ascertain because of publication bias, challenges in definitions, and limitations in test interpretation, particularly those that are qualitative or subjective.[8] Because of the heterogeneous presentations and absence of well-validated diagnostic criteria, the diagnosis of overlap syndrome requires prompt pattern recognition, careful interpretation of serologic and radiologic findings, exclusions of other causes, and histologic evaluation by an experienced

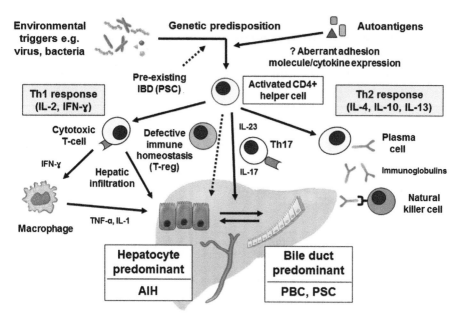

Fig. 1. Pathogenesis of autoimmune liver diseases. IFN, interferon; IL, interleukins; TNF, tumor necrosis factor. (*Adapted from* Trivedi PJ, Hirschfield GM. Review article: overlap syndromes and autoimmune liver disease. Aliment Pharmacol Ther 2012;36:520; with permission.)

pathologist. Without large therapeutic trials, treatment of overlap syndrome is largely empiric and extrapolated from data derived from the primary autoimmune liver diseases. Thus, treatment responses and outcomes are highly variable.

TYPES AND DIAGNOSIS OF OVERLAP SYNDROMES

The key clinical characteristic and serologic markers of the 3 classical phenotypes of autoimmune liver diseases, AIH, PBC, and PSC, are summarized in **Tables 1** and **2**.[1–4] In almost all cases, the so-called overlap syndromes are between AIH and PBC or AIH and PSC (**Fig. 2**). The overlapping features include symptoms, clinical findings, biochemical tests, serologic findings, and liver histology. In addition, the overlap features between AIH and other variants of indeterminate autoimmune cholestatic syndromes, such as autoimmune cholangitis, small-duct PSC, and AMA-negative PBC, have also been described as AIH-cholestatic overlap syndrome.[9] Because PBC and PSC have highly disease-specific features, the overlap syndrome between PBC and PSC is very rare and has been reported in only few patients to date.[10–13] The frequency of PBC-PSC overlap has been estimated as 0.7% in a cohort of 261 patients with autoimmune liver disease followed up prospectively over a 20-year period.[13]

The diagnosis of AIH and its overlap syndromes can be challenging because of many clinical, biochemical, immunologic, and histologic findings. The original diagnosis criteria of AIH were proposed by the International Autoimmune Hepatitis Group (IAIHG) in 1993, then were revised in 1999 in an attempt to standardize the diagnosis.[14] However, these criteria are complex and can be cumbersome in clinical practice. In 2008, the IAIHG decided to devise a simplified scoring system to facilitate the bedside diagnosis of AIH.[15] These scoring systems have been validated in several

Table 1
Clinical features of the 3 classical phenotypes of autoimmune liver diseases

	AIH	PBC	PSC
Age of onset	All ages (bimodal; peak 10–20 y and 40–50 y)	Middle age (>40 y)	All ages (often <40 y)
Gender	Female >male (4:1)	Female >male (9:1)	Male >female (2:1)
Clinical presentation	Acute and chronic hepatitis	Pruritus, fatigue, elevated ALP	RUQ discomfort, pruritus, features of cholangitis
Concurrent autoimmune disease(s)	17%–40%: thyroiditis, synovitis, IBD	~20%: thyroiditis, CREST syndrome, sicca symptoms	~80%: IBD
Cholangiography	Usually normal	Normal	Multifocal strictures throughout the biliary tree
Liver histology	Interface hepatitis, lymphoplasmacytic infiltrate in the portal area, rosette formation	Florid duct lesion, lymphocytic infiltrate in the portal area	Onion skin periductal fibrosis, lymphocytic infiltrate in the portal area
Response to treatment	Good response to corticosteroids ± AZA	Good response to UDCA	No or minimal response to immunosuppressive drugs or UDCA

Abbreviation: RUQ, right upper quadrant.

Table 2
Serologic markers of the 3 classical phenotypes of autoimmune liver diseases

	AIH	PBC	PSC
Immunoglobulins	IgG elevated	IgM elevated in most cases	IgG elevated and 45% IgM elevated
Specific autoantigen(s)	F-actin for ASMA CYP2D6 for LKM-1	PDC-E2 for AMA	Not identified
ANA	70%–80% (significant titer ≥1:40)	20%–50% (anti-GP210 and anti-SP100 are highly specific)	8%–70%
ASMA	70%–80%	0%–10%	0%–83%
Anti-LKM1	3%–5%	—	—
Anti SLA/LP	10%–30%	Few	Few
p-ANCA	60%–90% (often atypical p-ANNA)	0%–10%	26%–94%
AMA	AMA in low titer occasionally seen (0%–9%) (AMA anti–PDC-E2 pattern rarely detected)	AMA in 90%–95% (AMA anti-PDC-E2 pattern is highly specific)	Few

Abbreviations: Anti-GP210, antibody against nuclear pore membrane glycoprotein; anti-SLA/LP, anti-soluble liver antigen/liver pancreas; anti-SP100, antibody against nuclear protein SP100; LKM, liver kidney microsomal antibodies; p-ANCA, perinuclear antineutrophil cytoplasmic antibodies; p-ANNA, perinuclear antineutrophil antibody; PDC-E2, pyruvate dehydrogenase complex-E2.

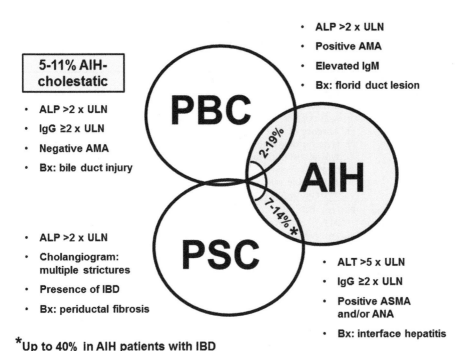

- ALP >2 x ULN
- Positive AMA
- Elevated IgM
- Bx: florid duct lesion

5-11% AIH-cholestatic

- ALP >2 x ULN
- IgG ≥2 x ULN
- Negative AMA
- Bx: bile duct injury

2-19%

AIH

PBC

- ALP >2 x ULN
- Cholangiogram: multiple strictures
- Presence of IBD
- Bx: periductal fibrosis

PSC

7-14%*

- ALT >5 x ULN
- IgG ≥2 x ULN
- Positive ASMA and/or ANA
- Bx: interface hepatitis

*Up to 40% in AIH patients with IBD

Fig. 2. Prevalence and features of overlap syndromes.

series for their ability to reliably diagnose or exclude AIH[15,16] and are endorsed by the American Association for the Study of Liver Diseases (AASLD).[2]

In clinical practice, overlap syndromes should be considered in the differential diagnosis when a patient with autoimmune liver disease deviates from the normal clinical course, classical biochemical and serologic findings, and expected response to therapy, but it is important that we not overdiagnose, or consider overlap syndrome, at presentation of a predominant disease process as a means of justifying nonstandard therapy.[8] Unlike AIH, the diagnosis criteria of the overlap syndromes have been less defined, and the taxonomy of these variants is still controversial. Without standardization of diagnostic criteria, overlap syndrome may perhaps be a much overused descriptive term in hepatology.[6] However, the critical importance of having the prominent features of classical AIH and secondary objective findings of PBC or PSC has been highlighted by the IAIHG,[17] the AASLD,[2–4] and the European Association for the Study of the Liver (EASL).[6] The presence of an AIH component must be satisfactorily defined based on clinical features and codified diagnostic criteria as defined by the original or the simplified AIH scores.[7] The definite or probable diagnosis of AIH according to these criteria is mandatory, and the prominent histologic findings should be interface hepatitis with or without plasma cells (Table 3).[6,7,17] Serum AMA and cholangiography are helpful to define the type of overlap syndrome.[18] Traditionally, endoscopic retrograde cholangiography (ERC) has been considered as the gold standard for the diagnosis of PSC. However, ERC is invasive and is associated with risk of complications requiring hospitalization (ie, cholangitis, pancreatitis) in more than 10% of PSC patients despite antibiotic prophylaxis.[19] Given its noninvasive nature, magnetic resonance cholangiography (MRC) has become a diagnostic procedure of choice for PSC, whereas ERC should be reserved for those patients who require endoscopic therapeutic intervention or when MRC view is suboptimal (Fig. 3).[3,18,20]

Table 3	
Diagnostic criteria and diagnostic features of AIH and its overlap syndromes	
	Diagnostic Criteria or Features
AIH (simplified IAIHG criteria)	I. Autoantibodies: ANA or ASMA $\geq$1:40 = 1 point; $\geq$1:80 = 2 points; or LKM $\geq$1:40 = 2 points; or SLA positive = 2 points. (Addition of points achieved for all autoantibodies is limited to 2 points) II. IgG: >ULN = 1 point; >1.1 × ULN = 2 points III. Absence of viral hepatitis = 2 points IV. Liver histology: compatible with AIH (interface hepatitis) = 1 point; typical AIH (interface hepatitis, emperipolesis and rosettes) = 2 points Scoring: $\geq$6: Probable AIH (88% sensitivity, 97% specificity) $\geq$7: Definite AIH (81% sensitivity, 99% specificity)
AIH-PBC overlap (Paris criteria)	PBC criteria I. ALP $\geq$2 × ULN or GGT $\geq$5 × ULN II. Positive AMA $\geq$1:40 III. Liver biopsy showing florid bile duct lesion AIH criteria I. ALT $\geq$5 × ULN II. IgG $\geq$2 × ULN or positive ASMA III. Liver biopsy with moderate or severe periportal or periseptal lymphocytic piecemeal necrosis Scoring At least 2 of 3 accepted criteria of PBC and AIH must be present for a diagnosis, and the presence of interface hepatitis is required
AIH-PSC overlap	I. Probable or definite for AIH by IAIHG criteria (interface hepatitis should be present) II. Cholangiography: multifocal bile duct strictures Other supportive features Negative for AMA, concurrent IBD is common
AIH-cholestatic syndrome	I. Probable or definite for AIH by IAIHG criteria (Interface hepatitis should be present) II. Negative for AMA III. Normal cholangiography IV. Liver histology: features of bile duct injury or loss

Abbreviations: anti-SLA/LP, anti-soluble liver antigen/liver pancreas; LKM, liver kidney microsomal antibodies.

AUTOIMMUNE HEPATITIS–PRIMARY BILIARY CIRRHOSIS OVERLAP
Epidemiology and Diagnostic Features

PBC and AIH are the most frequent autoimmune liver disease with a prevalence of 25 to 40/100,000 and 17/100,000, respectively, based on epidemiologic studies from Europe and North America.[21–23] Patients with overlapping features between PBC and AIH have long been recognized in a small subgroup of patients. The prevalence of AIH-PBC overlap is estimated to be 4.3% to 9.2% among patients with PBC and 2% to 19% among patients with AIH (when the revised IAIHG criteria were applied).[17,24–26] The diagnosis of AIH-PBC overlap is based on the presence of classical features of both AIH and PBC. AMAs have a very high specificity and positive predictive value for the diagnosis of PBC.[4] Most patients who are determined to have positive AMA, even with normal hepatic biochemical tests, have the full clinical picture of PBC over time.[27] However, in approximately 5% to 10% of the patients, AMA antibodies are absent or present only in low titer ($\leq$1:80), on conventional immunofluorescence testing,[4] and AMA can be found in up to 8% of patients with AIH.[28] In

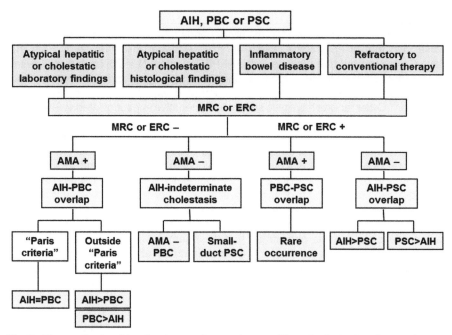

Fig. 3. Diagnostic algorithm for the overlap syndromes. (*From* Czaja AJ. Overlap syndromes. Clin Liver Dis 2014;3(1):3; with permission.)

some PBC patients, antinuclear antibodies (ANA), particularly anti-GP210 or anti-SP100 are present and may correlate with prognosis.[4,29] The Paris criteria can be used to provide an objective basis and to ensure uniformity of making diagnosis of AIH-PBC overlap (see **Table 3**).[7,24,30] These criteria have been incorporated in the EASL guidelines for management of cholestatic liver diseases and in the IAIHG position statement, while highlighting that histologic evidence of interface hepatitis is mandatory for the diagnosis.[6,17] The sensitivity and specificity of the Paris criteria for diagnosing the AIH-PBC overlap syndrome were 92% and 97%, respectively, when using experts' clinical judgment as the gold standard.[30]

The most commonly identified presentation in such a situation is the simultaneous presence of both diseases, although less commonly, the onset of AIH and PBC is sequentially encountered, often with PBC presenting first.[1,17] In a large series of 282 PBC patients, AIH later developed in 12 (4.3%) patients after a variable interval of 6 months to 13 years.[31] The subsequent development of AIH cannot be predicted by baseline characteristics and initial response to ursodeoxycholic acid (UDCA) in those with PBC.[31] In rarer circumstances, PBC may occur after the diagnosis of AIH.[32] A change in diagnosis from one condition to the other during follow-up has also been reported. In a series of patients from Sweden with variant forms of PBC, transitions between the variant forms of PBC (25 AIH-PBC overlap, 8 autoimmune cholangitis, and 2 AMA-negative PBC) over time were observed, but the diagnosis remained unchanged in most AIH-PBC overlap cases (16 out of 25).[33] In contrast, in a study from Japan, most patients with AIH-PBC overlap evolved to have either classical AIH or PBC, with only 0.8% having AIH-PBC overlap by stringent criteria.[34] Additionally, overlap of AMA-negative PBC with AIH has also been reported.[24]

Management and Outcomes

The prognosis of AIH-PBC overlap mainly depends on AIH activity and seems to be worse than that of PBC alone (**Table 4**).[1,6,9,17] A 6-year follow-up study from the Mayo Clinic reported that patients with AIH-PBC overlap (N = 26) have more severe disease and worse clinical outcomes, such as esophageal varices, ascites, need for liver transplantation (LT), and death, compared with patients with PBC alone (N = 109).[35] Other reports have also supported a negative impact of interface hepatitis and serum aminotransferase levels on prognosis in PBC.[36,37] However, when Joshi and colleagues[26] evaluated data from 331 patients enrolled in the Canadian and Mayo Clinic multicenter, randomized controlled trials of UDCA for PBC (16 patients had features of AIH; 12 UDCA, 4 placebo), the biochemical response and survival rates were similar in patients with PBC with or without features of AIH, and little change in histologic features of AIH was observed over a 2-year period. Thus, it remains unclear whether the clinical outcome of AIH-PBC overlap is different from that of isolated AIH.

The low prevalence of AIH-PBC overlap syndrome has made controlled therapeutic trials not feasible in these patients so that the treatment recommendations rely on retrospective studies and the experience in the treatment of either PBC or AIH. Treatment with UDCA is recommended for PBC and has shown the ability to reduce progression of the disease and the need for LT.[4] For AIH, immunosuppressive treatment (with either corticosteroids alone or in combination with azathioprine [AZA]) is recommended when serum aspartate aminotransferase (AST) or alanine aminotransferase (ALT) levels are ≥10-fold the upper limit of normal (ULN), ≥5-fold ULN in conjunction with a serum gamma-globulin levels ≥2-fold ULN, or histologic features of bridging necrosis or multilobular necrosis.[2] Whether AIH-PBC overlap syndrome requires immunosuppressive therapy in addition to UDCA is somewhat of a

Table 4
Suggested treatment and outcomes of AIH and its overlap syndromes

	Treatment	Outcomes
AIH-PBC overlap	• Immunosuppressive agents[a] plus UDCA, 13–15 mg/kg/d • In patients with mild activity of AIH, an alternative approach is to start with UDCA only and to add immunosuppressive agents if inadequate response in 3 mo	• Biochemical response achieved in most patients • Overall prognosis: depends mainly on AIH activity, worse than classical PBC, and may be slightly worse than AIH alone
AIH-PSC overlap	• Immunosuppressive agents[a] with or without UDCA, 13–15 mg/kg/d	• Biochemical response: variable (20%–100%) • Most patients progress to cirrhosis/ESLD after 10 y • Overall prognosis: better than classical PSC and worse than AIH alone
AIH-cholestatic overlap	• Immunosuppressive agents[a] and/or UDCA 13–15 mg/kg/d, depending on the predominant manifestations	• Biochemical response: rare • Approximately 33% progress to ESLD • Overall prognosis: worse than AIH alone, nearly similar to AIH-PSC

[a] Immunosuppressive therapy: prednisolone 60 mg/d × 1 wk → 40 mg/d × 1 wk → 30 mg/d × 2 wk → 20 mg or less/d until endpoint or prednisolone (half dose of monotherapy) plus azathioprine 50 mg/d (or 1–2 mg/kg/d in Europe). Second-line treatment options are mycophenolate mofetil (2 g/d) mainly to maintain remission, and cyclosporine.

controversial issue. Although UDCA therapy alone may induce biochemical responses in some patients with AIH-PBC overlap,[26] most patients may require a combination of UDCA and immunosuppressive therapy to obtain a complete response.[24,38,39] In the largest series, 17 strictly defined patients with concurrent form of AIH-PBC overlap patients who received either UDCA alone or in combination with immunosuppressive therapy were followed up for an average of 7.5 years.[39] In the UDCA group (N = 11), biochemical response was observed in 3 patients (27%) together with stable or decreased fibrosis, whereas the other 8 (73%) were biochemical nonresponders, and 4 had increased fibrosis.[39] Seven of these 8 nonresponders subsequently received combined therapy for 3 years, and biochemical response was achieved in 6 of 7 together with no further increase of fibrosis being noted. The overall fibrosis progression in noncirrhotic patients occurred more frequently under UDCA monotherapy (4 of 8) than under combined therapy (0 of 6; $P = .04$), suggesting that combined therapy may be the best option.[39] Therefore, the EASL and the IAIHG guidelines recommend a combination of UDCA and corticosteroids (with or without azathioprine) as the first-line therapy in patients with AIH-PBC overlap.[6,17] As an alternative approach for patients with relatively mild activity of AIH, it has been suggested to start with UDCA only and corticosteroids be added if an adequate biochemical response has not been obtained within a timeframe of 3 months.[6,17] Steroid-sparing agents would be ideal in patients requiring long-term immunosuppression.[6] Mycophenolate mofetil (MMF) has been effective as second-line treatment in most patients with AIH[2] and in patients with overlap syndromes, irrespective of prior response to AZA.[40] In a cohort study from the Netherlands, 45 patients treated with MMF included overlap syndromes (30 AIH, 11 AIH-PBC, and 4 AIH-PSC overlap).[40] In patients with overlap syndromes, biochemical response or remission, after the use of MMF, was achieved in 83% in the AZA-nonresponse group and 63% of the AZA-intolerant group (P value not significant); 33% had side effects and 13% discontinued MMF. In patients with AIH, remission was achieved in 20% in the AZA-nonresponse group compared with 73% in the AZA-intolerant group ($P = .008$).[40] Additionally, a case report has suggested a beneficial effect of cyclosporine A in a patient with overlap syndrome not responsive to UDCA plus corticosteroids.[41] Liver transplantation is reserved for patients who have end-stage liver disease (ESLD).

Patients with AIH or PBC who exhibit features that are suspicious for overlap syndrome, but do not meet the Paris criteria, should be treated according to the clinically predominant disease.[7] Immunosuppressive therapy is indicated for AIH-predominant patients, and UDCA is indicated for PBC-predominant patients.

AUTOIMMUNE HEPATITIS–PRIMARY SCLEROSING CHOLANGITIS OVERLAP
Epidemiology and Diagnostic Features

AIH-PSC overlap is a rare syndrome that has mainly been described in children, adolescents, and young adults.[42–44] The diagnostic criteria described for the overlap syndrome of AIH with PSC are more uniform compared with the overlap syndrome of AIH with PBC. It is a syndrome characterized by overt cholangiographic or histologic findings typical of PSC, together with robust histologic features of AIH concurrently or historically.[1,6] Notably, typical cholangiographic changes of PSC include multifocal, short, annular strictures with intervening segments of normal or dilated ducts involving the intrahepatic or extrahepatic biliary tree, or both, resulting in the characteristic "beads-on-a-string" or "beadedlike" appearance.[20]

The development of AIH-PSC overlap syndrome in adults often occurs in sequential manner, typically presenting with features of AIH first and PSC being diagnosed several years later in some cases.[1,45,46] AIH is more rarely diagnosed in patients with an original diagnosis of PSC.[17] When the revised IAIHG criteria were applied to large series of PSC patients, the prevalence of AIH-PSC overlapping features ranged from 7% to 14%.[17,44,47] On the other hand, abnormal cholangiographic appearance suggesting PSC can be found in a proportion of AIH patients with the prevalence varying according to the group of patients evaluated: 2% to 10% of adults with classical AIH,[48,49] 41% of adults with AIH and ulcerative colitis,[50] and up to 50% in children with AIH.[42]

Unlike AIH, PSC is strongly associated with inflammatory bowel disease (IBD). The prevalence of IBD in patients with overlap AIH-PSC has been reported to be higher than in patients with AIH only and corresponding to that in PSC.[17,25] IBD is present in about 16% of adults with AIH, and its presence raises the possibility of concurrent PSC, which then compels a cholangiographic assessment in such patients.[5] In addition, the possibility for AIH-PSC overlap should also be considered in AIH patients with younger age, pruritus, cholestatic liver tests (elevated alkaline phosphatase [ALP] or bilirubin levels), and histologic bile duct changes and in those with a poor response to therapy.[17,49]

Management and Outcomes

Similar to AIH-PBC overlap, controlled therapeutic trials are impossible to conduct in AIH-PSC overlap because of the rarity of the syndrome (see **Table 4**). In classical PSC, several medical treatments targeting to alleviate inflammation and cholestasis have extensively been investigated; however, the results have been disappointing.[3,6] UDCA has been used widely in the treatment of PSC, although long-term efficacy remains unproven so far. High-dose UDCA (>25 mg/kg/d) may be harmful and is not recommended.[3,6,51] Several immunosuppressive, anti-inflammatory, and antifibrotic agents have also been studied in PSC, but none has shown a consistent benefit on overall or transplant-free survival.[3,6] Because of the progressive nature of the disease and the lack of an effective therapy in PSC (most who develop ESLD approximately 17 years after diagnosis with 10-year survival of approximately 65%),[1,3] one would speculate that individuals with AIH-PSC overlap will also have poor, or even poorer, outcomes. However, unlike the classical PSC, patients with AIH-PSC overlap seem to derive some benefit from UDCA and immunosuppressive agents, and the survival rates are apparently better than in classical PSC, but with a poorer outcome than classical AIH and AIH-PBC overlap.[46,52]

In a prospective Italian study, 41 consecutive PSC patients (7 fulfilled the criteria for AIH-PSC overlap syndrome) were treated either with immunosuppressive agents plus UDCA in those with AIH-PSC overlap or with UDCA in those with classical PSC.[46] Over 5 years of follow-up, death (9 of 34) and neoplasms (8 of 34) were recorded only in the classical PSC group. Liver transplantation was performed in 6 of 34 of classical PSC patients and in 1 of 7 of AIH-PSC overlap patients.[46] In patients with AIH-PSC overlap, a 5-year treatment with immunosuppressive agents plus UDCA was significantly effective in improving AST ($r^2 = 0.7591$, $P<.05$); a drop in serum ALT, gamma-glutamyl transferase (GGT), and ALP was also obtained, albeit without reaching a statistical significance.[46] The Mayo score prognostic index did not change significantly during the follow-up in AIH-PSC overlap patients, whereas it noted a progressive and significant increase in the classical PSC group.[46] A biochemical response to immunosuppressive therapy in AIH-PSC overlap patients has also been reported in another study from Sweden (N = 26; 7 were small duct–type PSC)[53] and in a study in children.[42]

It should be noted that, unlike in PBC and AIH, biochemical improvement in PSC or AIH-PSC overlap may not necessarily translate into better long-term clinical outcome, nor does it predict survival free of liver-related complications or death.[1,44] Data from case series of 16 AIH-PSC overlap patients from Germany show that although immunosuppressive therapy improved biochemical markers, fibrosis was observed to progress in almost all of the patients during a median observation period of 12 years.[54] In this series, 3 patients initially presented with cirrhosis, 12 of 16 patients had cirrhosis at the end of the observation period, and 3 had complications of cirrhosis.[54]

The EASL guideline recommend that patients with AIH-PSC overlap syndrome be treated with UDCA and immunosuppressive therapy but emphasizes that this is not evidence based.[6] The AASLD guideline on PC recommends the use of corticosteroids and other immunosuppressive agents in those with an AIH-PSC overlap.[3]

Management of other complications of PSC should also be emphasized in patients with AIH-PSC overlap syndrome. The current guidelines for the management of pruritus recommend cholestyramine as first-line therapy, and rifampicin, naltrexone, and sertraline, respectively, as second-, third-, and fourth-line treatments.[6,55] Clinically significant dominant strictures should be managed by balloon dilatation with or without stenting.[3,20] Surveillance for cholangiocarcinoma, gallbladder cancer, and colorectal cancer (in patients with IBD) should also be performed as suggested for PSC,[3,20] although the development of these cancers in AIH-PSC overlap have not been reported so far.[46,54] Liver transplantation is indicated in end-stage disease. Other unique indications for LT in those with PSC (may also be applied for AIH-PSC overlap) include intractable pruritus, recurrent bacterial cholangitis, and cholangiocarcinoma.[3,20]

AUTOIMMUNE HEPATITIS–CHOLESTATIC OVERLAP SYNDROME
Epidemiology and Diagnostic Features

The overlap between AIH and indeterminate cholestasis, so-called AIH-cholestatic overlap syndrome, may have been categorized previously as autoimmune cholangitis, and they may constitute a heterogeneous category that includes patients with AMA-negative PBC and small-duct PSC.[5] The indeterminate cholestatic features are not uncommonly seen in patients with AIH with the estimated overall frequency of 5% to 11%, which is nearly similar to the frequency of PBC overlap and PSC overlap in AIH patients.[5,56,57] The features of AIH-cholestatic overlap syndrome have been described by Czaja,[5,7,25] in which the diagnosis of this syndrome is implied in patients with clinical diagnoses of AIH with cholestatic pictures (either clinical, biochemical, or histologic) in the absence of a positive AMA and the presence of histologic features of bile duct injury or loss and normal cholangiography. It typically presents around of the age 40 to 50 years.[58] The serum ALP level is typically greater than 2-fold of ULN, and histologic findings may comprise portal fibrosis, portal edema, and ductopenia reminiscent of PSC or a dense lymphoplasmacytic portal infiltrate with interface hepatitis and bile duct injury suggestive of PBC.[5,58,59] Patients with AIH-cholestatic overlap are distinguished from AIH by lower levels of AST, gamma-globulin, and immunoglobulin G (IgG); higher levels of ALP; and lower frequency of autoantibodies.[58] They are distinguished from PBC by higher levels of AST and bilirubin, lower serum IgM, and greater occurrence of autoantibodies.[58] Their female predominance, lower levels of ALP, higher frequency of autoantibodies, and absence of inflammatory bowel disease differentiated them from PSC.[58]

Management and Outcomes

Treatment with immunosuppressive agents or UDCA is generally ineffective in patients with AIH-cholestatic overlap syndrome (see **Table 4**). In cohorts of AIH-cholestatic overlap patients treated with corticosteroids or UDCA, 88% to 100% failed to achieve biochemical remission, and 33% eventually required LT.[25,53,58] The overall response rates to immunosuppressive therapy is significantly poorer than that of classical AIH, slightly poorer than that of AIH large-duct PSC overlap, and somewhat similar to AIH small-duct PSC overlap.[7,25,53] There have been no treatment recommendations for AIH-cholestatic overlap from the EASL or AASLD. Empiric therapy usually involves corticosteroids alone, UDCA alone, or corticosteroids in combination with UDCA depending on the patient risk, predominant manifestation, and intensity of the cholestasis.[5,7]

DIFFERENTIAL DIAGNOSIS
Immunoglobulin G4–Associated Cholangitis

IgG4-associated cholangitis (I4AC) disease is a systemic disorder of unknown nature that may cause both sclerosing cholangitis and hepatitis, which, in turn, may be mistaken for PSC-AIH overlap syndrome.[6,60–62] It presents with biochemical and cholangiographic features indistinguishable from classical PSC, frequently involves the extrahepatic bile ducts, and is characterized by elevated serum IgG4 and infiltration of IgG4-positive plasma cells in bile ducts and liver tissue. IgG4-associated cholangitis is often associated with autoimmune pancreatitis and fibrosing disorder in other organs, such as salivary glands, retroperitoneum, gastrointestinal tract, lymph nodes, kidneys, and lungs.[6,60,62]

The possibility for I4AC should be raised in suspected AIH-PSC patients with older age, male gender, absence of IBD, and presenting with jaundice, biliary strictures predominantly in the distal common bile duct, abnormal pancreatic imaging (pancreatic mass/enlargement without pancreatic duct dilatation), multiorgan involvement, and substantial response after corticosteroid therapy. Notably, the AASLD guideline recommends measuring serum IgG4 levels in all patients with suspected PSC to exclude this condition.[3] Modest increases of IgG4 levels (>140 mg/dL) have a moderate sensitivity of 70% to 80% for diagnosing autoimmune pancreatitis (AIP), but also have been described in 9% to 22% of patients with classical PSC.[20,63,64] Serum IgG4 levels greater than 2 × ULN provided a high specificity for I4AC, albeit at a decreased sensitivity.[62] It should also be noted that an elevated serum IgG4 level is found in most, but not all, patients with I4AC, and in such patients, identification of the IgG4 plasma cells in the diseased tissue may be needed to establish a definitive diagnosis.[6,60,61] Corticosteroids are regarded as the initial treatment of choice in this disease, and azathioprine should be considered in those with proximal and intrahepatic stenoses and those after relapse during or after corticosteroid therapy.[60]

Drug-Induced Liver Disease

Several medications and herbs can be associated with mixed hepatitis and cholestatic pattern of biochemical and histologic liver injury and the presence of serum autoantibodies. It is important to exclude drug-induced liver injury in patients with suspicion of overlap syndrome, either presenting as concurrent (acute and chronic mixed cholestatic hepatitis) or in a superimposed fashion (cholestasis on of top chronic hepatitis or hepatitis on top of chronic cholestasis). Medications that are known to cause chronic hepatitis and autoantibodies mimicking AIH are minocycline, nitrofurantoin, hydralazine, methyldopa, halothane, diclofenac, isoniazid acid, propylthiouracil, and infliximab.[65] Commonly prescribed medications that are known to be associated with mixed cholestasis and hepatocellular injury are antibiotics (eg, amoxicillin-clavulanate, cloxacillin, trimethoprim-sulfamethoxazole, sulfasalazine, erythromycin, fluoroquinolones, tetracyclines), antifungals (eg, ketoconazole, itraconazole), antivirals (eg, stavudine, didanosine, nevirapine), anti-inflammatory (eg, piroxicam, diclofenac, ibuprofen, sulindac, penicillamine, azathioprine), psychotropes (eg, chlorpromazine, fluphenazine, risperidone, imipramine, amitriptyline), and others (eg, methyldopa, propylthiouracil, glibenclamide, captopril, phenytoin).[66] Despite discontinuation, liver injury from some of these medications may progress to a rare form of drug-induced chronic intrahepatic cholestasis mimicking PBC, so-called vanishing bile duct syndrome, and characterized by chronic bile duct injury, bile duct loss, and subsequent cirrhosis.[66] In addition, several herbs and dietary supplements can exhibit hepatitis or mixed cholestatic hepatitis features with or without serum autoantibodies, such as Chinese herbs (eg, Jin Bu Huan, Dai-saiko-to), black cohosh, green tea, germander, greater celandine, chaparral, and some forms of Hydroxycut and Herbalife products.[67]

LIVER TRANSPLANTATION FOR OVERLAP SYNDROMES

Currently in the United States, autoimmune liver diseases are the primary indication for approximately 1 of 4 LTs (approximately 12% for PBC, approximately 8% for PSC, and approximately 4% for AIH).[68] Overall, graft and patient survival rates after LT for autoimmune liver diseases are excellent, but recurrent diseases can negatively impact both.[68] The prevalence of recurrent disease tends to increase with time after LT and at 5 to 10 years post-LT; the frequency of recurrent disease has been reported to range from 12% to 46% in patients with AIH,[2,68] 20% to 25% in those with PBC[4,68] and 20% to 30% in those with PSC.[3,68] Because overlap syndromes are rare, studies documenting outcomes for recurrent disease post-LT in this population are limited. The largest series from Canada evaluated 231 adult patients who underwent LT for autoimmune liver diseases and included 12 patients with overlap syndromes (7 AIH-PBC and 5 AIH-PSC).[69] Patients with overlap syndromes had a higher probability of recurrence (at 5 years, 53% vs 17%; at 10 years, 69% vs 29%; $P = .001$), and the median time to recurrence in overlap syndrome was shorter (67 $\pm$ 20 vs 172 $\pm$ 9 months; $P = .001$) when compared with those with single autoimmune liver disease.[69] The overall median graft (123 $\pm$ 16 months vs 180 $\pm$ 8 months; $P = .9$) and patient survival (135 $\pm$ 13 months vs 193 $\pm$ 8 months; $P = .6$) were comparable between the 2 groups. When the authors did a subanalysis comparing patients with recurrent disease as overlap syndrome (1 AIH-PBC and 1 AIH-PSC) with those who had recurrence of a single autoimmune liver disease, graft survival was significantly lower in these patients (43 months vs 208 months; $P = .004$).[69] Another report from Japan reported that survival rates after living-donor LT for AIH (N $=$ 12) and AIH-PBC overlap syndrome (N $=$ 4) were excellent, and there was no evidence of clinical recurrence during 6 years of follow-up.[70]

SUMMARY

Overlapping features between AIH and cholestatic disorders (PBC, PSC, or indeterminate cholestasis), so-called overlap syndromes, are not uncommon and usually have a progressive course toward cirrhosis and liver failure without adequate treatment. Overlap syndromes should be considered in the differential diagnosis when a patient with autoimmune liver disease deviates from the normal clinical course, classical biochemical and serologic findings, and expected response to therapy. AIH-PSC overlap is increasingly common in patients with young age and IBD. The diagnosis of overlap syndrome requires the prominent features of classic AIH (positive ANA or antismooth muscle antibody [ASMA], elevated IgG, and interface hepatitis) and secondary objective findings of PBC (positive AMA, elevated IgM, and florid duct lesion) or PSC (abnormal cholangiography). The simplified IAIHG criteria, the Paris criteria, and cholangiography are helpful to diagnose overlap syndrome. The possibility for IgG4-associated cholangitis and drug-induced liver injury should also be excluded in patients with possible AIH-PSC and AIH-PBC overlap, respectively. Empiric treatment for patients with AIH-PBC overlap is immunosuppressive therapy plus UDCA, and the response is nearly similar to classical AIH. Empiric treatment for patients with AIH-PSC and AIH-cholestatic overlap is immunosuppressive therapy with or without UDCA. However, the clinical responses are highly variable, and most patients eventually progress to cirrhosis. Liver transplantation is indicated for patients with overlap syndrome who have ESLD. After LT, such patients tend to have a higher recurrence rate and relatively aggressive disease recurrence when compared with patients who have single autoimmune liver disorders, but the overall survival seems comparable.

REFERENCES

1. Trivedi PJ, Hirschfield GM. Review article: overlap syndromes and autoimmune liver disease. Aliment Pharmacol Ther 2012;36(6):517–33.
2. Manns MP, Czaja AJ, Gorham JD, et al. Diagnosis and management of autoimmune hepatitis. Hepatology 2010;51(6):2193–213.
3. Chapman R, Fevery J, Kalloo A, et al. Diagnosis and management of primary sclerosing cholangitis. Hepatology 2010;51(2):660–78.
4. Lindor KD, Gershwin ME, Poupon R, et al. Primary biliary cirrhosis. Hepatology 2009;50(1):291–308.
5. Czaja AJ. Cholestatic phenotypes of autoimmune hepatitis. Clin Gastroenterol Hepatol 2013;12(9):1430–8.
6. European Association for the Study of the Liver. EASL clinical practice guidelines: management of cholestatic liver diseases. J Hepatol 2009;51(2):237–67.
7. Czaja AJ. Diagnosis and management of the overlap syndromes of autoimmune hepatitis. Can J Gastroenterol 2013;27(7):417–23.
8. Haldar D, Hirschfield GM. Overlap syndrome: a real syndrome? Clin Liver Dis 2014;3(3):43–7.
9. Czaja AJ. The overlap syndromes of autoimmune hepatitis. Dig Dis Sci 2013; 58(2):326–43.
10. Burak KW, Urbanski SJ, Swain MG. A case of coexisting primary biliary cirrhosis and primary sclerosing cholangitis: a new overlap of autoimmune liver diseases. Dig Dis Sci 2001;46(9):2043–7.
11. Rubel LR, Seeff LB, Patel V. Primary biliary cirrhosis-primary sclerosing cholangitis overlap syndrome. Arch Pathol Lab Med 1984;108(5):360–1.
12. Jeevagan A. Overlap of primary biliary cirrhosis and primary sclerosing cholangitis - a rare coincidence or a new syndrome. Int J Gen Med 2010;3: 143–6.
13. Kingham JG, Abbasi A. Co-existence of primary biliary cirrhosis and primary sclerosing cholangitis: a rare overlap syndrome put in perspective. Eur J Gastroenterol Hepatol 2005;17(10):1077–80.
14. Alvarez F, Berg PA, Bianchi FB, et al. International autoimmune hepatitis group report: review of criteria for diagnosis of autoimmune hepatitis. J Hepatol 1999; 31(5):929–38.
15. Hennes EM, Zeniya M, Czaja AJ, et al. Simplified criteria for the diagnosis of autoimmune hepatitis. Hepatology 2008;48(1):169–76.

16. Wiegard C, Schramm C, Lohse AW. Scoring systems for the diagnosis of autoimmune hepatitis: past, present, and future. Semin Liver Dis 2009;29(3):254–61.
17. Boberg KM, Chapman RW, Hirschfield GM, et al. Overlap syndromes: the International Autoimmune Hepatitis Group (IAIHG) position statement on a controversial issue. J Hepatol 2011;54(2):374–85.
18. Czaja A. Overlap syndromes. Clin Liver Dis 2014;3(1):2–5.
19. Bangarulingam SY, Gossard AA, Petersen BT, et al. Complications of endoscopic retrograde cholangiopancreatography in primary sclerosing cholangitis. Am J Gastroenterol 2009;104(4):855–60.
20. Bunchorntavakul C, Tanwandee T, Charatcharoenwitthaya P, et al. Primary sclerosing cholangitis: from pathogenesis to medical management. N A J Med Sci 2012;5(2):82–93.
21. Boberg KM. Prevalence and epidemiology of autoimmune hepatitis. Clin Liver Dis 2002;6(3):635–47.
22. Kim WR, Lindor KD, Locke GR 3rd, et al. Epidemiology and natural history of primary biliary cirrhosis in a US community. Gastroenterology 2000;119(6):1631–6.
23. Prince MI, James OF. The epidemiology of primary biliary cirrhosis. Clin Liver Dis 2003;7(4):795–819.
24. Chazouilleres O, Wendum D, Serfaty L, et al. Primary biliary cirrhosis-autoimmune hepatitis overlap syndrome: clinical features and response to therapy. Hepatology 1998;28(2):296–301.
25. Czaja AJ. Frequency and nature of the variant syndromes of autoimmune liver disease. Hepatology 1998;28(2):360–5.
26. Joshi S, Cauch-Dudek K, Wanless IR, et al. Primary biliary cirrhosis with additional features of autoimmune hepatitis: response to therapy with ursodeoxycholic acid. Hepatology 2002;35(2):409–13.
27. Metcalf JV, Mitchison HC, Palmer JM, et al. Natural history of early primary biliary cirrhosis. Lancet 1996;348(9039):1399–402.
28. Czaja AJ, Carpenter HA, Manns MP. Antibodies to soluble liver antigen, P450IID6, and mitochondrial complexes in chronic hepatitis. Gastroenterology 1993;105(5):1522–8.
29. Nakamura M, Kondo H, Mori T, et al. Anti-gp210 and anti-centromere antibodies are different risk factors for the progression of primary biliary cirrhosis. Hepatology 2007;45(1):118–27.
30. Kuiper EM, Zondervan PE, van Buuren HR. Paris criteria are effective in diagnosis of primary biliary cirrhosis and autoimmune hepatitis overlap syndrome. Clin Gastroenterol Hepatol 2010;8(6):530–4.
31. Poupon R, Chazouilleres O, Corpechot C, et al. Development of autoimmune hepatitis in patients with typical primary biliary cirrhosis. Hepatology 2006;44(1):85–90.
32. Horsmans Y, Piret A, Brenard R, et al. Autoimmune chronic active hepatitis responsive to immunosuppressive therapy evolving into a typical primary biliary cirrhosis syndrome: a case report. J Hepatol 1994;21(2):194–8.
33. Lindgren S, Glaumann H, Almer S, et al. Transitions between variant forms of primary biliary cirrhosis during long-term follow-up. Eur J Intern Med 2009;20(4):398–402.
34. Suzuki Y, Arase Y, Ikeda K, et al. Clinical and pathological characteristics of the autoimmune hepatitis and primary biliary cirrhosis overlap syndrome. J Gastroenterol Hepatol 2004;19(6):699–706.
35. Silveira MG, Talwalkar JA, Angulo P, et al. Overlap of autoimmune hepatitis and primary biliary cirrhosis: long-term outcomes. Am J Gastroenterol 2007;102(6):1244–50.

36. Corpechot C, Carrat F, Poupon R, et al. Primary biliary cirrhosis: incidence and predictive factors of cirrhosis development in ursodiol-treated patients. Gastroenterology 2002;122(3):652–8.

37. Huet PM, Vincent C, Deslaurier J, et al. Portal hypertension and primary biliary cirrhosis: effect of long-term ursodeoxycholic acid treatment. Gastroenterology 2008;135(5):1552–60.

38. Lohse AW, zum Buschenfelde KH, Franz B, et al. Characterization of the overlap syndrome of primary biliary cirrhosis (PBC) and autoimmune hepatitis: evidence for it being a hepatitic form of PBC in genetically susceptible individuals. Hepatology 1999;29(4):1078–84.

39. Chazouilleres O, Wendum D, Serfaty L, et al. Long term outcome and response to therapy of primary biliary cirrhosis-autoimmune hepatitis overlap syndrome. J Hepatol 2006;44(2):400–6.

40. Baven-Pronk AM, Coenraad MJ, van Buuren HR, et al. The role of mycophenolate mofetil in the management of autoimmune hepatitis and overlap syndromes. Aliment Pharmacol Ther 2011;34(3):335–43.

41. Duclos-Vallee JC, Hadengue A, Ganne-Carrie N, et al. Primary biliary cirrhosis-autoimmune hepatitis overlap syndrome. Corticoresistance and effective treatment by cyclosporine A. Dig Dis Sci 1995;40(5):1069–73.

42. Gregorio GV, Portmann B, Karani J, et al. Autoimmune hepatitis/sclerosing cholangitis overlap syndrome in childhood: a 16-year prospective study. Hepatology 2001;33(3):544–53.

43. McNair AN, Moloney M, Portmann BC, et al. Autoimmune hepatitis overlapping with primary sclerosing cholangitis in five cases. Am J Gastroenterol 1998; 93(5):777–84.

44. van Buuren HR, van Hoogstraten HJ, Terkivatan T, et al. High prevalence of autoimmune hepatitis among patients with primary sclerosing cholangitis. J Hepatol 2000;33(4):543–8.

45. Abdo AA, Bain VG, Kichian K, et al. Evolution of autoimmune hepatitis to primary sclerosing cholangitis: a sequential syndrome. Hepatology 2002;36(6): 1393–9.

46. Floreani A, Rizzotto ER, Ferrara F, et al. Clinical course and outcome of autoimmune hepatitis/primary sclerosing cholangitis overlap syndrome. Am J Gastroenterol 2005;100(7):1516–22.

47. Kaya M, Angulo P, Lindor KD. Overlap of autoimmune hepatitis and primary sclerosing cholangitis: an evaluation of a modified scoring system. J Hepatol 2000; 33(4):537–42.

48. Lewin M, Vilgrain V, Ozenne V, et al. Prevalence of sclerosing cholangitis in adults with autoimmune hepatitis: a prospective magnetic resonance imaging and histological study. Hepatology 2009;50(2):528–37.

49. Abdalian R, Dhar P, Jhaveri K, et al. Prevalence of sclerosing cholangitis in adults with autoimmune hepatitis: evaluating the role of routine magnetic resonance imaging. Hepatology 2008;47(3):949–57.

50. Perdigoto R, Carpenter HA, Czaja AJ. Frequency and significance of chronic ulcerative colitis in severe corticosteroid-treated autoimmune hepatitis. J Hepatol 1992;14(2–3):325–31.

51. Lindor KD, Kowdley KV, Luketic VA, et al. High-dose ursodeoxycholic acid for the treatment of primary sclerosing cholangitis. Hepatology 2009;50(3):808–14.

52. Al-Chalabi T, Portmann BC, Bernal W, et al. Autoimmune hepatitis overlap syndromes: an evaluation of treatment response, long-term outcome and survival. Aliment Pharmacol Ther 2008;28(2):209–20.

53. Olsson R, Glaumann H, Almer S, et al. High prevalence of small duct primary sclerosing cholangitis among patients with overlapping autoimmune hepatitis and primary sclerosing cholangitis. Eur J Intern Med 2009;20(2):190–6.
54. Luth S, Kanzler S, Frenzel C, et al. Characteristics and long-term prognosis of the autoimmune hepatitis/primary sclerosing cholangitis overlap syndrome. J Clin Gastroenterol 2009;43(1):75–80.
55. Bunchorntavakul C, Reddy KR. Pruritus in chronic cholestatic liver disease. Clin Liver Dis 2012;16(2):331–46.
56. Gheorghe L, Iacob S, Gheorghe C, et al. Frequency and predictive factors for overlap syndrome between autoimmune hepatitis and primary cholestatic liver disease. Eur J Gastroenterol Hepatol 2004;16(6):585–92.
57. Muratori L, Cassani F, Pappas G, et al. The hepatitic/cholestatic "overlap" syndrome: an Italian experience. Autoimmunity 2002;35(8):565–8.
58. Czaja AJ, Carpenter HA, Santrach PJ, et al. Autoimmune cholangitis within the spectrum of autoimmune liver disease. Hepatology 2000;31(6):1231–8.
59. Czaja AJ, Carpenter HA. Histological features associated with relapse after corticosteroid withdrawal in type 1 autoimmune hepatitis. Liver Int 2003;23(2):116–23.
60. Ghazale A, Chari ST, Zhang L, et al. Immunoglobulin G4-associated cholangitis: clinical profile and response to therapy. Gastroenterology 2008;134(3):706–15.
61. Mayo MJ. Cholestatic liver disease overlap syndromes. Clin Liver Dis 2013;17(2): 243–53.
62. Silveira MG. IgG4-associated cholangitis. Clin Liver Dis 2013;17(2):255–68.
63. Alswat K, Al-Harthy N, Mazrani W, et al. The spectrum of sclerosing cholangitis and the relevance of IgG4 elevations in routine practice. Am J Gastroenterol 2012;107(1):56–63.
64. Mendes FD, Jorgensen R, Keach J, et al. Elevated serum IgG4 concentration in patients with primary sclerosing cholangitis. Am J Gastroenterol 2006;101(9): 2070–5.
65. Czaja AJ. Drug-induced autoimmune-like hepatitis. Dig Dis Sci 2011;56(4): 958–76.
66. Bhamidimarri KR, Schiff E. Drug-induced cholestasis. Clin Liver Dis 2013;17(4): 519–31, vii.
67. Bunchorntavakul C, Reddy KR. Review article: herbal and dietary supplement hepatotoxicity. Aliment Pharmacol Ther 2013;37(1):3–17.
68. Ilyas JA, O'Mahony CA, Vierling JM. Liver transplantation in autoimmune liver diseases. Best Pract Res Clin Gastroenterol 2011;25(6):765–82.
69. Bhanji RA, Mason AL, Girgis S, et al. Liver transplantation for overlap syndromes of autoimmune liver diseases. Liver Int 2013;33(2):210–9.
70. Yamashiki N, Sugawara Y, Tamura S, et al. Living-donor liver transplantation for autoimmune hepatitis and autoimmune hepatitis-primary biliary cirrhosis overlap syndrome. Hepatol Res 2012;42(10):1016–23.

The Ins and Outs of Liver Imaging

Erin K. O'Neill, MD[a], Jonathan R. Cogley, MD[b], Frank H. Miller, MD[c],*

KEYWORDS

- Liver • Imaging • Elastography • Hemangioma • Focal nodular hyperplasia
- Hepatic adenoma • Hepatocellular carcinoma • Cholangiocarcinoma

KEY POINTS

- Dedicated contrast-enhanced liver magnetic resonance (MR) imaging or computed tomography (CT) can often definitively characterize many lesions as benign or malignant.
- Dedicated liver CT and MR imaging are accurate for the diagnosis of hemangioma due to its characteristic enhancement pattern. Other lesions such as focal nodular hyperplasia and hepatic adenoma can also be diagnosed based on imaging alone. MR imaging with a hepatobiliary contrast agent may prove helpful in some cases.
- Evolving MR techniques including diffusion-weighted imaging and MR elastography will have a greater role in evaluating the liver in the future.
- Optimal protocols are essential and preferences for certain examinations over others may be institutionally dependent, but it is important to work closely with radiologists to improve patient care.

LIVER IMAGING

The use of radiology in the evaluation of diffuse and focal liver disease has dramatically increased in recent years, in part because of advances in imaging technology. Imaging of the liver can be performed with a variety of modalities, and is used as both a screening and a diagnostic tool. In certain instances, imaging can help avoid the use of invasive procedures, making it a valuable clinical tool.

ULTRASONOGRAPHY

Ultrasonography is often the initial imaging study for the evaluation of suspected liver disease secondary to its low cost, ready availability, and lack of radiation exposure.

Disclosures: No financial disclosures related to activity for any of authors.
[a] Department of Radiology, Northwestern Memorial Hospital, Northwestern University Feinberg School of Medicine, 676 North Saint Clair Street, Suite 800, Chicago, IL 60611, USA; [b] Department of Radiology, VA Western New York Healthcare System, 3495 Bailey Avenue, Buffalo, NY 14215, USA; [c] Body Imaging Section, Department of Radiology, Northwestern Memorial Hospital, Northwestern University Feinberg School of Medicine, 676 North Saint Clair Street, Suite 800, Chicago, IL 60611, USA
* Corresponding author.
E-mail address: fmiller@northwestern.edu

Typical indications for the use of ultrasonography include detection and evaluation of hepatomegaly, elevated liver function tests, hepatic steatosis, cirrhosis, biliary obstruction, and hepatic lesions.[1–5] Drawbacks include difficulty with imaging the entire liver particularly near the diaphragm, interobserver variability, less accuracy in the detection of mild diffuse liver disease, limitations in patients with large body habitus or poor acoustic windows, and in the setting of fatty or fibrofatty infiltration of the liver secondary to decreased penetration of the sound beam.[1,3,5,6] It has lower sensitivity and specificity for liver masses, especially in the setting of cirrhosis.

Ultrasonography is particularly useful in evaluating the hepatic vasculature. The liver has a dual blood supply from the portal vein and hepatic artery. The portal vein supplies most of the blood supply to the liver. Normal physiologic portal venous flow is termed hepatopetal, or antegrade, with blood flowing through the portal vein from the central portion of the liver toward the periphery. The opposite process, termed hepatofugal, or retrograde, occurs when blood flows from the periphery of the liver centrally. Hepatofugal flow commonly occurs in the setting of liver disease, including cirrhosis with portal hypertension.[7] Direction of portal venous flow is readily detected on ultrasonography with color Doppler interrogation and waveform analysis.

COMPUTED TOMOGRAPHY

Computed tomography (CT) offers many advantages including its wide availability, moderate cost, speed, and its ability to detect and characterize diffuse liver disease and focal liver lesions. Depending on the clinical scenario and indication for the study, CT of the liver can be conducted using a variety of protocols, including unenhanced and single-phase, dual-phase, or triphasic contrast-enhanced CT examination.

Unenhanced CT of the liver can be used to evaluate diffuse or focal hepatic steatosis, hepatic deposition of iron, detection of calcifications in the setting of calcified metastases or postinflammatory processes, and in the evaluation of Lipiodol distribution after treatment with chemoembolization.[8,9]

Single-phase contrast-enhanced CT typically is performed when a specific hepatic disorder is not anticipated, or the entire abdomen and pelvis is imaged in the evaluation of systemic disorders such as metastatic disease. This study is generally performed during the portal venous phase of imaging because during this phase the liver demonstrates maximal enhancement, making it the most useful phase in which to detect hypovascular liver lesions such as those seen with a large number of metastases.[8,10]

Dual-phase contrast-enhanced CT can be performed in the evaluation for hypervascular metastases, such as breast, renal cell, or thyroid carcinomas, in addition to melanoma and endocrine tumors. In this setting, the scan is usually performed in the late hepatic arterial and portal venous phases. Another application of dual-phase CT would be in the setting of preoperative evaluation for partial liver resection, where detailed information regarding the vascular anatomy (assessed in the hepatic arterial phase) and imaging of the liver (assessed in the portal venous phase) is required.[8]

Triphasic contrast-enhanced CT is typically used in the setting of either known or suspected cirrhosis or hepatocellular carcinoma (HCC), and in the evaluation of focal liver lesions. In this protocol, an unenhanced phase is followed by hepatic arterial and portal venous phases.[8] The term triphasic has also been used to describe imaging in the arterial, venous, and delayed phases without unenhanced imaging. A hepatic arterial-phase sequence is performed in the setting of cirrhosis to best detect HCCs, which are supplied by the hepatic arterial system rather than the portal venous system. These lesions characteristically demonstrate hypervascular enhancement during the hepatic arterial phase and become isodense or hypodense to the adjacent liver parenchyma in the portal venous phase.[10–12] Therefore, these lesions can be difficult to detect if a routine CT scan of the abdomen is done, whereby only portal venous-phase imaging is acquired. Several studies have shown increased detection of HCC when both an arterial phase and a portal venous phase are acquired.[11,13–16]

Sometimes a delayed phase is performed 5 to 15 minutes after contrast administration. The rationale of the delayed-phase acquisition is the concept that equilibrium of contrast material between the vascular space and interstitial space nears equality during the delayed phase. The liver attenuation mainly depends on the volume of the interstitial space, as this is larger than the vascular space. Most tumors, including HCCs, demonstrate hypoenhancement on delayed images because they have increased cellularity, and therefore decreased interstitial space, in comparison with the adjacent liver parenchyma. Some lesions, such as hemangiomas, have a large interstitial space, and therefore demonstrate relative hyperenhancement to the adjacent liver parenchyma on delayed images.[10]

Some studies have reported that the use of arterial and portal venous phases of imaging is adequate for the detection of HCC and that the routine use of delayed-phase imaging is not needed.[17] Other studies have shown that HCCs may be better detected and characterized with the use of delayed-phase imaging, as lesions can be more conspicuous.[10,18–21] This presentation can be particularly true in the case of small HCCs, which may not demonstrate hypervascular enhancement on arterial-phase images secondary to a poor arterial blood supply.[10,15,19,22–24] Another useful application of triphasic contrast-enhanced CT is in the evaluation of cholangiocarcinoma or confluent hepatic fibrosis. In this setting, the protocol differs and includes a nonenhanced phase, a portal venous phase, and a 10- to 15-minute delayed phase.[8] Cholangiocarcinomas typically demonstrate hyperenhancement on the delayed images secondary to abundant fibrous tissue.[25,26]

MRI

Magnetic resonance (MR) imaging offers many advantages over CT and ultrasonography, including lack of ionizing radiation, higher spatial resolution, ability to use both extracellular and hepatocyte-specific contrast media, detailed evaluation of the biliary tree with magnetic resonance cholangiopancreatography (MRCP), characterization of occasional problematic pseudolesions on ultrasonography or CT such as focal fatty infiltration or focal fatty sparing, and better accuracy in the detection and characterization of focal lesions.[27] The potential of MR imaging to definitively characterize a lesion as benign (eg, cyst, hemangioma, focal nodular hyperplasia, or adenoma) and distinguish it from malignancy makes it the best imaging method for lesion characterization. Disadvantages include its higher cost, longer imaging time, the need for patient cooperation such as participation in breath-holding techniques to minimize motion artifact and obtain high-quality images in many instances, occasional patient claustrophobia, and its contraindications in certain patients, such as those with pacemakers or with poor renal function because of concern for nephrogenic systemic fibrosis.

MR has advantages over CT, as it is able to characterize liver lesions based on using multiple sequences, including its signal intensity on T1-weighted and T2-weighted images and the presence of fat (which loses signal intensity on the opposed-phase images relative to the in-phase images), and the contrast enhancement pattern. Fluid-containing structures such as cysts and hemangiomas are typically of low signal intensity on T1-weighted images and high signal intensity on T2-weighted images because of long T1 and T2 relaxation times, similarly to water.

The 2 main types of contrast agents used in MR imaging are (1) standard agents with extracellular distribution and (2) hepatocyte-specific contrast material. The extracellular agents are the most widely used and best documented, having been in clinical use the longest. Use of these agents follows the same principle as for the iodine-based contrast agents used for CT, as they rely on blood flow differential between liver parenchyma and liver lesions for detection and characterization. The timing of initial postcontrast images on MR imaging is similar to that of CT, with arterial and portal venous-phase images obtained. A major difference is that more delayed postcontrast images are routinely performed with MR imaging, whereas with CT they may or may not be performed depending on the institution, protocoling radiologist, and clinical indication, given the potential risks of added radiation exposure.

Hepatocyte-specific contrast agents provide information similar to that obtained by extracellular agents plus unique functional information on more delayed images, because they are also taken up by hepatocytes and excreted through the biliary system. The primary example of this type of contrast agent is gadoxetate disodium (Eovist; Bayer Health Care, Leverkusen, Germany), which has approximately 50% biliary excretion. Delayed hepatocyte-phase images are generally obtained at 20 minutes. These agents have the ability to differentiate tumors of hepatocellular origin that have functioning hepatocytes and biliary excretion from those that lack the same properties or are nonhepatocellular in origin. Current roles include differentiation of focal nodular hyperplasia (FNH) from hepatic adenoma, and improved detection of small liver metastases in the hepatocyte phase that could potentially be missed otherwise. Disadvantages of hepatocyte-specific agents include higher cost, some challenges obtaining peak arterial-phase enhancement including the effect of an Food and Drug Administration–approved manufacturer recommended dose that is one-fourth that of extracellular agents, longer imaging time required (eg, 20-minute delayed images), and impaired hepatic uptake and excretion in patients with obstructive jaundice or hepatocyte dysfunction. In some instances it may be difficult to distinguish a benign liver lesion from a well-differentiated HCC, as hepatocytes in well-differentiated HCC may retain enough function to take up hepatocyte-specific agents and appear isointense or even hyperintense to liver on delayed images.[28,29]

Diffusion-weighted (DW) imaging is a technique that has been increasingly applied to abdominal MR imaging protocols in recent years. DW imaging derives image contrast from differences in random motion of water molecules between biological tissues, and does not rely on intravenous contrast. The degree of random water motion is inversely correlated with the degree of tissue cellularity and cell membrane integrity. For instance, diffusion of water is more restricted in areas of high cellularity such as tumors. The ability of DW imaging to depict such areas allows for improved detection and characterization of lesions, and may also help in monitoring treatment response.[30] Common benign liver masses, such as cysts or hemangiomas, generally show a lesser degree of restricted diffusion than malignant lesions.[31–35] However, considerable overlap limits the ability of DW imaging to differentiate solid benign and malignant lesions at present.

MR elastography is a technique used to quantify the elasticity of the liver parenchyma, which in turn allows for the assessment of hepatic fibrosis. Elastography was originally described and used in ultrasonography, and is a relatively new application in MR imaging. As the liver becomes more fibrotic, the elastic properties of the tissues decrease; this can be measured with MR elastography and is more reliable than anatomic assessment for cirrhosis alone.[36] During early-stage cirrhosis, the liver may appear morphologically normal on routine imaging.[37] It has been shown that the liver stiffness measured on MR elastography correlates with and parallels the degree of fibrosis, and has both high sensitivity and specificity in characterizing the severity of fibrosis.[38] Therefore, MR elastography can be used as a noninvasive alternative to liver biopsy for measuring and quantifying hepatic fibrosis (**Fig. 1**). In addition, MR elastography can allow for more of the liver to be "sampled" than a liver biopsy, which can at times be fraught with sampling error. MR elastography is safe with no known complications, and may be helpful in guiding management, especially in hepatitis and nonalcoholic fatty liver disease, to assess the degree of fibrosis.[8,39–41] Ultrasonographic techniques including transient elastography (Fibroscan) and acoustic radiation force impulse imaging (ARFI) can be used to assess fibrosis but are more limited in the setting of obesity and ascites. MR elastography has higher sensitivity and specificity than ARFI.[42]

With conventional MR imaging, specific protocols allow for dedicated evaluation of the liver parenchyma. The hepatic vasculature can be assessed on a routine examination, but detail may be suboptimal depending on specific sequences performed, type of contrast material used, and timing of the postcontrast sequences. When specific questions arise in regard to the hepatic vasculature rather than the liver parenchyma, MR angiography and MR venography can be performed. These modalities can provide detailed information about the hepatic artery, hepatic veins, portal vein, splenic vein, inferior vena cava, and transplant vasculature with a single contrast injection in

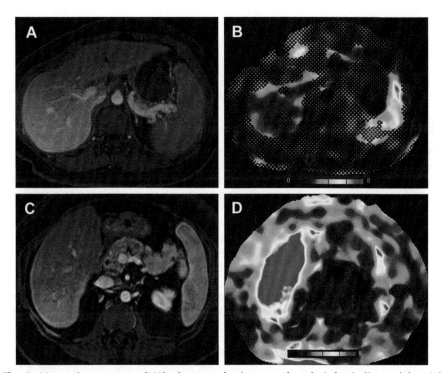

Fig. 1. Magnetic resonance (MR) elastography in normal and cirrhotic livers. (*A*) Axial T1-weighted postcontrast image shows homogeneous enhancement of the liver. (*B*) MR elastography shows normal pressures of the liver seen as blue color on elastogram. (*C*) Axial T1-weighted postcontrast image in a different patient shows homogeneous enhancement of the liver with only mild surface nodularity. (*D*) MR elastography shows markedly elevated pressures with high stiffness values from cirrhosis (*red color*).

a noninvasive manner, in contrast to conventional angiography or portal venography. MR angiography and MR venography can be performed as an adjunct to ultrasonography and can be used before angiography, percutaneous interventional procedures, or surgery as a guide or road map for the interventionist or surgeon.[43,44]

FOCAL LIVER LESIONS

Focal liver lesions are often detected during imaging studies performed for other reasons. In the general population, most of these lesions are benign and of no clinical consequence, yet many cannot be categorized as such when they are first encountered (eg, incidental findings on ultrasonography, noncontrast CT, or single-phase contrast-enhanced CT). The ability to definitively characterize a lesion as benign by dynamic contrast-enhanced MR imaging or CT helps avoid costly follow-up imaging and potential biopsy, and alleviates patient anxiety. Conversely, distinguishing classic benign "don't touch" lesions from malignant or potentially malignant lesions by imaging alone has obvious implications.

HEPATIC CYSTS

Hepatic cysts are commonly found, and can be solitary and multiple. Most are asymptomatic. It is important to not confuse hepatic cysts with more significant abnormality. On ultrasonography, cysts are well characterized as anechoic with increased through-transmission. On CT, they are generally seen as water density (0–10 Hounsfield units [HU]) and do not enhance following contrast. Fluid content is readily seen on MR imaging, with cysts showing low signal intensity on T1-weighted images and high signal intensity on T2-weighted images. These cysts are generally able to be distinguished from abscesses based on clinical history. In addition, abscesses appear more complicated, showing peripheral wall enhancement and restricted diffusion.

HEMANGIOMA

Hemangiomas are the most common benign hepatic tumor. These lesions are composed of numerous vascular channels, occur more frequently in women than in men (ratio 2:1 to 5:1), and are often multiple (>50%).[45,46] Hemangiomas are usually asymptomatic, discovered incidentally, and can be left alone. Therefore, it is essential to make a confident imaging diagnosis.

The most common ultrasonographic appearance of hemangioma is a circumscribed, rounded, or slightly lobulated lesion that is uniformly hyperechoic to liver and demonstrates posterior acoustic enhancement (**Fig. 2**). Hemangiomas often lack detectable internal vascular flow on color Doppler assessment. Although they occur anywhere, they are often peripheral and located in the posterior segments of the right hepatic lobe. A frequent atypical appearance of hemangioma on ultrasonography is a lesion with an isoechoic or hypoechoic core and a peripheral hyperechoic rim.[46] Hemangiomas can also appear hypoechoic to the liver in the setting of diffuse steatosis.

[99m]Tc-labeled red blood cell (RBC) scanning can play a role in determining whether a lesion is a hemangioma in select cases, such as patients who cannot undergo MR imaging. Activity from tagged RBCs accumulates within hemangiomas, whereas other lesions will appear photopenic relative to adjacent liver. Single-photon emission CT imaging may be helpful for improved contrast resolution and lesion localization. Unlike MR imaging, tagged RBC scans expose the patient to ionizing radiation and are unable to characterize other lesions.

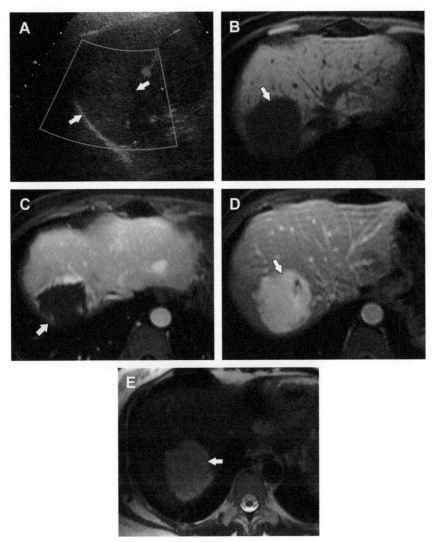

Fig. 2. Hemangioma in a patient with hepatitis B. (*A*) Color Doppler ultrasonography shows an echogenic mass in the posterior right hepatic lobe (*arrows*). (*B*) Precontrast T1-weighted fat-suppressed image shows the mass to be well circumscribed and hypointense to the liver (*arrow*). (*C*) Early postgadolinium image shows peripheral nodular enhancement of hemangioma (*arrow*). (*D*) On delayed images, the hemangioma completely fills in (*arrow*). (*E*) T2-weighted image shows typical hyperintense signal of hemangioma (*arrow*).

On noncontrast CT, hemangiomas are of low attenuation, similarly to blood vessels (~30–40 HU) but do not approach simple fluid density. With hepatic steatosis, they may become less conspicuous or even appear hyperdense to liver on noncontrast CT.[47] The typical enhancement pattern of discontinuous peripheral nodular enhancement with progressive centripetal filling on dynamic contrast-enhanced CT or MR imaging is diagnostic.[48] MR imaging is the preferred modality for diagnosis, in part owing to the characteristic hyperintense signal displayed on T2-weighted images, attributed to the long T2 relaxation times of its blood-filled spaces but also because of the ability to obtain multiple phases after contrast without requiring radiation (see **Fig. 2**).

Some small hemangiomas (usually <2 cm) may fill completely during arterial phase. These hemangiomas can be differentiated from other hypervascular lesions by their T2 hyperintense signal and retention of contrast on delayed images, remaining similar in signal intensity to that of blood pool. An adjacent wedge-shaped region of transient arterial hyperenhancement or arterioportal shunting can be associated with hemangiomas, and is more commonly seen with this smaller "flash-filling" variety.[47,48] Giant hemangiomas larger than 5 cm can appear more heterogeneous on T2-weighted images, with areas of thrombosis or scarring resulting in incomplete filling centrally on delayed postcontrast images.[49]

Sclerosed hemangiomas are those that undergo degeneration and fibrous replacement of their vascular channels. Because typical imaging features are lost, a prospective diagnosis of a sclerosed or sclerosing hemangioma is challenging. Findings that may suggest the diagnosis are T2 hyperintense signal, well-defined margins, associated volume loss/capsular retraction, internal nodular foci of arterial hyperenhancement, adjacent wedge-shaped arterial hyperenhancement, and presence of other hemangiomas with typical features.[50]

There are some potential pitfalls when it comes to diagnosing hemangioma. Some malignant lesions can also be T2 hyperintense and/or mimic peripheral nodular enhancement, including hypervascular metastases from neuroendocrine tumors or breast cancer, cystic-appearing metastases from mucinous subtypes of colon and ovarian cancer, metastatic or primary sarcoma, and cystic subtype of HCC. In these clinical scenarios, it is necessary to scrutinize the lesion for the presence of a continuous (rather than discontinuous) rim of arterial enhancement and other features such as washout on delayed postcontrast images that would ordinarily dismiss the diagnosis of hemangioma. When in doubt, short-term follow-up to assess stability or biopsy may be warranted.

There can be apparent differences in behavior of hemangiomas when a hepatocyte-specific contrast agent is used for liver MR imaging. Hemangiomas appear hypointense to liver on 20-minute delayed hepatocyte-phase images because they lack hepatocytes. However, contrast begins to be taken up by hepatocytes of the background liver and removed from vascular spaces even earlier. Pseudo-washout of a flash-filling hemangioma can be observed on postcontrast images obtained before the delayed hepatocyte phase, potentially mimicking a hypervascular metastasis unless one notices a similar decrease in signal intensity of the blood pool.[51] Some small hemangiomas lack early enhancement. Delayed filling of this particular subset that would ordinarily establish the diagnosis of hemangioma can be masked when a hepatocyte-specific contrast agent is used.[52] Thus, conventional extracellular contrast agents are preferred when liver MR imaging is performed to answer the question of whether a lesion is a hemangioma or not.

FOCAL NODULAR HYPERPLASIA

FNH is the second most common benign hepatic tumor, most often seen in young and middle-aged women and usually a solitary lesion. FNH is generally thought to reflect a hyperplastic response to a developmental or acquired vascular anomaly, and occurs in a liver that is otherwise histologically normal or near normal.[53] Key components are densely packed functioning hepatocytes, an enlarged feeding artery, central scar of fibrous tissue, and malformed bile ductules. Like hemangioma, FNH is asymptomatic and can be left alone in most cases.

FNH can appear slightly hypoechoic, isoechoic, or slightly hyperechoic relative to liver on ultrasonography (**Fig. 3**). Lesion conspicuity may improve with a relativity large or prominent central scar, although this is not often seen.[53] Sometimes called a stealth lesion, FNH may blend in with the surrounding liver on noncontrast CT and even MR images. On MR imaging, it is usually isointense or faintly hyperintense on T2-weighted images and isointense or slightly hypointense on precontrast T1-weighted images. FNH is best seen during the arterial phase, when it typically shows intense enhancement given its arterial-predominant blood supply.[54] FNH generally "fades" to become similar in signal intensity to background liver on subsequent postcontrast images. A central scar, if present, is classically T2 hyperintense and shows delayed enhancement (see **Fig. 3**), and helps in the diagnosis to increase specificity. On occasion, atypical features such as lesion heterogeneity may be misleading. One should not always rush to a diagnosis of FNH based on presence of a central scar, as this feature can also be seen in malignancies such as HCC and fibrolamellar carcinoma.[55] Sulfur colloid scintigraphy can sometimes aid in the diagnosis of FNH and distinction from adenomas, but is less frequently used given further developments in MR imaging. Kupffer cells allow FNH to take up ^{99m}Tc sulfur colloid. FNH shows greater uptake than adjacent liver in about 10% of patients and normal uptake in almost 50% of patients, and shows a photopenic or cold defect in up to 40% of patients.[56] Lack of uptake is not specific and can be seen in many lesions. Adenomas are usually seen as cold defects, but can occasionally show uptake-limiting effectiveness in diagnosis.

The most common differential diagnosis for FNH is hepatic adenoma, given overlapping imaging features and similar patient demographics. Liver MR imaging using the hepatocyte-specific contrast agent gadoxetate disodium can be helpful in distinguishing these 2 lesions. Gradual contrast accumulation and delayed biliary excretion owing to densely packed functioning hepatocytes and malformed blind-ending biliary ductules usually results in FNH being hyperintense or at least isointense to liver on delayed hepatocyte phase. A smaller proportion of FNH may demonstrate a hyperintense rim but may appear hypointense centrally. If present, the central scar of FNH does not typically retain contrast during the hepatocyte phase. Although adenomas also have functioning hepatocytes, they lack bile ductules and usually appear uniformly hypointense to liver on the hepatocyte phase, allowing for distinction from FNH in most cases.[57] Adenomas may also contain intracellular fat, which is not seen in FNH except on rare occasions in the setting of diffuse hepatic steatosis.

HEPATIC ADENOMA

Hepatic adenomas are less common benign tumors that are most often found in women of childbearing age, and have a known association with oral contraceptives. A recent better understanding of these lesions has led to classification into 3 main subtypes of adenoma: (1) inflammatory, (2) hepatocyte nuclear factor 1α (HNF-1α)-inactivated, and (3) β-catenin–activated.

Inflammatory adenoma is the most common subtype (40%–50%) and includes lesions that were formerly called telangiectatic FNH or adenoma. These lesions are characterized at histopathology by inflammatory infiltrates, sinusoidal dilatation, and dystrophic vessels.[58] The next most common subtype (30%–35%) results from inactivation of the HNF-1α tumor-suppressor gene, ultimately promoting lipogenesis, hepatocellular proliferation, and intracellular fat deposition. HNF-1α–inactivated adenomas occur only in women and have a high association with oral contraceptives. β-Catenin–activated adenoma is the least common subtype (10%–15%), resulting from uncontrolled hepatocyte formation arising from sustained activation of the

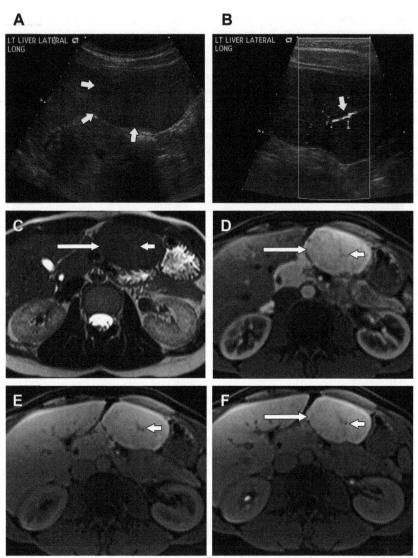

Fig. 3. Focal nodular hyperplasia (FNH). (*A*) Ultrasonography shows a large exophytic lesion (*arrows*) of the left hepatic lobe that is nearly isoechoic to the liver. (*B*) Color Doppler image shows the characteristic flow seen in the central scar (*arrow*) of FNH. (*C*) T2-weighted image shows the lesion (*long arrow*) is isointense to the liver. There is a subtle T2 hyperintense scar (*short arrow*). (*D*) Arterial phase image following gadoxetate disodium shows arterial hyper-enhancement of the lesion (*long arrow*) but not the scar (*short arrow*). (*E*) Subsequent post-contrast image shows the lesion fades to become isointense to liver with central scar now better visualized (*arrow*). (*F*) Twenty-minute delayed-phase image following gadoxetate disodium shows the lesion (*long arrow*) to be isointense to slightly hyperintense to liver with exception of the central scar (*short arrow*).

β-catenin gene. This last subtype occurs more frequently in men and may be associated with male hormone administration, glycogen storage disease, or familial adenomatosis polyposis.[59]

The 2 most important complications of hepatic adenoma are bleeding with associated rupture and malignant transformation. Different subtypes have varying complication rates. Intratumoral bleeding has been reported to occur in 20% to 25% of adenomas, although this percentage seems high. Inflammatory adenomas are most prone to bleed, owing to the presence of dilated sinusoids and abnormal arteries; a larger size (>5 cm) and subcapsular location increase the risk of bleeding and rupture.[59] The overall risk of malignant transformation of adenoma to HCC is about 4%.[60] Risk factors include male sex, glycogen storage disease, anabolic steroid use, and larger size (>5 cm). Of the different subtypes, β-catenin–activated adenomas are at greatest risk, but inflammatory adenomas can also develop HCC.

As a group, hepatic adenomas have a variable appearance at imaging. However, some studies have shown distinguishing features on MR imaging that could allow for subtype differentiation. Diffuse intralesional fat deposition, as detected on chemical shift imaging, is characteristic of the HNF-1α–inactivated subtype.[58] Although intralesional fat can also be seen in inflammatory adenoma, it occurs much less commonly and is usually more patchy and heterogeneous rather than uniform.[58,61] Other features associated with inflammatory adenomas are a greater degree of T2 hyperintense signal, especially peripherally, and avid enhancement during arterial phase that persists on more delayed images (**Fig. 4**).[58] Vaguely defined T2 hyperintense areas within a lesion could be associated with β-catenin activation, but this has not been clearly proved, and biopsy remains the best way to diagnosis this subtype.[62]

In young healthy patients, the most common differential diagnosis for an arterial hyperenhancing solid hepatic lesion is FNH. Lesion heterogeneity and intralesional fat are distinguishing features of adenoma. Adenomas also rarely contain central scars. In cases where it proves difficult to distinguish adenoma from atypical FNH, gadoxetate disodium–enhanced MR imaging may prove to be helpful. Hepatic adenomas also share features with HCC, including occasional washout or appearance of a capsule. Review of patient demographics and the absence of risk factors for liver disease and cirrhotic morphology should allow for the correct diagnosis.

HEPATOCELLULAR CARCINOMA

HCC is the most common primary liver malignancy (85%–90%). It is usually seen in patients with cirrhosis, and those with chronic hepatitis B or C viral infection and high alcoholic intake are at greatest risk.[63] HCC can also develop in patients without cirrhosis in the setting of chronic hepatitis B, toxin exposure, or other chronic liver disease such as hemochromatosis.[64] The incidence of HCC is growing and is expected to continue to increase. An increase in recent years can be partly attributed to rising rates of obesity and diabetes and their association with nonalcoholic fatty liver disease.[63] HCC is associated with a poor prognosis and is the third leading cause of cancer-related death worldwide. Several treatment options exist including surgical resection, local ablative procedures, and chemoembolization, but liver transplantation offers the best chance of long-term survival in patients with cirrhosis and early-stage HCC.[65] Thus, early detection and accurate staging are critical for successful treatment outcomes.

Surveillance for those at risk for developing HCC is recognized to increase the chances of early detection and long-term survival. According to the American Association

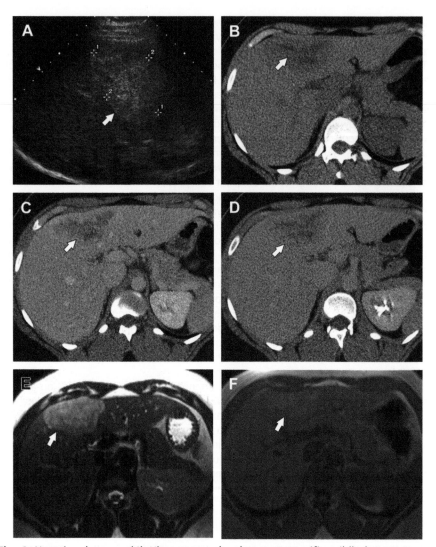

Fig. 4. Hepatic adenoma. (*A*) Ultrasonography shows nonspecific mildly heterogeneous hyperechoic lesion (*arrow*). (*B*) Unenhanced computed tomography (CT) shows heterogeneous low attenuating lesion in the left hepatic lobe (*arrow*). (*C*) Following contrast there is predominately peripheral contrast enhancement (*arrow*). (*D*) Delayed image shows persistent heterogeneous enhancement (*arrow*) without findings to suggest hemangioma. (*E*) Axial T2-weighted image shows the lesion to be hyperintense to liver (*arrow*). (*F*) Axial T1-weighted in-phase image shows mild T1 signal hyperintensity related to fat (*arrow*). (*G*) Axial T1-weighted opposed-phase image of the lesion (*arrow*) shows areas of signal loss consistent with the presence of fat, accounting for the low attenuation on CT and hyperechoic appearance on ultrasonography. (*H*) Early postcontrast axial image shows heterogeneous hyperenhancement of the lesion (*arrow*). (*I*) Delayed postcontrast axial image shows heterogeneous enhancement, with hypoenhancement noted within the regions of fat (*arrow*).

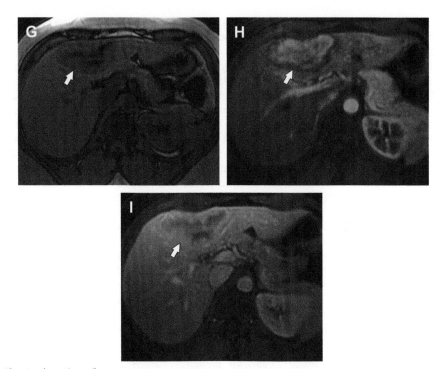

Fig. 4. (*continued*)

for the Study of Liver Disease (AASLD) Practice Guidelines, routine surveillance is considered cost-effective when the expected risk for development of HCC exceeds 1.5% per year in patients with hepatitis C and 0.2% per year in patients with hepatitis B.[66] Determination of α-fetoprotein lacks adequate sensitivity and specificity to be considered effective for surveillance.[66–68] Therefore, patients with cirrhosis should be screened with ultrasonography every 6 months.[66,69] Additional persons at increased risk for HCC who should also be screened include those with hepatitis B and 1 of the following risk factors: Asian men older than 40 years, Asian women older than 50 years, African Americans, or people who have a strong family history of HCC.[69]

According to the AASLD guidelines, when a subcentimeter nodule is detected by ultrasonography, this nodule should be followed by ultrasonography every 3 months until the nodule is no longer visualized, is stable for 18 to 24 months, or grows larger than 1 cm in size. Once the nodule is greater than 1 cm in size, further evaluation with contrast-enhanced MR imaging or CT is recommended for more accurate character-ization.[66,69] In everyday practice, many radiologists will recommend dedicated MR imaging or CT once a nodule is detected at ultrasonography, even if it is smaller than 1 cm. Many physicians, including liver specialists and radiologists, prefer dy-namic contrast-enhanced MR imaging to CT and ultrasonography, given its higher sensitivity and specificity.[69] According to the American College of Radiology (ACR) Appropriateness Criteria, dynamic contrast-enhanced MR imaging is given the high-est score to help characterize liver masses.[70] MR imaging clearly has advantages in the detection and characterization of hepatic masses as HCC in the setting of cirrhosis. Ultrasonography has limitations in the detection of small or infiltrating HCCs, given the heterogeneity and coarsened echotexture of the background liver parenchyma in the setting of cirrhosis. As a result, transplant centers rely on contrast-enhanced MR imaging or CT to detect and characterize liver masses depending on institutional preference.

Findings of HCC at ultrasonography may vary depending on individual lesion, size, and appearance of the background liver. Appearance of HCC may also vary at CT or MR imaging, but the ability to assess its enhancement pattern provides the best measure for diagnosis. Arterial-phase hyperenhancement of a nodule or mass is the single most consistently seen feature in patients with HCC.[63] This appearance reflects the stepwise process whereby HCC develops in a cirrhotic liver, with neoangiogenesis of arteries supplying a nodule and replacing portal venous blood supply. Classic HCC is a mass that demonstrates arterial-phase hyperenhancement and subsequent washout on portal venous or more delayed phase, with appearance of a capsule or pseudocapsule (**Fig. 5**). On MR imaging, HCC may have variable T2 signal intensity, and many small HCCs (<2 cm) can be occult on T2-weighted images.[65] When typical imaging features of HCC are demonstrated, these lesions should be treated without the need for biopsy to confirm the diagnosis.

There has been a recent effort to improve the consistency in interpretation and reporting of imaging findings by radiologists in academic and community settings. The Liver Imaging-Reporting and Data System (LI-RADS) is an initiative supported and endorsed by the ACR to provide a system of standardized terminology and criteria in the interpretation and reporting of liver imaging studies done in patients with cirrhosis or at risk for HCC. This evolving document can be accessed online at the

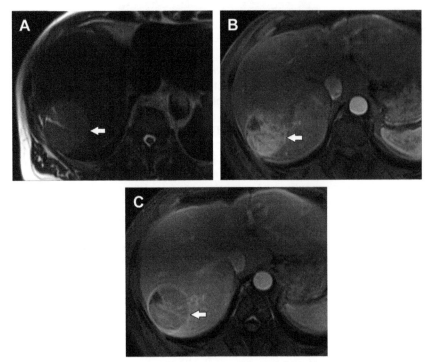

Fig. 5. Hepatocellular carcinoma. (*A*) Axial T2-weighted image shows a heterogeneous T2 hyperintense lesion in the posterior right lobe (*arrow*). (*B*) Arterial-phase image shows hypervascular enhancement of the lesion (*arrow*). (*C*) Venous-phase image shows classic findings of washout and capsular enhancement (*arrow*).

ACR Web site (www.acr.org).[71] Goals of LI-RADS include reducing variability in lesion interpretation, standardizing report content and structure, improving communication with clinicians, and facilitating decision making and outcome monitoring.[63] LI-RADS categorizes observations on a scale of 1 to 5 based on degree of suspicion of HCC in patients at risk, with LR1 definite benign and LR5 definite HCC. Remaining categories are LR4 (probable HCC), LR3 (indeterminate), and LR2 (probable benign).

A detailed summary of LI-RADS is beyond the scope of this article. Major features that currently would place a mass into the LR5 (definite HCC) category are: arterial phase hyperenhancement plus at least 1 other major feature (washout, capsule appearance, or threshold interval growth) if the mass is at least 20 mm in size; arterial-phase hyperenhancement plus at least 2 other major features (washout, capsule, threshold growth) if the mass is between 10 and 19 mm in size; or presence of tumor in vein (LR5V category). Tumor thrombus needs to be differentiated from bland thrombus, which can develop from portal hypertension and venous stasis in cirrhotic livers. Tumor thrombus may show arterial-phase hyperenhancement with or without an associated parenchymal mass, or even arterial-phase hypoenhancement or isoenhancement. Creation of subtraction images (whereby the unenhanced image is subtracted from the enhanced image) may be helpful to confirm enhancing tumor thrombus in the lumen of the vein. Conversely, nontumoral bland thrombus does not enhance and usually does not expand the lumen to the same degree as tumor thrombus (**Fig. 6**).[63,71] Ancillary features that may favor HCC over other masses include mild to moderate T2 hyperintensity, restricted diffusion, corona pattern of perilesional enhancement, mosaic architecture, nodule-in-nodule appearance, intralesional fat, focal lesional iron sparing (eg, in setting of hemochromatosis), blood products, and interval growth but less than "threshold growth" criteria (eg, less than doubling of size over a period of >6 months).[71]

CHOLANGIOCARCINOMA

Cholangiocarcinomas are malignancies that arise from bile duct epithelium, originating within the liver or more often along the extrahepatic bile ducts. Histologically, most of these tumors are adenocarcinomas. Intrahepatic cholangiocarcinoma is the second most common primary hepatic malignancy (10%–20%).[25] It can be further classified into 3 types based on gross morphologic features: (1) mass-forming (most common), (2) periductal infiltrating, or (3) intraductal growth pattern.[72] Of note, hilar cholangiocarcinoma, or Klatskin tumor, should be classified as extrahepatic cholangiocarcinoma or a separate entity.[25]

Risk factors for cholangiocarcinoma are processes that result in chronic inflammation of the biliary tree. Infection with liver flukes and intrahepatic stone disease (recurrent pyogenic cholangitis) are common risk factors for cholangiocarcinoma in endemic regions such as eastern Asia. Primary sclerosing cholangitis, cirrhosis, chronic hepatitis, heavy alcohol use, and diabetes are risk factors in Western countries.[25] The best treatment option for intrahepatic cholangiocarcinoma is curative resection, although this is possible in less than half of patients.[73] Imaging has a major role in diagnosis, tumor staging, and treatment planning.

Each morphologic type of intrahepatic cholangiocarcinoma has its own imaging characteristics. Mass-forming cholangiocarcinoma has irregular but well-defined margins, and is often large at discovery. Ancillary imaging features include peripheral bile duct dilatation, capsular retraction, and presence of satellite nodules (**Fig. 7**). Tumor may encase adjacent vessels, but visualization of intraluminal tumor thrombus is rare with cholangiocarcinoma. Appearance is variable at ultrasonography, ranging

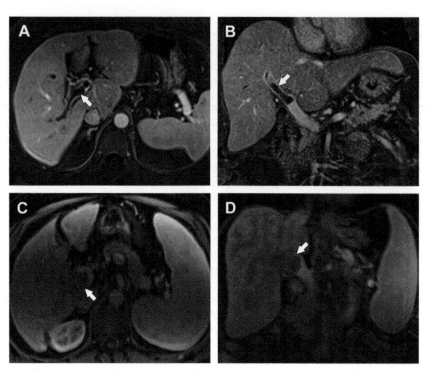

Fig. 6. Bland versus tumor thrombus. (*A*) Axial venous-phase image shows the bland thrombus (*arrow*) as hypointense within the right portal vein. Unlike tumor thrombus, there is no enhancement of the thrombus and the thrombus is not expansile. (*B*) Coronal image in the same patient nicely shows bland thrombus in the main portal vein (*arrow*). (*C*) Axial venous-phase image in a patient with infiltrating HCC shows tumor thrombus (*arrow*) in the main portal vein with enhancement of the thrombus and expansion of the vein. The thrombus is contiguous with the tumor within the right hepatic lobe. (*D*) Coronal image shows the tumor thrombus (*arrow*) extending into and expanding the portal vein.

from hypoechoic to hyperechoic, but usually well defined. A peripheral hypoechoic rim may be seen in approximately 35% of lesions.[25] On CT, the most common appearance is a hypoattenuating mass that shows irregular peripheral enhancement during the arterial phase with centripetal or gradual progression. This initial peripheral enhancement is circumferential, not to be confused with the discontinuous nodular peripheral enhancement seen with hemangioma. If delayed images are obtained, substantial late enhancement of the mass greater than adjacent liver is often observed because of abundant fibrous stroma.[74] MR imaging shows typically increased T2 signal of the mass and may better demonstrate peripheral and gradual centripetal enhancement than CT.[25] If gadoxetic acid–enhanced MR imaging is performed, a similar enhancement pattern has been described during early phases, but with improved lesion conspicuity and detection of satellite nodules or intrahepatic metastases on delayed hepatocyte-phase images.[75]

Some mass-forming cholangiocarcinomas show heterogeneous or more uniform internal enhancement or hyperenhancement during the arterial phase, nearly 30% in one series.[76] Furthermore, a percentage of these hypervascular cholangiocarcinomas may appear lower in attenuation to adjacent liver during portal venous phase (washout appearance). These arterial-enhancing lesions are often smaller than those with the

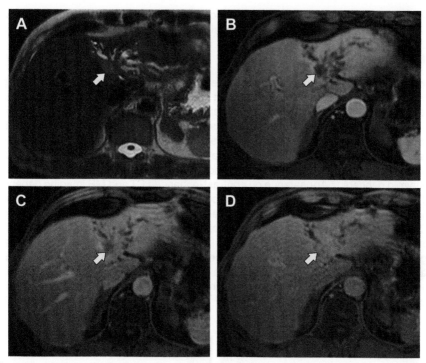

Fig. 7. Intrahepatic cholangiocarcinoma. (*A*) T2-weighted image shows biliary ductal dilatation and atrophy of the left hepatic lobe lateral segment with underlying mildly T2 hyperintense lesion more centrally (*arrow*). (*B*) Venous-phase image shows the lesion (*arrow*) is hypointense to the liver. (*C*) Equilibrium phase shows progressive enhancement of the lesion (*arrow*). (*D*) Delayed-phase image shows delayed complete enhancement of the lesion (*arrow*).

more typical enhancement pattern, and have been found to have larger cellular areas and less central fibrous stroma and necrosis at pathology.[76] Owing to various overlapping features, differential diagnosis may include HCC, combined HCC-cholangiocarcinoma, metastatic disease, and abscess.

Periductal infiltrating cholangiocarcinoma refers to a pattern of tumor growth along a bile duct without mass formation. On CT or MR imaging, this manifests as diffuse periductal thickening and increased enhancement along an irregularly dilated or narrowed bile duct. This type is rarely seen in intrahepatic cholangiocarcinoma but accounts for most hilar cholangiocarcinomas.[25] During early stages, it is difficult to distinguish periductal infiltrating cholangiocarcinoma from a benign stricture based on imaging alone. In patients with known extrahepatic malignancies, periportal lymphangitic metastatic disease is another consideration, but this may involve the liver more diffusely and also tends not to be associated with biliary ductal dilatation.

Lastly, intraductal cholangiocarcinoma is a slow-growing tumor with variable appearance on imaging and a relatively favorable prognosis. Most are papillary adenocarcinomas and are usually small, sessile, or polypoid.[72] Imaging patterns include diffuse and marked duct ectasia with or without a visible mass, intraductal polypoid mass causing localized biliary dilatation, intraductal cast-like lesions within a mildly dilated duct, and focal stricture-like lesion with mild upstream biliary ductal dilatation.[25] Cholangiocarcinoma can be differentiated from intraductal stone disease by demonstrating soft-tissue enhancement, accomplished with MR imaging or inclusion of initial noncontrast images during triphasic CT.

METASTASES

Liver metastases occur at a much greater frequency than primary hepatic malignancies, and have various appearances at imaging. Most often multiple masses are present, but sometimes a solitary or larger confluent mass is seen at presentation. At ultrasonography, they can manifest as uniform or heterogeneous hypoechoic, isoechoic, or hyperechoic masses. A hypoechoic halo is more often seen with metastases than with benign lesions.[77] Calcification may be associated with metastases from mucinous gastrointestinal tumors and from some breast, ovarian, lung, renal, or thyroid cancers.[78] Appearance on contrast-enhanced CT and MR imaging depends on the degree of hepatic artery supply. Hypovascular metastases enhance to a lesser degree than background liver, are best seen during portal venous phase, and may show delayed enhancement. Colon, lung, prostate, gastric, and transitional cell carcinomas are some primary tumors that result in hypovascular metastases.[79] By comparison, hypervascular metastases are best seen during the arterial phase and often show washout on delayed images (**Fig. 8**). These metastases typically result from neuroendocrine tumors (eg, pancreatic islet cell and carcinoid tumor), renal cell carcinoma, melanoma, sarcoma, and thyroid cancer.[80] Hypervascular metastases are often T2

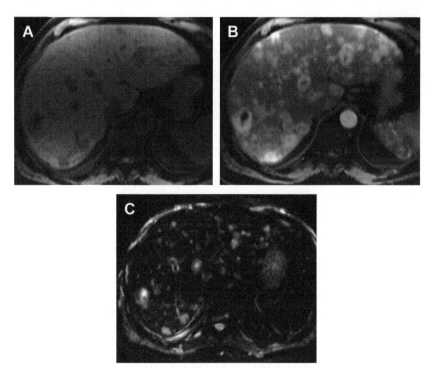

Fig. 8. Metastases (plasmacytoma). (*A*) Axial T1-weighted fat-suppressed image shows numerous heterogeneous hypointense lesions. (*B*) Postgadolinium image shows ring-enhancing lesions from metastases. (*C*) Diffusion-weighted image shows the lesions as hyperintense on low b-value image. Diffusion MR improves detection of certain lesions, including small metastases.

hyperintense and T1 hypointense on MR imaging. T1 hyperintense signal may be seen with hemorrhagic metastases and melanoma. Cystic change and necrosis is observed in hypervascular metastases that display rapid growth. Cystic-appearing metastases may also result from mucinous subtypes of adenocarcinomas. MR imaging with the use of gadoxetic acid hepatocyte-specific contrast agent and DW imaging allows for improved detection of small metastases.[81]

SUMMARY

The ability of imaging studies to detect and characterize liver lesions and disease has improved significantly in recent years. In many patients it has helped to avoid biopsies and surgery for diagnosis. Optimal protocols are essential, and preferences for certain examinations over others may be institutionally dependent, but it is important to work closely with radiologists to improve patient care.

REFERENCES

1. Needleman L, Kurtz AB, Rifkin MD, et al. Sonography of diffuse benign liver disease: accuracy of pattern recognition and grading. AJR Am J Roentgenol 1986; 146:1011–5.
2. Quinn SF, Gosink BB. Characteristic sonographic signs of hepatic fatty infiltration. AJR Am J Roentgenol 1985;145:753–5.
3. Dasarathy S, Dasarathy J, Khiyami A, et al. Validity of real time ultrasound in the diagnosis of hepatic steatosis: a prospective study. J Hepatol 2009;51:1061–7.
4. Ribeiro R, Sanches J. Fatty liver characterization and classification by ultrasound. In: Pattern recognition and image analysis. Berlin Heidelberg: Springer; 2009. p. 354–61.
5. Harbin WP, Robert NJ, Ferrucci JT Jr. Diagnosis of cirrhosis based on regional changes in hepatic morphology: a radiological and pathological analysis. Radiology 1980;135:273–83.
6. Tchelepi H, Ralls PW, Radin R, et al. Sonography of diffuse liver disease. J Ultrasound Med 2002;21:1023–32.
7. McNaughton DA, Abu-Yousef MM. Doppler US of the liver made simple. Radiographics 2011;31:161–88.
8. Boll D, Merkle E. Diffuse liver disease: strategies for hepatic CT and MR imaging. Radiographics 2009;29:1591–614.
9. Kodama Y, Ng CS, Wu TT. Comparison of CT methods for determining the fat content of the liver. AJR Am J Roentgenol 2007;185:1307–12.
10. Monzawa S, Ichikawa T, Nakajima H, et al. Dynamic CT for detecting small hepatocellular carcinoma: usefulness of delayed phase imaging. AJR Am J Roentgenol 2007;188:147–53.
11. Laghi A, Iannaccone R, Rossi P, et al. Hepatocellular carcinoma: detection with triple-phase multi-detector row helical CT in patients with chronic hepatitis. Radiology 2003;226:543–9.
12. Lee KH, O'Malley ME, Haider MA, et al. Triple-phase MDCT of hepatocellular carcinoma. AJR Am J Roentgenol 2004;182:643–9.
13. Oliver JH 3rd, Baron RL, Federle MP, et al. Detecting hepatocellular carcinoma: value of unenhanced or arterial phase CT imaging or both used in conjunction with conventional portal venous phase contrast-enhanced CT imaging. AJR Am J Roentgenol 1996;167:71–7.
14. Baron RL, Oliver JH 3rd, Dodd GD 3rd, et al. Hepatocellular carcinoma: evaluation with biphasic, contrast-enhanced, helical CT. Radiology 1996;199:505–11.

15. Ohashi I, Hanafusa K, Yoshida T. Small hepatocellular carcinomas: two-phase dynamic incremental CT in detection and evaluation. Radiology 1993;189: 851–5.

16. Hollett MD, Jeffrey RB Jr, Nino-Murcia M, et al. Dual-phase helical CT of the liver: value of arterial phase scans in the detection of small (< or = 1.5 cm) malignant hepatic neoplasms. AJR Am J Roentgenol 1995;164:879–84.

17. Choi BI, Lee HJ, Han JK, et al. Detection of hypervascular nodular hepatocellular carcinomas: value of triphasic helical CT compared with iodized-oil CT. AJR Am J Roentgenol 1997;168:219–24.

18. Mitsuzaki K, Yamashita Y, Ogata I, et al. Multiple-phase helical CT of the liver for detecting small hepatomas in patients with liver cirrhosis: contrast-injection protocol and optimal timing. AJR Am J Roentgenol 1996;167:753–7.

19. Hwang GJ, Kim MJ, Yoo HS, et al. Nodular hepatocellular carcinomas: detection with arterial-, portal-, and delayed-phase images at spiral CT. Radiology 1997; 202:383–8.

20. Kim T, Murakami T, Takahashi S, et al. Optimal phases of dynamic CT for detecting hepatocellular carcinoma: evaluation of unenhanced and triple-phase images. Abdom Imaging 1999;24:473–80.

21. Lim JH, Choi D, Kim SH, et al. Detection of hepatocellular carcinoma: value of adding delayed phase imaging to dual-phase helical CT. AJR Am J Roentgenol 2002;179:67–73.

22. Choi BI, Takayasu K, Han MC. Small hepatocellular carcinomas and associated nodular lesions of the liver: pathology, pathogenesis, and imaging findings. AJR Am J Roentgenol 1993;160:1177–87.

23. Takayasu K, Furukawa H, Wakao F, et al. CT diagnosis of early hepatocellular carcinoma: sensitivity, findings, and CT-pathologic correlation. AJR Am J Roentgenol 1995;164:885–90.

24. Matsui O, Kadoya M, Kameyama T, et al. Benign and malignant nodules in cirrhotic livers: distinction based on blood supply. Radiology 1991;178:493–7.

25. Chung YE, Kim MJ, Park YN, et al. Varying appearances of cholangiocarcinoma: radiologic-pathologic correlation. Radiographics 2009;29:683–700.

26. Keogan MT, Seabourn JT, Paulson EK, et al. Contrast-enhanced CT of intrahepatic and hilar cholangiocarcinoma; delay time for optimal imaging. AJR Am J Roentgenol 1997;169:1493–9.

27. Tanimoto A, Lee JM, Murakami T, et al. Consensus report of the 2nd international forum for liver MRI. Eur Radiol 2009;19:S975–89.

28. Cogley JR, Miller FH. MR Imaging of benign focal liver lesions. Radiol Clin North Am 2014;52:657–82.

29. Seale MK, Catalano OA, Saini S, et al. Hepatobiliary-specific MR contrast agents: role in imaging the liver and biliary tree. Radiographics 2009;29:1725–48.

30. Koh DM, Collins DJ. Diffusion-weighted MRI in the body: applications and challenges in oncology. AJR Am J Roentgenol 2007;188:1622–35.

31. Bruegel M, Holzapfel K, Gaa J, et al. Characterization of focal liver lesions by ADC measurements using a respiratory triggered diffusion-weighted single-shot echo-planar MR imaging technique. Eur Radiol 2008;18:477–85.

32. Taouli B, Vilgrain V, Dumont E, et al. Evaluation of liver diffusion isotropy and characterization of focal hepatic lesions with two single-shot echo-planar MR imaging sequences: prospective study in 66 patients. Radiology 2003;226:71–8.

33. Miller FH, Hammond N, Siddiqi AJ, et al. Utility of diffusion-weighted MRI in distinguishing benign and malignant hepatic lesions. J Magn Reson Imaging 2010; 32:138–47.

34. Parikh T, Drew SJ, Lee VS, et al. Focal liver lesion detection and characterization with diffusion-weighted MR imaging: comparison with standard breath-hold T2-weighted imaging. Radiology 2008;246:812–22.

35. Agnello F, Ronot M, Valla DC, et al. High-b-value diffusion-weighted MR imaging of benign hepatocellular lesions: quantitative and qualitative analysis. Radiology 2012;262:511–9.

36. Rustogi R, Horowitz J, Harmath C, et al. Accuracy of MR elastography and anatomic MR imaging features in the diagnosis of severe hepatic fibrosis and cirrhosis. J Magn Reson Imaging 2012;35:1356–64.

37. Brancatelli G, Federle MP, Ambrosini R, et al. Cirrhosis: CT and MR imaging evaluation. Eur J Radiol 2007;61:57–69.

38. Wang Y, Ganger DR, Levitsky J, et al. Assessment of chronic hepatitis and fibrosis: comparison of MR elastography and diffusion-weighted imaging. AJR Am J Roentgenol 2011;196:553–61.

39. Foucher J, Chanteloup E, Vergniol J, et al. Diagnosis of cirrhosis by transient elastography (FibroScan): a prospective study. Gut 2006;55:403–8.

40. Ganne-Carrié N, Ziol M, de Ledinghen V, et al. Accuracy of liver stiffness measurement for the diagnosis of cirrhosis in patients with chronic liver diseases. Hepatology 2006;44:1511–7.

41. Carey E, Carey WD. Noninvasive tests for liver disease, fibrosis, and cirrhosis: is liver biopsy obsolete? Cleve Clin J Med 2010;77:519–27.

42. Guo Y, Parthasarathy S, Goyal P, et al. Magnetic resonance elastography and acoustic radiation force impulse for staging hepatic fibrosis: a meta-analysis. Abdom Imaging 2014. [Epub ahead of print].

43. Stafford-Johnson DB, Hamilton BH, Dong Q, et al. Vascular complications of liver transplantation: evaluation with gadolinium-enhanced MR angiography. Radiology 1998;207:153–60.

44. Strovski E, Liu D, Scudamore C, et al. Magnetic resonance venography and liver transplant complications. World J Gastroenterol 2013;19:6110–3.

45. Vilgrain V, Boulos L, Vullierme MP, et al. Imaging of atypical hemangiomas of the liver with pathologic correlation. Radiographics 2000;20:379–97.

46. Caseiro-Alves F, Brito J, Araujo AE, et al. Liver haemangioma: common and uncommon findings and how to improve the differential diagnosis. Eur Radiol 2007;17:1544–54.

47. Jang HJ, Kim TK, Lim HK, et al. Hepatic hemangioma: atypical appearances on CT, MR imaging, and sonography. AJR Am J Roentgenol 2003;180:135–41.

48. Jeong MG, Yu JS, Kim KW. Hepatic cavernous hemangioma: temporal peritumoral enhancement during multiphase dynamic MR imaging. Radiology 2000;216:692–7.

49. Prasanna PM, Fredericks SE, Winn SS, et al. Best cases from the AFIP: giant cavernous hemangioma. Radiographics 2010;30:1139–44.

50. Doyle DJ, Khalili K, Guindi M, et al. Imaging features of sclerosed hemangioma. AJR Am J Roentgenol 2007;189:67–72.

51. Doo KW, Lee CH, Choi JW, et al. "Pseudo washout" sign in high-flow hepatic hemangioma on gadoxetic acid contrast-enhanced MRI mimicking hypervascular tumor. AJR Am J Roentgenol 2009;193:W490–6.

52. Goshima S, Kanematsu M, Watanabe H, et al. Hepatic hemangioma and metastasis: differentiation with gadoxetate disodium-enhanced 3-T MRI. AJR Am J Roentgenol 2010;195:941–6.

53. Hussain SM, Terkivatan T, Zondervan PE, et al. Focal nodular hyperplasia: findings at state-of-the-art MR imaging, US, CT, and pathologic analysis. Radiographics 2004;24:3–17 [discussion: 18–9].

54. Buetow PC, Pantongrag-Brown L, Buck JL, et al. Focal nodular hyperplasia of the liver: radiologic- pathologic correlation. Radiographics 1996;16:369–88.
55. Blachar A, Federle MP, Ferris JV, et al. Radiologists' performance in the diagnosis of liver tumors with central scars by using specific CT criteria. Radiology 2002; 223:532–9.
56. Welch TJ, Sheedy PF II, Johnson CM, et al. Focal nodular hyperplasia and hepatic adenoma: comparison of angiography, CT, US and scintigraphy. Radiology 1985;156:593–5.
57. van Kessel CS, de Boer E, Kate FJ, et al. Focal nodular hyperplasia: hepatobiliary enhancement patterns on gadoxetic-acid contrast-enhanced MRI. Abdom Imaging 2013;38:490–501.
58. Laumonier H, Bioulac-Sage P, Laurent C, et al. Hepatocellular adenomas: magnetic resonance imaging features as a function of molecular pathological classification. Hepatology 2008;48:808–18.
59. Katabathina VS, Menias CO, Shanbhogue AK, et al. Genetics and imaging of hepatocellular adenomas: 2011 update. Radiographics 2011;31:1529–43.
60. Stoot JH, Coelen RJ, De Jong MC, et al. Malignant transformation of hepatocellular adenomas into hepatocellular carcinomas: a systematic review including more than 1600 adenoma cases. HPB (Oxford) 2010;12:509–22.
61. Ronot M, Bahrami S, Calderaro J, et al. Hepatocellular adenomas: accuracy of magnetic resonance imaging and liver biopsy in subtype classification. Hepatology 2011;53:1182–91.
62. van Aalten SM, Thomeer MG, Terkivatan T, et al. Hepatocellular adenomas: correlation of MR imaging findings with pathologic subtype classification. Radiology 2011;261:172–81.
63. Purysko AS, Remer EM, Coppa CP, et al. LI-RADS: a case-based review of the new categorization of liver findings in patients with end-stage liver disease. Radiographics 2012;32:1977–95.
64. Khatri G, Merrick L, Miller FH. MR imaging of hepatocellular carcinoma. Magn Reson Imaging Clin N Am 2010;18:421–50.
65. Hecht EM, Holland AE, Israel GM, et al. Hepatocellular carcinoma in the cirrhotic liver: gadolinium-enhanced 3D T1-weighted MR imaging as a stand-alone sequence for diagnosis. Radiology 2006;239:438–47.
66. Bruix J, Sherman M, American Association for Study of Liver Diseases. Management of hepatocellular carcinoma: an update. Hepatology 2011;53:1020–2.
67. El-Serag HB, Mason AC. Rising incidence of hepatocellular carcinoma in the United States. N Engl J Med 1999;340:745–50.
68. Deuffic S, Poynard T, Buffat L, et al. Trends in primary liver cancer. Lancet 1998; 351:214–5.
69. Barr DC, Hussain HK. Magnetic resonance imaging in cirrhosis. What's new? Top Magn Reson Imaging 2014;23:129–49.
70. Lalani T, Rosen MP, Blake MA, et al. ACR appropriateness criteria liver lesion – initial characterization. American College of Radiology. Available at: https://acsearch. acr.org. Accessed July 2, 2014.
71. American College of Radiology. Liver imaging reporting and data system version 2013.1. Available at: http://www.acr.org/Quality-Safety/Resources/LIRADS/. Accessed July 12, 2014.
72. Lim JH. Cholangiocarcinoma: morphologic classification according to growth pattern and imaging findings. AJR Am J Roentgenol 2003;181:819–27.
73. Kim SJ, Lee JM, Han JK, et al. Peripheral mass-forming cholangiocarcinoma in cirrhotic liver. AJR Am J Roentgenol 2007;189:1428–34.

74. Lacomis JM, Baron RL, Oliver JH, et al. Cholangiocarcinoma: delayed CT contrast enhancement patterns. Radiology 1997;203:98–104.

75. Kang Y, Lee JM, Kim SH, et al. Intrahepatic mass-forming cholangiocarcinoma: enhancement patterns on gadoxetic acid-enhanced MR images. Radiology 2012;264:751–60.

76. Kim SA, Lee JM, Lee KB, et al. Intrahepatic mass-forming cholangiocarcinomas: enhancement patterns at multiphasic CT, with special emphasis on arterial enhancement pattern—correlation with clinicopathologic findings. Radiology 2011;260:148–57.

77. Wernecke K, Vassallo P, Bick U, et al. The distinction between benign and malignant liver tumors on sonography: value of a hypoechoic halo. AJR Am J Roentgenol 1992;159:1005–9.

78. Sica GT, Ji H, Ros PR. CT and MR imaging of hepatic metastases. AJR Am J Roentgenol 2000;174:691–8.

79. Elsayes KM, Narra VR, Yin Y, et al. Focal hepatic lesions: diagnostic value of enhancement pattern approach with contrast-enhanced 3D gradient-echo MR imaging. Radiographics 2005;25:1299–320.

80. Silva AC, Evans JM, McCullough AE, et al. MR imaging of hypervascular liver masses: a review of current techniques. Radiographics 2009;29:385–402.

81. Shimada K, Isoda H, Hirokawa Y, et al. Comparison of gadolinium-EOB-DTPA enhanced and diffusion-weighted liver MRI for detection of small hepatic metastases. Eur Radiol 2010;20:2690–8.

Contemporary Assessment of Hepatic Fibrosis

Alan Bonder, MD, Elliot B. Tapper, MD, Nezam H. Afdhal, MD*

KEYWORDS

- Liver biopsy • Cirrhosis • Hepatitis • Non-alcoholic fatty liver disease

KEY POINTS

- Noninvasive tests now enable the clinician to successfully stage and monitor a wide variety of liver diseases and have significantly reduced the need for liver biopsy.
- The evaluation of liver fibrosis is of major importance for the management of chronic liver disease and the prediction of prognosis, as complications occur in patients with advanced fibrosis stages.
- Progression to cirrhosis is associated with a risk of liver-related complications, hepatocellular carcinoma, and mortality.

INTRODUCTION

The evaluation of liver fibrosis is of major importance for the management of chronic liver disease and the prediction of prognosis, as complications occur in patients with advanced fibrosis stages. Progression to cirrhosis is associated with a risk of liver-related complications, hepatocellular carcinoma (HCC), and mortality.

Liver biopsy is currently the gold standard in assessing liver histology. Although percutaneous liver biopsy is in general a safe procedure, it is costly and does carry a small risk for complication. In addition, there could be sampling error, because only 1/50,000 of the organ is sampled.[1] Furthermore, inter- and intraobserver discrepancies are around 10% to 20% in assessing hepatic fibrosis, which may lead to understaging of cirrhosis.[2] Noninvasive approaches to assess histology in patients with chronic liver diseases include clinical symptoms and signs, routine laboratory tests, serum markers of fibrosis and inflammation, quantitative assays of liver function, and radiologic imaging studies. However, at present, none of these tests or markers alone is accurate or reliable in predicting histology, in particular, liver fibrosis. An ideal noninvasive diagnostic test for hepatic fibrosis should be simple, readily available,

Disclosure: Nezam H. Afdhal is an unpaid investigator for EchoSens.
Liver Center, Beth Israel Deaconess Medical Center, Harvard Medical School, Boston, MA, USA
* Corresponding author. Department of Medicine, Liver Center, Beth Israel Deaconess Medical Center, Harvard Medical School, 110 Francis Street, Suite 8E, Boston, MA 02215.
E-mail address: nafdhal@bidmc.harvard.edu

inexpensive, and accurate. Herein, are reviewed the serologic tests such as AST (aspartate aminotransferase)-to-Platelet Ratio Index (APRI), Fibrometer, FibroTest, HepaScore, FIB-4 and the radiologic tests inclusive of vibration-controlled transient elastography (VCTE) and magnetic resonance elastography.

NONINVASIVE TESTS FOR HEPATIC FIBROSIS
Aspartate Aminotransferase-to-Platelet Ratio Index

The APRI is clinically best applied for the diagnosis or exclusion of cirrhosis alone. It does not give a linearity of scale allowing for intermediate disease staging. APRI is derived from the following formula: (AST/[AST upper limit of normal])/platelet count (10^9/L) × 100. Patients with APRI of 0.50 or less are unlikely to have significant cirrhosis, while in those with an APRI greater than 1.50, significant fibrosis is much more likely.[3] The area under the receiver operating curve (AUROC) of APRI for predicting significant fibrosis and cirrhosis is 0.80 and 0.89, respectively.

FIB-4

FIB-4 is a freely available test that utilizes the following formula: age (years) x AST [U/L]/platelets [10^9/L] x ALT (alanine aminotransferase) [U/L $^1/_2$].[4] FIB-4 correctly identifies patients with severe fibrosis (F3-F4) and cirrhosis with an AUROC of 0.85 (95% confidence interval [CI] 0.82–0.89) and 0.91 (95% CI 0.86–0.93). A threshold value of less than 1.45 has a negative predictive value for the exclusion of extended fibrosis (F4-F6 in the Ishak classification) of 90%. Similar issues of lack of linearity with FIB-4 as compared to APRI are applicable.

Nonalcoholic Fatty Liver Disease Fibrosis Score

The NAFLD (nonalcoholic fatty liver disease) Fibrosis Score is a freely available algorithm derived from an international validation study of 733 patients with NAFLD.[5] This score is based on a formula that incorporates age, hyperglycemia, body mass index (BMI), platelet count, albumin, and AST/ALT ratio. Using an online calculator, clinicians may input these variables to generate a continuous score. By applying a cutoff of -1.455, advanced fibrosis may be excluded, with a negative predictive value (NPV) of 88%. Conversely, by applying a cutoff of 0.676, the presence of advanced fibrosis may be predicted, with a positive predictive value (PPV) of 82%.

Fibrometer

The Fibrometer is a patented test that incorporates into an algorithm the following parameters: alpha-2-macroglobulin, ALT, AST, gamma glutamyl transpeptidase (GGT), prothrombin index, and urea.[6] The AUROC discerning fibrosis stage (F2-F4) is 0.892. It is reported as a value between 0 and 1 corresponding to the probability of advanced fibrosis and demonstrates a linearity of score across fibrosis stages.

FibroTest/Fibrosure

Developed by Poynard and colleagues,[7] FibroTest/Fibrosure (Biopredictive, Paris, France) is a patented algorithm using the combination of 5 serum biochemical parameters (α-2-macroglobulin, apolipoprotein A1, haptoglobin, L-glutamyltranspeptidase, and bilirubin). This test is reported as a linear score. As a result, it can risk stratify patients for mild disease F0-1 and for cirrhosis. Additionally, the probability of having any stage of disease is also given with the test result, so it may be used for making treatment decisions for direct-acting antiviral (DAA) therapy. Clear advantages of FibroTest/Fibrosure include widespread availability, interlaboratory reproducibility, and limited contraindications (<5%). The AUROC ranges from 0.73 to 0.87 for stages

F2, F3, and F4 for most chronic liver disease. At a cut-off of 0.31, the FibroTest/ Fibrosure NPV for excluding significant fibrosis (prevalence 0.31) was 91%.[7,8]

HepaScore

HepaScore is another patented test that combines serum bilirubin, hyaluronic acid (HA), α-2-macroglobulin (A2M) levels, and GGT with age and sex.[9,10] The precise formula is as follows: years/(1 + y) with y = exp [− 4.185818 − (0.0249 age (years)) + (0.7464 sex (M = 1, F = 0) + (1.0039 A2M (g/L)) + (0.0302 HA (µg/L)) + (0.0691 bilirubin (µmol/L)) − (0.0012 GGT (U/L)))]. HepaScore's AUROC is 0.85, 0.96, and 0.94 for significant fibrosis, advanced fibrosis, and cirrhosis, respectively. In the validation set, a score of at least 0.5 (range, 0.0–1.0) was 89% specific and 63% sensitive for significant fibrosis. A score less than 0.5 was 74% specific and 88% sensitive for advanced fibrosis.[10]

Vibration-Controlled Transient elastography

Noninvasive liver stiffness measurement (LSM), or elastography, by ultrasound-based VCTE using FibroScan (Echosens; Paris, France) is a US-Food and Drug Administration (FDA)-approved technique that has revolutionized the management of liver disease. It is the simplest and most rapid point-of-care test to measure liver fibrosis. LSM is particularly effective as a surrogate marker of advanced fibrosis (F3) and cirrhosis (F4). Elastography calculates liver stiffness expressed in kilopascals (kPa), which, in turn, correlates closely with liver fibrosis. VCTE often outperforms serologic tests in head-to-head evaluations, particularly for the diagnosis of cirrhosis.[11] VCTE is also predictive of the complications of chronic liver disease such as the development of portal hypertension, esophageal varices, and long-term outcomes of liver disease such as HCC, liver failure, and death. The precise LSM cutoffs and confounders vary by disease state and will be discussed seperately.[12,13]

Magnetic Resonance Elastography

Magnetic resonance elastography uses propagating mechanical shear waves (range, 20–200 Hz) to probe the mechanical properties of various organs during an MRI examination. Shear waves propagate more rapidly in stiffer tissue and more slowly in softer tissue. Although not yet FDA approved and of limited availability, this technique can be readily implemented on a conventional magnetic resonance system with added hardware to generate mechanical waves, and special software for acquisition and processing. Normal liver parenchyma has shear stiffness values less than 3 kPa.[14]

HEPATITIS C

Our approach to the patient with hepatitis C virus (HCV) must change in the era of highly efficacious antiviral therapy with direct-acting antiviral agents (DAAs). The efficacy of the present generation of anti-HCV therapy, combined with the Centers for Disease Control and Prevention (CDC) recommendation for baby-boomer cohort screening,[15] means that the volume of patients presenting for management of HCV will rise steeply. American Association for the Study of Liver Diseases (AASLD) guidelines suggest, and insurance approval for this therapy often requires, clinicians to determine the risk of their patients with chronic HCV for advanced liver disease.[16] Risk assessment allows the clinician to prioritize treatment for those with advanced fibrosis and pursue appropriate screening strategies for patients with cirrhosis. However, in this therapeutic context, the cost and risk of liver biopsy, not to mention the patient preference to avoid invasive procedures, have raised the profile of noninvasive markers of liver fibrosis.

No marker can effectively discern each stage of fibrosis as well as a biopsy, but this may not be important for patients with HCV. Indeed, the burden for fibrosis assessment in HCV is essentially to determine whether the patient has advanced fibrosis. To that end, there are many reliable noninvasive markers of fibrosis available to aid clinicians.

When using noninvasive tests in order to avoid liver biopsy, the key for patients with HCV is to seek concordance. One could obtain both a serologic and imaging test for advanced fibrosis in a single clinic visit. Thereafter, clinicians could immediately divide their patient population into 3 groups: concordant low and high risk and conflicting or intermediate results.[12,17] One could choose to repeat the tests or pursue liver biopsy for the group with mixed or equivocal results depending on how the results might change patient management.

The choice of serologic test is mainly related to availability in one's center. The key is consistency within a given practice to streamline comparisons and decision making. The most extensively studied serologic tests for patients with chronic HCV are the FibroTest and APRI. In a meta-analysis that pooled 6378 subjects with both FibroTest and biopsy (3501 HCV patients), the mean standardized AUROC for diagnosing significant fibrosis was 0.84 (95% CI, 0.83–0.86).[7] A different meta-analysis, which pooled 4266 HCV patients from 22 studies, showed that APRI could discern significant fibrosis and cirrhosis with mean AUROC of 0.76 (0.74–0.79) and 0.82 (0.79–0.86), respectively.[18] In a recent prospective study, FibroTest, HepaScore, and FibroMeter were compared and found to be equally effective.[9]

The imaging techniques employed in the noninvasive determination of fibrosis include ultrasound and magnetic resonance-based LSM. The FDA-approved option for patients with chronic HCV who are candidates for LSM is ultrasound-based VCTE, commonly delivered by FibroScan. It is helpful to keep a range of LSMs in mind to maximize the clinical import of the finding. For example, in the authors' study, a cutoff of 7.3 kPa offered excellent (near perfect) NPV, excluding patients without advanced liver disease.[19] Elsewhere, a cutoff of 12.5 kPa displayed a PPV of 77% and an NPV of 98%.[20,21]

The combination of VCTE and serologic tests leads to clinically meaningful results. Poynard and colleagues,[22] for example, showed how VCTE and FibroSure can be used to group all patients with chronic HCV into risk categories. Although higher cutoffs captured the patients at highest risk, 12.5 kPa predicted the development of hepatic decompensation and HCC. Furthermore, the rate of change in noninvasive metrics over time predicted clinical outcomes. In a cohort of patients undergoing anti-HCV therapy, baseline measurements and serial VCTE were predictive of overall survival. In a multivariate model of mortality risk that adjusted for demographic factors, baseline VCTE (per kPa) was associated with a hazard ratio (HR) of 5.76 (95% CI 3.74–8.87); increased LSM on follow-up had an HR of 1.19 (95% CI 1.11–1.28), and sustained virological response (SVR) had an HR of 0.19 (95% CI 0.05–0.80). In this study, SVR at any LSM or a baseline LSM of less than 7 kPa was associated with a good outcome. The patients with bad outcomes, on the other hand, were those with a 14 kPa or greater at baseline with any LSM increase on follow-up.[23]

HUMAN IMMUNODEFICIENCY VIRUS-HEPATITIS C VIRUS COINFECTED PATIENTS

One-third of patients infected with the human immunodeficiency virus (HIV) in the United States and Europe are also infected with HCV. HCV appears to have a more severe and progressive course in coinfected patients than in those with HCV mono-infection. Rates of liver disease-related death are increasing in the HIV population.

HCV-associated chronic liver disease accounts from 12% to 45% of overall mortality in HIV-infected patients in most recent reports.[24] Fortunately, noninvasive indices of fibrosis also perform well in this population.

In a large cohort of 272 HIV-HCV coinfected patients, Cacoub and colleagues[25] compared multiple tests including FibroTest, HepaScore, Fibrometer, FIB-4, APRI, and Serum Hyaluronic Acid, AST, Albumin (SHASTA)[26] to differentiate patients with mild-to-moderate fibrosis (<F2) from those with advanced fibrosis (>F3). The SHASTA, which has utility for patients with HIV-HCV coinfection, is a formula that includes serum hyaluronidase, albumin, and AST.[26] The AUROCs for >F2 fibrosis were of 0.78, 0.84 and 0.89 for FibroTest, HepaScore, and Fibrometer respectively. Elsewhere, in a cohort of 137 patients, hyaluronic acid levels were even more discriminating for low amounts of fibrosis when combined with albumin and AST results. SHASTA's AUROC for patients with Ishak scores less than 3 was 0.878.[26] The SHASTA index in HIV-HCV patients had similar accuracy to FibroTest and significantly better accuracy than the APRI test.

In 2010, Sánchez-Conde and colleagues[27] published a prospective study of 100 patients with documented HIV-HCV coinfection undergoing liver biopsy and VCTE. This study showed that the optimal LSM cutoffs are within the ranges seen for patients with HCV monoinfection. With a cutoff of 11 kPa for F3 fibrosis, the NPV is 96.3%, with a PPV of 60.0%. A cutoff of 14 kPa for cirrhosis has an NPV of 100% and a PPV of 57.1%. This study confirmed VCTE as an efficient technique for the exclusion of advanced liver fibrosis and cirrhosis in this unique population.

HEPATITIS B

The determination of fibrosis stage for patients with chronic hepatitis B virus (HBV) defines both the role for treatment and screening for complications of cirrhosis. AASLD guidelines for the consideration of HBV treatment and screening include a straightforward algorithm based on surface and e antigen expression, viral load, inflammation, and fibrosis burden.[28] It may be reasonable, however, to supplant liver biopsy with noninvasive tests. However, without a biopsy—without a gold standard, the authors recommend a strategy that relies on concordance between 2 or more tests.[12] For chronic HBV, as for most other chronic liver diseases, the clinician interested in noninvasive metrics of fibrosis has many options. These include serologic indices, both simple and advanced, and imaging-based techniques, namely VCTE.

Among the simple serologic indices fibrosis, FIB-4 is the best studied for patients with chronic HBV. In their prospective validation study of 668 South Korean patients with chronic HBV, Kim and colleagues[29] found an FIB-4 cutoff of 1.6 provided a 93.2% NPV. Beyond that, the AUROC was 0.910 and 0.926 for severe (F$\geq$3) fibrosis and cirrhosis (F = 4), respectively. Subsequently, Li and colleagues[30] validated FIB-4 in 284 US patients. Here, FIB-4 distinguished F3–F4 from F0–F2, with an AUROC of 0.86 (95% CI 0.80–0.92). This group found that the optimal cutoff for F4 fibrosis was 5.17.

The advanced serologic markers of fibrosis are of roughly equivalent clinical value for patients with chronic HBV. The best available study to compare these tests, namely FibroTest, FibroMeter, and HepaScore, came from Leroy and colleagues[9] in 2014. Examining 255 French, mostly (72.2%) male patients aged 39.9 plus or minus 13.6 years with chronic HBV, this group compared the fibrosis score values generated with those from patients with HCV. Their goal was a set of validated cutoffs applicable to patients with chronic HBV or HCV. Each test possessed an AUROC of 0.82 to 0.85 for F of at least 3 and 0.84 to 0.87 for F4. FibroTest, with cutoffs of 0.59 and 0.79 had an NPV of 84.0% and 91.0% for F of at least 3 and F4, respectively. FibroMeter yielded an NPB of 91% and 92% for F of at least 3 and F4 using respective cutoffs of 0.57 and 0.84. Finally, HepaScore, with a cutoffs of 0.84, yielded an NPV of 94%. The choice of test is largely based on personal experience and availability.

Experience with VCTE in HBV is growing rapidly. VCTE may be more accurate than serologic indices of fibrosis in this population.[11] Often derived from local experience or with reference to HCV studies, VCTE cutoffs vary from study to study. In their early study of VCTE paired with liver biopsy, Marcellin and colleagues[31] evaluated 202 patients with chronic HBV. Cutoffs of 7.2 and 11.0 kPa for greater than F2 and F 4, yielded AUROC of 0.81 and 0.93, respectively. A cutoff of 11.0 kPa for cirrhosis had an NPV for cirrhosis 99%, which was confirmed elsewhere.[20,31] In a meta-analysis of published studies comprising 2772 patients evaluated the performance of VCTE in chronic HBV, optimal cutoffs for F3–F4 and F4 were 8.8 kPa and 11.7 kPa respectively. 11.7 kPa had a sensitivity of 84.6% and a specificity of 81.5% for the detection of cirrhosis, while 8.8 kPa was 74.3% sensitive and 78.3% specific for greater than or equal to F3 fibrosis.[32]

It is important to consider the limitations of these tests. In contrast to the serologic tests, the confounders of VCTE are well described. Most important for patients with HBV is the relative contribution to liver stiffness from necroinflammatory activity.[33–35]

For this reason, the authors agree with the strategy proposed by Chan to interpret the results of VCTE in the context of the ALT level.[36] Although the precise effect of ALT on VCTE test characteristics is yet to be determined, one should think in terms of relatively broad ranges. Chan, for example, suggests that when patients with a normal ALT score above or below VCTE cutoffs for significant fibrosis (in their study ≤ 5 kPa vs ≥ 9.0 kPa), one can make treatment decisions without reference to other evaluations. However, for patients with elevated ALT (greater than the upper limit of normal), further evaluation (in their case, liver biopsy) was employed in an expanded indeterminate zone of 7 to 12 kPa.

NONALCOHOLIC FATTY LIVER DISEASE

NAFLD is the most common liver disease in the United States of America. Given the volume of patients with NAFLD who seek (and will seek) care from gastroenterologists, it will be increasingly important to safely, efficiently, and inexpensively discern which patients are at the highest risk. To this end, several noninvasive indices of hepatic fibrosis are available to support clinicians. Routinely employing risk scores in clinical practice allows clinicians to divide their NAFLD patients into 2 populations first those at lowest risk for advanced liver disease who may avoid liver biopsy, and second those who would benefit from further evaluation and novel therapeutic agents.

The best-studied indices of hepatic fibrosis are risk scores derived from standard, readily available blood tests. These scores include the NAFLD fibrosis score FIB-4 and APRI. The principle advantage of such scores is that they provide the clinician with an immediate estimate of their patient's risk for advanced liver disease using calculators found on the Internet.

Many studies have evaluated multiple fibrosis risk scores head-to-head in the NAFLD population.[37–39] The Nonalcholic Steatohepatitis (NASH) Clinical Research network, for example, assessed fibrosis markers in a prospective American cohort of 541 adults.[40] In this study, both the FIB-4 and NAFLD fibrosis score performed similarly well in the diagnosis of advanced fibrosis with respective AUROCs of 0.8 and 0.76. Crucially, assuming a population prevalence of 10%, the NPV for advanced fibrosis (F3–F4) using FIB-4 is 96%, with a liberal cutoff of 1.3, and it barely falls to 93% with a more stringent cutoff (2.67). The NAFLD fibrosis score has similar test characteristics. In a separate international validation study of 733 patients (aged 47.7 years on average and 53% male) with biopsy-confirmed NALFD, a cutoff of -1.455 had an NPV of 88% for excluding the presence of advanced fibrosis with an AUROC of 0.84.[5] The validity of an FIB-4 cutoff of 1.3 and NAFLD fibrosis score of -1.455 has been reproduced in multiple settings.[17,37]

Diagnostic tests using more complicated metrics and proprietary algorithms such as FibroSure and FibroMeter have been evaluated in NAFLD. In 1 study of 225 patients, FibroMeter has demonstrated a marginally lower misclassification rate for F3 fibrosis than the NAFLD fibrosis score. However, there was no difference in test performance in patients with F4 fibrosis.[39] In general, for patients with NAFLD, the more complicated serum tests have not demonstrated value over and above the simple, universally available metrics.[41]

Still, the principle worry when assessing patients without the histologic gold stand is the possibility of a false-negative result in serologic testing, which is unfortunately not rare.[41] As for other diseases, one ought to seek concordance between a serologic test and another modality for the noninvasive evaluation of advanced fibrosis.[12] To that end, the best available option is VCTE.

In the largest study of VCTE in NAFLD to date, Wong and colleagues[42] prospectively enrolled 246 consecutive patients from centers in China and France. Employing a 10.3 kPa cutoff, this group found a 99% NPV and 46% PPV for the diagnosis of cirrhosis. Given the effect of BMI on VCTE performance, valid complaints about the reliability of VCTE in NAFLD have been raised, especially for patients with morbid obesity.[43,44] To overcome differences in chest wall depth in obese patients, a novel probe, the XL probe, was developed and appears to restore the efficacy of this modality. However, even with the XL probe, the reliability of VCTE decreases for patients with a BMI greater than 30 kg/m^2.[45] For this reason, combination with other noninvasive tests of fibrosis is critical.

Recent studies show that the combination of VCTE and serologic tests is a winning strategy. This is a strategy that the authors and others support.[12,41] In a prospective trial, Petta and colleagues[17] validated this approach in 2 Italian cohorts. The optimal combination in their hands was VCTE with the NAFLD Fibrosis Score, yielding a 0% false-positive and 7.3% false-negative rate.

A promising tool that can be combined with VCTE is termed controlled attenuation parameter (CAP). CAP allows for estimation of steatosis. This tool uses the same radio frequency data as VCTE and is only appraised if the LSM acquisition is valid. In the original report, CAP paired with histology has an AUROC of 0.91, 0.95, and 0.89 for steatosis stages 1, 2 and 3, respectively.[46] When later assessed in 615 patients with chronic HCV by the same group, CAP had an AUROC of 0.80, 0.86, and 0.88 for stages 1, 2 and 3, respectively.[47] As steatosis is a reversible marker reflecting the potential for further liver injury, CAP is a promising investigational tool for clinicians to advise patients on future risks and therapeutic strategies.

CHOLESTATIC DISEASES

VCTE is the best studied noninvasive approach to the evaluation of fibrosis and histologic stages in chronic cholestatic diseases. Corpechot and colleagues[48] studied 101 patients, 73 patients with Primary Biliary Cirrhosis (PBC) and 28 with Primary Sclerosing Cholangitis (PSC). In their hands, AUROCs (95% CI) were 0.88 (0.81–0.95), 0.91 (0.85–0.97), and 0.96 (0.93–1.00) for predicting fibrosis of stage greater than or equal to 2, greater than or equal to 3 and 4, respectively. The optimal LSM cutoff values were 7.3 kPa, 9.8 kPa, and 17.3 kPa for fibrosis stage greater than 2, greater than 3, and 4, respectively.

The most recent study to asses degree of fibrosis with VCTE and the correlation with outcomes for only patients with PSC was published Corpechot and colleagues.[49] Seventy-three patients with a liver biopsy underwent transient elastography no more than 6 months after the biopsy. Cutoff values for fibrosis stages greater than or equal to F1, greater than or equal to F2, greater than or equal to F3, and F4 were 7.4 kPa, 8.6 kPa, 9.6 kPa, and 14.4 kPa, respectively. The adjusted diagnostic accuracy values for severe fibrosis and cirrhosis were 0.83 and 0.88, respectively. In this cohort of patients, VCTE was able to differentiate severe from nonsevere liver fibrosis with high levels of confidence.

PUTTING IT ALL TOGETHER—RECOMMENDATIONS FOR CLINICAL PRACTICE

The clinician needs to first ask the question how will knowledge of fibrosis stage effect the management of the individual patients liver disease? There are usually 3 major considerations. First, is there cirrhosis to commence HCC and varices screening? Second, is the patient a candidate for therapy? Third, what is the long-term prognosis? Each of these questions can be answered using the simple algorithms and combinations of tests listed for individual diseases (**Fig. 1**).

The authors prefer VCTE for cirrhosis diagnosis, and if the LSM is greater than 12.5kPA, then they suggest a diagnosis of cirrhosis and appropriate screening. If VCTE is not available, then serum tests and magnetic resonance elastography can be used. For decision making for therapy, the authors use a combination of

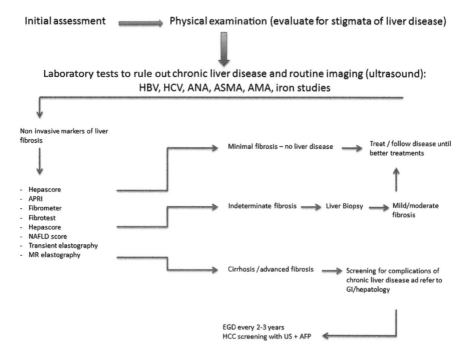

Fig. 1. Putting it together. AFP, alpha fetoprotein; AMA, antimitochrondial antibody; ANA, antinuclear antibody; APRI, AST-to-platelet ratio index; ASMA, antismooth muscle antibody; EGD, esophagogastric duodenoscopy; GI, gastroenterology; HBV, hepatitis B virus; HCV, hepatitis C virus; MR, magnetic resonance; NAFLD, nonalcoholic fatty liver disease.

VCTE and biomarkers. If there is concordance and the fibrosis stage is significant, therapy can be initiated. When there is discordance, the authors usually repeat in 3 months and if still discordant perform a liver biopsy. Finally, the prognosis of liver disease over the intermediate term of 5 years is also confirmed by LSM where patients with a liver stiffness less than 11.5 are 99% unlikely to have a liver-related outcome.[13]

Many clinicians will also ask how often to repeat the tests. This has been less well studied and is again dependent on the clinical scenario. For patients who are being monitored without treatment, the authors recommend no more frequently than annual evaluations and no less frequently than every 2 years. For patients who have had a successful treatment (eg, SVR after HCV treatment), the authors usually repeat the LSM at 1 year and if less than 8.5 kPA, they will discharge from the clinic. For monitoring cirrhosis, the authors recommend annual examinations, and this includes following patients with SVR to see if there is regression of cirrhosis, which should always be confirmed prior to stopping any HCC screening.

In summary, noninvasive tests now enable the clinician to successfully stage and monitor a wide variety of liver diseases and have significantly reduced the need for liver biopsy.

REFERENCES

1. Bravo AA, Sheth SG, Chopra S. Liver biopsy. N Engl J Med 2001;344(7):495–500.
2. Bedossa P. Intraobserver and interobserver variations in liver biopsy interpretation in patients with chronic hepatitis C. Hepatology 1994;20(1):15–20.
3. Wai CT, Greenson JK, Fontana RJ, et al. A simple noninvasive index can predict both significant fibrosis and cirrhosis in patients with chronic hepatitis C. Hepatology 2003;38(2):518–26.
4. Vallet-Pichard A, Mallet V, Nalpas B, et al. FIB-4: an inexpensive and accurate marker of fibrosis in HCV infection. Comparison with liver biopsy and FibroTest. Hepatology 2007;46(1):32–6.
5. Angulo P, Hui JM, Marchesini G, et al. The NAFLD fibrosis score: a noninvasive system that identifies liver fibrosis in patients with NAFLD. Hepatology 2007; 45(4):846–54.
6. Cales P, Oberti F, Michalak S, et al. A novel panel of blood markers to assess the degree of liver fibrosis. Hepatology 2005;42(6):1373–81.
7. Poynard T, Morra R, Halfon P, et al. Meta-analyses of FibroTest diagnostic value in chronic liver disease. BMC Gastroenterol 2007;7(1):40.
8. Poynard T, Imbert-Bismut F, Munteanu M, et al. Overview of the diagnostic value of biochemical markers of liver fibrosis (FibroTest, HCV FibroSure) and necrosis (ActiTest) in patients with chronic hepatitis C. Comp Hepatol 2004;3(1):8.
9. Leroy V, Sturm N, Faure P, et al. Prospective evaluation of FibroTest®, FibroMeter®, and HepaScore® for staging liver fibrosis in chronic hepatitis B: comparison with hepatitis C. J Hepatol 2014;61:28–34.
10. Adams LA, Bulsara M, Rossi E, et al. Hepascore: an accurate validated predictor of liver fibrosis in chronic hepatitis C infection. Clin Chem 2005;51(10):1867–73.
11. Degos F, Perez P, Roche B, et al. Diagnostic accuracy of FibroScan and comparison to liver fibrosis biomarkers in chronic viral hepatitis: a multicenter prospective study (the FIBROSTIC study). J Hepatol 2010;53(6):1013–21.
12. Tapper EB, Castera L, Afdhal NH. FibroScan (vibration controlled transient elastography): where does it stand in the US practice. Clin Gastroenterol Hepatol 2014. [Epub ahead of print].

13. Bonder A, Afdhal N. Utilization of FibroScan in clinical practice. Curr Gastroenterol Rep 2014;16(2):1–7.
14. Venkatesh SK, Ehman RL. Magnetic resonance elastography of liver. Magn Reson Imaging Clin N Am 2014;22(3):433–46.
15. Smith BD, Morgan RL, Beckett GA, et al. Recommendations for the identification of chronic hepatitis C virus infection among persons born during 1945-1965. MMWR Recomm Rep 2012;61(RR–4):1–32.
16. Diseases AAftSoL, America IDSo. Recommendations for testing, managing, and treating hepatitis C. 2014. Available at: http://www.hcvguidelines.org.
17. Petta S, Vanni E, Bugianesi E, et al. The combination of liver stiffness measurement and NAFLD fibrosis score improves the noninvasive diagnostic accuracy for severe liver fibrosis in patients with nonalcoholic fatty liver disease. Liver Int 2014. [Epub ahead of print].
18. Shaheen AA, Myers RP. Diagnostic accuracy of the aspartate aminotransferase-to-platelet ratio index for the prediction of hepatitis C-related fibrosis: a systematic review. Hepatology 2007;46(3):912–21.
19. Tapper EB, Cohen EB, Patel K, et al. Levels of alanine aminotransferase confound use of transient elastography to diagnose fibrosis in patients with chronic hepatitis C virus infection. Clin Gastroenterol Hepatol 2012;10(8):932–7.e1.
20. Cardoso AC, Carvalho-Filho RJ, Stern C, et al. Direct comparison of diagnostic performance of transient elastography in patients with chronic hepatitis B and chronic hepatitis C. Liver Int 2012;32(4):612–21.
21. Castéra L, Vergniol J, Foucher J, et al. Prospective comparison of transient elastography, Fibrotest, APRI, and liver biopsy for the assessment of fibrosis in chronic hepatitis C. Gastroenterology 2005;128(2):343–50.
22. Poynard T, Vergniol J, Ngo Y, et al. Staging chronic hepatitis C in seven categories using fibrosis biomarker (FibroTest™) and transient elastography (FibroScan®). J Hepatol 2014;60(4):706–14.
23. Vergniol J, Boursier J, Coutzac C, et al. The evolution of non-invasive tests of liver fibrosis is associated with prognosis in patients with chronic hepatitis C. Hepatology 2014;60:65–76.
24. Sherman KE, Rouster SD, Chung RT, et al. Hepatitis C virus prevalence among patients infected with human immunodeficiency virus: a cross-sectional analysis of the US adult AIDS Clinical Trials Group. Clin Infect Dis 2002;34(6):831–7.
25. Cacoub P, Carrat F, Bédossa P, et al. Comparison of non-invasive liver fibrosis biomarkers in HIV/HCV co-infected patients: the fibrovic study–ANRS HC02. J Hepatol 2008;48(5):765–73.
26. Kelleher TB, Mehta SH, Bhaskar R, et al. Prediction of hepatic fibrosis in HIV/HCV co-infected patients using serum fibrosis markers: the SHASTA index. J Hepatol 2005;43(1):78–84.
27. Sánchez-Conde M, Montes-Ramírez M, Miralles P, et al. Comparison of transient elastography and liver biopsy for the assessment of liver fibrosis in HIV/hepatitis C virus-coinfected patients and correlation with noninvasive serum markers. J Viral Hepat 2010;17(4):280–6.
28. Lok AS, McMahon BJ. Chronic hepatitis B: update 2009. Hepatology 2009;50(3):661–2.
29. Kim S, Seo Y, Cheong J, et al. Factors that affect the diagnostic accuracy of liver fibrosis measurement by Fibroscan in patients with chronic hepatitis B. Aliment Pharmacol Ther 2010;32(3):498–505.
30. Li J, Gordon S, Rupp L, et al. The validity of serum markers for fibrosis staging in chronic hepatitis B and C. J Viral Hepat 2014. [Epub ahead of print].

31. Marcellin P, Ziol M, Bedossa P, et al. Non-invasive assessment of liver fibrosis by stiffness measurement in patients with chronic hepatitis B. Liver Int 2009;29(2):242–7.
32. Chon YE, Choi EH, Song KJ, et al. Performance of transient elastography for the staging of liver fibrosis in patients with chronic hepatitis B: a meta-analysis. PLoS One 2012;7(9):e44930.
33. Fung J, Lai CL, Chan SC, et al. Correlation of liver stiffness and histological features in healthy persons and in patients with occult hepatitis B, chronic active hepatitis B, or hepatitis B cirrhosis. Am J Gastroenterol 2010;105:1116–22.
34. Oliveri F, Coco B, Ciccorossi P, et al. Liver stiffness in the hepatitis B virus carrier: a non-invasive marker of liver disease influenced by the pattern of transaminases. World J Gastroenterol 2008;14(40):6154.
35. Viganò M, Massironi S, Lampertico P, et al. Transient elastography assessment of the liver stiffness dynamics during acute hepatitis B. Eur J Gastroenterol Hepatol 2010;22(2):180–4.
36. Chan HY, Wong GH, Choi PL, et al. Alanine aminotransferase-based algorithms of liver stiffness measurement by transient elastography (Fibroscan) for liver fibrosis in chronic hepatitis B. J Viral Hepat 2009;16(1):36–44.
37. Harrison SA, Oliver D, Arnold HL, et al. Development and validation of a simple NAFLD clinical scoring system for identifying patients without advanced disease. Gut 2008;57(10):1441–7.
38. Festi D, Schiumerini R, Marzi L, et al. Review article: the diagnosis of non-alcoholic fatty liver disease–availability and accuracy of non-invasive methods. Aliment Pharmacol Ther 2013;37(4):392–400.
39. Calès P, Lainé F, Boursier J, et al. Comparison of blood tests for liver fibrosis specific or not to NAFLD. J Hepatol 2009;50(1):165–73.
40. Shah AG, Lydecker A, Murray K, et al. Comparison of noninvasive markers of fibrosis in patients with nonalcoholic fatty liver disease. Clin Gastroenterol Hepatol 2009;7(10):1104–12.
41. Dowman JK, Tomlinson J, Newsome P. Systematic review: the diagnosis and staging of non-alcoholic fatty liver disease and non-alcoholic steatohepatitis. Aliment Pharmacol Ther 2011;33(5):525–40.
42. Wong VW, Vergniol J, Wong GL, et al. Diagnosis of fibrosis and cirrhosis using liver stiffness measurement in nonalcoholic fatty liver disease. Hepatology 2010;51(2):454–62.
43. Gaia S, Carenzi S, Barilli AL, et al. Reliability of transient elastography for the detection of fibrosis in non-alcoholic fatty liver disease and chronic viral hepatitis. J Hepatol 2011;54(1):64–71.
44. Petta S, Di Marco V, Cammà C, et al. Reliability of liver stiffness measurement in non-alcoholic fatty liver disease: the effects of body mass index. Aliment Pharmacol Ther 2011;33(12):1350–60.
45. de Lédinghen V, Wong VW, Vergniol J, et al. Diagnosis of liver fibrosis and cirrhosis using liver stiffness measurement: comparison between M and XL probe of FibroScan®. J Hepatol 2012;56(4):833–9.
46. Sasso M, Beaugrand M, De Ledinghen V, et al. Controlled attenuation parameter (CAP): a novel VCTE™ guided ultrasonic attenuation measurement for the evaluation of hepatic steatosis: preliminary study and validation in a cohort of patients with chronic liver disease from various causes. Ultrasound Med Biol 2010;36(11):1825–35.
47. Sasso M, Tengher-Barna I, Ziol M, et al. Novel controlled attenuation parameter for noninvasive assessment of steatosis using Fibroscan®: validation in chronic hepatitis C. J Viral Hepat 2012;19(4):244–53.

48. Corpechot C, El Naggar A, Poujol-Robert A, et al. Assessment of biliary fibrosis by transient elastography in patients with PBC and PSC. Hepatology 2006;43(5): 1118–24.

49. Corpechot C, Gaouar F, El Naggar A, et al. Baseline values and changes in liver stiffness measured by transient elastography are associated with severity of fibrosis and outcomes of patients with primary sclerosing cholangitis. Gastroenterology 2014;146(4):970–9 [quiz: e15–6].

Liver Transplantation for the Referring Physician

Ming-Ming Xu, MD, Robert S. Brown Jr, MD, MPH*

KEYWORDS

- Child-Turcotte-Pugh • Donation after cardiac death • Extended criteria donor
- Fulminant hepatic failure • Hepatic artery thrombosis • Hepatocellular carcinoma

KEY POINTS

- Liver transplantation is currently the treatment of choice for patients suffering from the complications of end-stage liver disease, acute liver failure, and primary hepatic malignancy. Over the last 2 decades, as the success of liver transplant increased, the number of patients seeking liver transplant has also steadily increased.
- Management of chronic medical conditions and their risk factor modifications are critical to ensure continued excellent graft function and overall survival of the recipient decades after transplant.
- Recurrence of the primary hepatic disease can occur for all autoimmune-based liver diseases and viral hepatitis, with the most challenging problem being recurrent hepatitis C virus.
- With newer direct-acting antiviral agents being developed, we should be optimistic that successful treatment of recurrent hepatitis C virus with interferon-free regimens will be accessible and feasible in the near future.

INTRODUCTION

Liver transplantation is currently the treatment of choice for patients suffering from the complications of end-stage liver disease, acute liver failure, and primary hepatic malignancy. Over the last 2 decades, as the success of liver transplant (LT) increased, the number of patients seeking LT has also steadily increased. In 2013, 6455 LTs were performed in the United States, with an additional 15,700 people currently active on the waiting list.[1] A persistent problem in LT has been the shortage of donor organs relative to the increasing demand for transplant, making appropriate recipient selection a critical part of the transplant process. The authors discuss the indications for transplant, candidate selection, transplant listing, methods of expanding the donor pool to address the shortage of donor organs, disease-specific issues as they relate to transplant outcomes and long-term management, and posttransplant care and complications.

Division of Digestive and Liver Diseases, Department of Medicine, Columbia University College of Physicians & Surgeons, 622 West 168th Street, PH14, New York, NY 10032, USA
* Corresponding author. Center for Liver Disease and Transplantation, 622 West 168th Street, PH14, New York, NY 10032.
E-mail addresses: rb464@columbia.edu; rb464@cumc.columbia.edu

Clin Liver Dis 19 (2015) 135–153
http://dx.doi.org/10.1016/j.cld.2014.09.008
1089-3261/15/$ – see front matter © 2015 Elsevier Inc. All rights reserved.

INDICATIONS FOR LIVER TRANSPLANTATION

Liver transplantation is indicated for the treatment of all causes of end-stage liver disease, complications of decompensated cirrhosis, fulminant hepatic failure, metabolic syndromes of hepatic origin, and primary hepatic malignancies (**Fig. 1, Box 1**).

PROGNOSTIC MODELS FOR LIVER TRANSPLANTATION ALLOCATION

Cirrhosis is the common end-stage form of all etiologies of chronic liver disease and accounts for most adult LTs performed. Cirrhosis is classified into compensated and decompensated stages, which portend significantly different chances of survival (**Fig. 2**). Compensated cirrhosis without manifestations of portal hypertension carries a low risk of death. Decompensation is marked by a rapidly progressive decline in hepatic function with the development of complications of portal hypertension: ascites, variceal bleeding, and hepatic encephalopathy.[2,3] Natural history studies of cirrhosis find that the development of decompensation is associated with a decreased median survival from greater than 12 years to 2 years (see **Fig. 2**).

The high mortality rate associated with decompensated cirrhosis and the scarcity of donor organs make it essential that our system of organ allocation prioritizes those with the greatest need for transplantation. The first prognostic model used in this capacity was the Child-Turcotte-Pugh (CTP) score, which was originally developed for risk stratification before surgical shunt procedures (**Table 1**). It

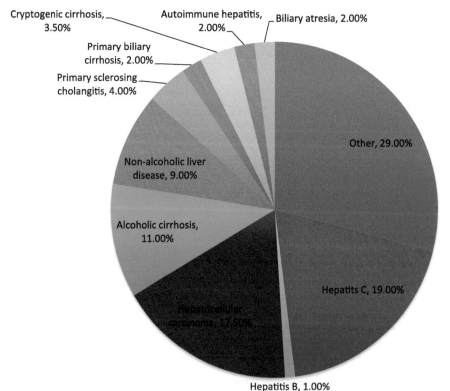

Fig. 1. Liver transplant by diagnosis, 2013. (*Data from* Organ procurement and Transplantation Network data as of July 8, 2014. Available at: http://optn.transplant.hrsa.gov. Accessed July 8, 2014.)

Box 1
Indications for liver transplantation
Fulminant hepatic failure
Complications of cirrhosis
Ascites
Chronic gastrointestinal blood loss caused by portal hypertensive gastropathy
Hepatic encephalopathy
Liver cancer
Recurrent variceal bleeding
Synthetic dysfunction
Liver-based metabolic conditions
Alpha 1 antitrypsin deficiency
Familial amyloidosis
Glycogen storage disease
Hemochromatosis
Primary oxaluria
Wilson disease
Tyrosinemia
Urea cycle enzyme deficiencies
Systemic complications of chronic liver disease
Hepatopulmonary syndrome
Portopulmonary hypertension
Adapted from Martin P, DiMartini A, Feng S, et al. Evaluation for liver transplantation in adults: 2013 practice guideline by the AASLD. Hepatology 2013;59:1144–65.

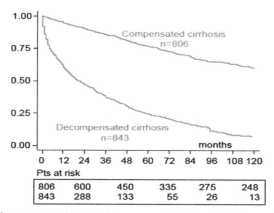

Fig. 2. Survival of compensated versus decompensated cirrhosis at diagnosis. (*From* D'Amico G, Garcia-Tsao G, Pagliaro L. Natural history and prognostic indicators of survival in cirrhosis: a systematic review of 118 studies. J Hepatol 2006;44:219; with permission.)

Table 1 The CPT scoring system			
Points	1	2	3
Total bilirubin (mg/dL)	<2.0	2–3	>3.0
Albumin (g/dL)	>3.5	2.8–3.5	<2.8
Prothrombin time prolongation (s)	1–4	5–6	>6
Encephalopathy	None	Minimal	Advanced
Ascites	None	Slight	Moderate

Data from Child CG, Turcotte JG. Surgery and portal hypertension. In: Child CG. The liver and portal hypertension. Philadelphia: Saunders; 1964. p. 50–64.

defined 3 classes of cirrhosis with increased mortality as disease progressed from one class to the next (**Table 2**). Before 2002, the CPT model was used to assess disease severity and, along with waiting time, became the primary determinant of transplant priority. The major limitation of the CPT scoring system was its inability to further stratify patients within the Child Class C and B patients. This limitation made waiting time the primary determinant of prioritization for organ allocation and led to transplants being performed in patients with less decompensated disease but longer time on the waiting list. Additionally, the use of 2 subjective parameters, the degree of ascites and encephalopathy, in the CPT led to questions of "gaming" the system. This activity led to a demand for a system for organ allocation that was based on an objective assessment of disease severity and the acuity of need for transplant.

In February 2002, the Model for End-Stage Liver Disease (MELD) system was adopted by the United Network of Organ Sharing (UNOS) as the standard scoring system for LT allocation.[4] The MELD is a prognostic model originally developed to predict survival after transjugular intrahepatic portosystemic shunt placement.[5] The MELD score is calculated from 3 biochemical variables that reflect hepatic and renal function: serum bilirubin level, creatinine level, and international normalized ratio of prothrombin time with score ranging from 6 to 40. This score has been validated in both retrospective and prospective studies of patients with chronic liver disease as a predictor of 90-day mortality (**Fig. 3**). Since the adoption of the MELD score, patients are prioritized for transplant based on disease severity regardless of the etiology of their liver disease or length of waiting time.

However, certain conditions are associated with end-stage liver disease that do not directly affect hepatic function (as reflected by the MELD score) but may affect mortality and would benefit from LT.[6] These conditions are specially recognized because of their increased risk of mortality and a high probability of cure with

Table 2 One- and 2-year survival based on CPT score		
Class	1 y	2 y
A (5–6 points)	100%	85%
B (7–9 points)	80%	60%
C (10–15 points)	45%	35%

Data from Child CG, Turcotte JG. Surgery and portal hypertension. In: Child CG. The liver and portal hypertension. Philadelphia: Saunders; 1964. p. 50–64.

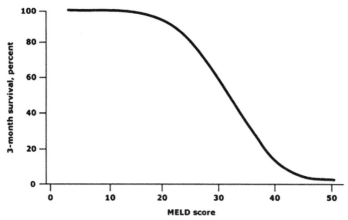

Fig. 3. Estimated 3-month survival as a function of MELD score. (*Data from* Wiesner R, Edwards E, Freeman R, et al. Model for end-stage liver disease (MELD) and allocation of donor livers. Gastroenterology 2003;124:91–6.)

transplant. These exceptional cases, most notably hepatocellular carcinoma (HCC), highlighted a deficiency in the MELD scoring system and led to the development of exception points to address these special conditions as they relate to transplant (**Box 2**). The provision of exception points to patients with these conditions allow for a more accurate assessment of their disease-related mortality risk and prioritization for transplant.

Box 2
Conditions for which MELD exception points may be allocated

HCC

Cholangiocarcinoma in select cases

Hepatopulmonary syndrome

Portopulmonary hypertension

Recurrent cholangitis

Budd-Chiari syndrome

Primary hyperoxaluria

Familial amyloidosis

Cystic fibrosis

Intractable pruritus

Polycystic liver disease

Hereditary hemorrhagic telangiectasia

Small-for-size syndrome

Data from Freeman RB, Gish RG, Harper A, et al. Model for end-stage liver disease (MELD) exception guidelines: results and recommendations from the MELD Exception Study Group and Conference (MESSAGE) for the approval of patients who need liver transplantation with diseases not considered by the standard MELD formula. Liver Transpl 2006;12:S128–36.

TRANSPLANT EVALUATION

Successful LT improves survival and enhances the quality of life of patients with end-stage liver disease. The selection of appropriate candidates for transplant is a balance between identifying patients sick enough to require transplant but without other medical or psychiatric comorbidities that would prohibit successful LT. Thus the approach to transplant evaluation is multidisciplinary with medical, psychosocial, and surgical evaluations (**Box 3**).

ABSOLUTE CONTRAINDICATIONS FOR TRANSPLANT

The contraindications for transplant have continued to evolve as advances in therapies and pretransplant protocols allow patients previously thought not to be candidates for transplant become potential recipients. However, certain medical conditions are considered absolute contraindications for transplant, these includes advanced cardiopulmonary comorbidities, active infections or sepsis, and extrahepatic malignancies that independently affect a patient's prognosis regardless of their liver disease. From a psychosocial standpoint, the lack of appropriate social support or a history of persistent medical noncompliance should also raise red flags during the evaluation process (**Table 3**). These psychosocial risk factors can be difficult to tease out because they can be subjective but are an essential part of the evaluation process to help identify barriers to medical compliance and patients' potential for relapse into high-risk behaviors that may lead to poor transplant outcomes. Ensuring there is an adequate social support system for the transplant recipient is critical because caregiver support is one of the major determinants of continued follow-up care.

RELATIVE CONTRAINDICATIONS

Relative contraindications for transplant are often center specific but raise important pretransplant consideration, including some that can be modified to improve posttransplant outcomes.

Age

There is no absolute age cutoff that precludes transplant, although this can vary in center-specific guidelines. In general, physiologic age is considered more important over chronologic age such that patients older than 70 with few extrahepatic comorbidities can be successful transplant candidates.

Obesity

The increasing prevalence of obesity in the general population has led to a concurrent increase in the number of LT candidates with obesity. Body mass index greater than 40 (morbid obesity) portends poor posttransplant outcomes with higher rates of primary graft nonfunction and 1-year, 2-year, and 5-year mortality.[7] Monitored weight loss should be recommended for obese patients being considered for LT. Some programs are also undertaking newer proposals including sleeve gastrectomy at the time of LT.

Pulmonary Hypertension

Portopulmonary hypertension (POPH) occurs when there is elevated main pulmonary artery pressure (MPAP) $\geq$25 mm Hg caused by portal hypertension. When POPH is suspected, a thorough evaluation to exclude other causes of primary pulmonary

Box 3
Typical diagnostic evaluation for transplant

Cardiac evaluation

- Electrocardiogram
- Echocardiogram
- Noninvasive stress test if risk factors present
- Coronary catheterization if stress test is abnormal or high risk for cardiac disease
- Right heart catheterization if suspected right heart failure or pulmonary hypertension
- Cardiology consultation as needed

Pulmonary evaluation

- Chest x-ray
- Pulmonary function testing
- Room air arterial blood gas if evidence of hypoxia
- Shunt study if evidence of intrapulmonary shunt

Surgical evaluation

- Identify technical challenges
- Discuss donor options

Infectious disease evaluation

- Latent tuberculosis (Tuberculosis skin test or Quantiferon gold)
- HIV testing
- Rapid plasma reagin (RPR)
- Cytomegalovirus, Epstein-Barr virus status

Nephrology evaluation

- Creatinine clearance
- Nephrology consultation if any evidence of renal dysfunction

Neurologic evaluation

- Carotid Doppler if age greater than 60
- Neurology consultation as needed

Laboratory studies

- Electrolytes
- Hepatic function panel
- Coagulation panel
- Hepatitis serologies
- Blood typing with antibodies
- Urine toxicology

Radiology evaluation

- Abdominal sonogram with Doppler
- Triple-phase computed tomography or gadolinium magnetic resonance imaging for HCC screening or tumor staging

Age-appropriate cancer screening

- PAP smear
- Mammogram
- Colonoscopy (age >50 or history of primary sclerosing cholangitis)

Social work evaluation

- Assess psychosocial issues
- Evaluate support base

Financial screening

Adapted from Martin P, DiMartini A, Feng S, et al. Evaluation for liver transplantation in adults: 2013 practice guideline by the AASLD. Hepatology 2013;59:1144–65.

hypertension should be performed, and the degree of POPH should be evaluated with right heart catheterization.[8] Greater-than-moderate POPH, defined as MPAP ≥35 mm Hg predicts increased mortality after LT, but vasodilatory therapy may improve outcomes in patients who respond.[9]

Hepatopulmonary Syndrome

Hepatopulmonary syndrome (HPS) occurs because of intrapulmonary vasodilation with shunting that leads to arterial hypoxemia. Severe HPS (Pao_2<50 mm Hg) is associated with high perioperative mortality, but LT can offer significant chance of reversal of HPS.[10] However, severe HPS may be a relative contraindication to transplant depending on the degree of hypoxemia and complications related to prolonged postoperative mechanical ventilation. Moderate HPS (with Pao_2<60 mm Hg and a high shunt fraction on macroaggregated albumin scan) is given MELD exception points in many regions.

Portal Vein or Superior Mesenteric Vein Thrombosis

Presence of portal vein thrombosis does not preclude LT but does increase the operative complexity of the case. Knowledge of the extent of portal vein thrombosis in the recipient allows for advanced surgical planning with options ranging from

Table 3
Contraindications to liver transplantation

Absolute Contraindications	Relative Contraindications
Extrahepatic malignancy	Age >75
Extensive HCC (macrovascular invasion, lymph node, metastatic or multifocal involvement)	Portopulmonary hypertension (MPAP between 35–50 mm Hg)
Cholangiocarcinoma (outside neoadjuvant protocols)	Hepatopulmonary syndrome (Pao_2 ≤50 mm Hg)
Uncontrolled sepsis	Morbid obesity with body mass index ≥35
Advanced cardiopulmonary disease	Extensive portal vein or superior mesenteric vein thrombosis
Active substance abuse	Previous malignancy
Poor social support	

thrombectomy to use of vascular grafts. Thrombosis of the entire mesenteric venous system may lead to the need for a multivisceral transplant or preclude LT.

LISTING AND MATCHING FOR TRANSPLANT

Once a patient is determined to be an appropriate candidate for LT by the multidisciplinary transplant team, they are placed on the UNOS waiting list. Status of patients on the transplant waiting list is dynamic as their disease progresses (or rarely improves) and clinical changes occur. Deactivation from the transplant list is usually because of clinical deterioration to the point at which the risk of transplant is outweighed by the potential benefit. Status 1A priority is given to patients with fulminant hepatic failure or retransplant for hepatic artery thrombosis and primary graft nonfunction within a week of the initial transplant. After status 1A, patients are prioritized based on their risk of mortality as estimated by the MELD score from a low of 6 to a maximum of 40 points. When a potential donor organ is available, the matching of the donor to the recipient depends on their ABO blood group compatibility and organ size compatibility as determined by the transplant surgeon; recipients are chosen in descending MELD order from within their matched blood group.

EXPANDING THE DONOR POOL

The shortage of deceased donor organs has been an ongoing problem since the inception of deceased donor LT (DDLT) and leads to the death of thousands of candidates on the waiting list annually. This finding has led to the development of several strategies to expand the donor pool using extended criteria donors (ECD), living donation, split liver grafts, and donation after cardiac death (DCD) with varying degrees of success and some attendant ethical considerations.

Extended Criteria Donors

ECD grafts come from donors with high-risk characteristics that make the graft a suboptimal but potentially viable option for transplant (**Box 4**). Risk factors that fall within the ECD category vary among transplant centers with no consensus definition but generally include factors that increase the risk for donor-transmitted disease or short- or long-term graft nonfunction or failure when compared with

---

Box 4
Extended criteria donor organs

History of hepatitis B (Hepatitis B core antibody positive)

History of hepatitis C

Older donor age (>60)

Graft steatosis (>30%)

Cold ischemia time greater than 12 hours

Abnormal liver enzymes in donor

History of treated malignancy

Split liver grafts

DCD

standard criteria donors. Some findings suggest that the effect of extended criteria characteristics on graft outcome may be cumulative such that presence of multiple risk factors (eg, older age and longer ischemic time) and urgency of transplant portend worse 1-year outcomes.[11] The donor risk index can quantify the risk of graft loss but does not include recipient factors or the risk of donor-transmitted disease.

Split Liver Grafts

Split liver graft allows the transplant of a single deceased adult donor liver to one adult (with right donor lobe) and one pediatric (or rarely another adult) recipient.[12,13] In adults, split graft survival is generally comparable to that of whole liver grafts with 5-year survival rate of close to 90%, except in the case of status 1A recipients and recipients with HCC exception points who are at higher risk of split graft failure.[14,15] Thus, expansion of split graft use in the appropriate recipients may be a viable method of addressing the shortage of organs, particularly in the pediatric pool, without sacrificing graft function.

Donation After Cardiac Death

Most DDLTs come from patients who suffer from brain death in which cardiac perfusion is maintained up to the time of organ procurement. DCD refers to organ procurement from a donor with severe, irreversible neurologic injury but not meeting criteria for brain death after they are removed from life support and meet the criteria for cardiac death resulting in longer ischemia time before organ procurement. Outcomes from DCD donors have generally been poorer with higher rates of primary graft nonfunction, biliary complications, hepatic artery strictures, and overall higher rates of retransplant.[16,17]

Living Donation

The first living-donor LTs (LDLTs) were performed in the pediatric population to address the disproportionate shortage of donor organs in that population. It was expanded to adults in 1998 after the safety and feasibility of LDLT were established. To date, there have been 3580 LDLT performed in the United States.[18] Since its beginning, LDLT has presented one of the biggest ethical dilemmas in liver transplantation, that of placing a perfectly healthy donor through a considerable operation with its inherent risks, including death, without any direct benefit to the donor. The benefit to the recipient, however, is substantial, most important being an expedited transplant at an earlier stage of disease with a lower MELD and decreased waiting time and overall mortality. If the donor is emotionally related to the recipient, they derive a benefit from providing that life-saving opportunity.

The outcomes after LDLT have generally been excellent. Data from the Adult-to-Adult Living Donor Liver Transplantation Cohort Study, a national consortium of 9 US transplant centers that collects data on outcomes of LDLT in both recipients and donors, show decreased mortality rates in patients awaiting LT who undergo LDLT versus awaiting deceased donor transplant.[18] This outcome does depend on center experience with an initial learning curve of about 20 LDLT after which the rate of serious complications (including death and need for retransplant) from LDLT is not different than that of DDLT.[19]

The most common recipient complications after LDLT are biliary stricture, leak, and vascular thrombosis, which occur at higher frequency in LDLT compared with DDLT.[19] Donor complications after LDLT are also an important aspect of LDLT and lie at the heart of ethical considerations in living donation. Data from the Adult-to-Adult Living Donor Liver Transplantation Cohort Study show an overall donor complication rate of 38% with the most common postoperative complications being infections, biliary leak, and incisional hernias.[20] There have been 4 donor deaths (0.11%) related to living donation in the United States,[21] which reinforces the need for a thorough evaluation and informed consent process for donor selection so there is a clear understanding of the donor-specific risks associated with the procedure.

DISEASE-SPECIFIC CONSIDERATIONS
Alcoholic Liver Disease

Alcohol-related liver disease is one of the most common causes for LT but has remained one of the most controversial indications because of concerns of recidivism, with a reported incidence of up to 30%.[22] Despite the absence of well-validated data on the length of abstinence needed to prevent recidivism, it is a nearly universal requirement of most transplant centers for candidates to show sobriety for 6 months before being listed for LT.[23] This 6-month period allows time to identify patients who are at high risk for short-term recidivism but also those who may have a reversible component to their alcoholic liver injury, which improves spontaneously with abstinence, sometimes to the point at which transplant is no longer needed. Despite the concerns surrounding alcoholic-related LT, the outcomes from these transplants are comparable to those done for other indications. Even in the setting of recidivism, graft function is generally well preserved with no difference in mortality or graft loss between recipients who have relapsed and those who remain abstinent.[24,25]

Hepatitis C

In the United States, chronic hepatitis C–related cirrhosis and HCC is the most common indication for LT (see **Fig. 1**). The challenge of LT in these patients is the nearly universal rate of recurrent hepatitis C virus (HCV) infection in the posttransplant setting if viral eradication was not achieved before transplant.[26,27] Recurrent hepatitis C in the setting of immunosuppression can lead to accelerated progression to cirrhosis, graft dysfunction, graft failure, possible need for retransplantation and increased mortality.[28-30] After the onset of graft failure, the estimated 3-year survival is less than 10%.[31] Retransplantation in the setting of recurrent HCV is fraught with inferior outcomes and is not even considered in some transplant centers.[32] In the era of interferon-based therapy for HCV, pretransplant viral suppression was significantly limited by poor patient tolerance of the treatment regimen, especially in the setting of decompensated cirrhosis. Posttransplant treatment with interferon and ribavirin achieved low sustained viral response rates, and the addition of first-generation protease inhibitors, boceprevir and telaprevir, had increased sustained virologic respond but increased toxicity and significant drug–drug interactions with calcineurin inhibitors used for immunosuppression. With the advent of multiple, newer potent direct-acting antiviral therapy for HCV, there is hope for successful interferon-free regimens for peritransplant viral suppression for prevention and treatment of recurrent HCV, even in those with the most severe manifestation of recurrent hepatitis C.[33]

Hepatitis B

Liver transplantation for chronic hepatitis B cirrhosis or acute fulminant infection is currently among the most successful of all indications for LT with 5-year graft survival rate of 85%.[34] Before the mid-1990s the high recurrence rate of hepatitis B infection

(HBV) of up to 80% was associated with poor posttransplant outcomes and significant mortality.[35] The use of hepatitis B immune globulin and oral antiviral therapy, initially with lamivudine, dramatically reduced HBV recurrence rates posttransplant to ≤10%.[36,37] In recent years, with the advent of the newer, highly efficacious, well-tolerated antivirals with low rates of viral resistance, tenofovir and entecavir, a hepatitis B immune globulin–free regimen of prophylaxis may be possible in select patients at low risk of HBV recurrence.[38,39] Regardless of the drug used for prevention of recurrence, the current standard of care is to continue posttransplant HBV prophylaxis indefinitely.

Hepatocellular Carcinoma

LT for HCC is steadily increasing and currently accounts for nearly 18% of all LTs performed (see **Fig. 1**). HCC is the most common indication for MELD exception points because of the increased risk of mortality associated with HCC independent of hepatic function. Currently, increased priority is only given to patients who meet the Milan criteria (1 lesion ≤5 cm or up to 3 lesions each ≤3 cm), which has been found to be associated with a low recurrence rate. Recent discussions focus on expanding these criteria to allow transplant in patients with an acceptably low risk of tumor recurrence but who fall outside the restrictive confines of the Milan criteria. The University of California, San Francisco criteria[40] (1 lesion ≤6.5 cm or 2–3 lesions each ≤4.5 cm with total tumor size ≤8 cm) is one expansion model derived from retrospective analysis of explant tumor pathology that has been independently validated with similar 5-year posttransplant survival rates compared with the Milan criteria (86% vs 81%).[41] However, independent prospective studies using the expanded criteria are still lacking; thus, the use of extended HCC criteria for transplant is not the current standard of care and will vary by center. The role of downstaging tumors with locoregional or systemic therapy also varies considerably in its application across centers but may allow for transplant in patients who are initially outside of the Milan criteria.

Cholangiocarcinoma

Cholangiocarcinoma (CCA) is an aggressive neoplasm of the biliary epithelium. Even when patients present at earlier resectable stages, the recurrence rate of the tumor is high with 5-year survival rates between 20% and 40%.[42,43] Patients with primary sclerosing cholangitis are at increased risk for CCA and were traditionally excluded from transplant evaluation if CCA developed. In 2004, the Mayo Clinic developed a protocol for select patients with perihilar CCA who underwent neoadjuvant external beam irradiation, brachytherapy, and chemotherapy before LT.[44] Outcomes from this single-center experience were promising with 5-year survival rate of 88% posttransplant. On the basis of this experience UNOS approved the allocation of MELD exception points for LT in these patients.[45] Later, a multicenter study of select patients who underwent LT with similar protocols showed a 5-year recurrence-free survival rate of 78% at 2 years and 65% at 5 years, showing the feasibility of wider application of the Mayo protocol to other experienced centers.[46]

Human Immunodeficiency Virus

With the advent of highly active antiretroviral therapy and immense improvement in the prognosis of patients with human immunodeficiency virus (HIV), it is no longer considered a contraindication for orthotopic LT (OLT). The main indications for LT in HIV-infected individuals are co-infection with HCV or HBV with an estimated prevalence of 30% and 10%, respectively, but can reach as high as 80% in hemophiliacs with HIV.[47,48] HIV/HCV co-infection leads to particularly aggressive liver disease with more rapid progression to hepatic fibrosis.[49] The generally accepted immunologic criteria for LT listing in HIV-infected patients is CD4 count greater than 100 cells per cubic millimeter, ideally without prior acquired immunodeficiency syndrome–defining opportunistic infections and an undetectable HIV viral load (<50 copies per milliliter) at the time of transplant.[50] The accumulated evidence has shown that HIV-infected patients with non–HCV-related end-stage liver disease have comparable survival rates after LT to those of other transplant recipients.[51] However, several studies have reported poorer posttransplant outcomes in HIV and HCV co-infected patients. Although short-term 1-year survival after OLT for HIV/HCV co-infected recipients is 88%, 5-year survival rates are significantly lower compared with HCV monoinfected patients at 54%.[52] These poorer outcomes are often attributable to recurrent HCV, including development of its most severe form, fibrosing cholestatic hepatitis. It is hopeful that with more effective post-LT HCV therapy, outcomes for HIV/HCV co-infected individuals will parallel that of HCV monoinfection.

Fulminant Hepatic Failure

Acute liver failure (ALF) or fulminant hepatic failure is granted the highest priority indication for LT. ALF is defined by severe hepatic dysfunction with evidence of coagulopathy (international normalized ratio, $\geq$1.5) and hepatic encephalopathy in a patient without prior liver disease.[53] It is differentiated from acute liver injury (hepatic injury, coagulopathy) by the presence of any degree of encephalopathy. Annually, there are about 2000 cases of ALF in the United States, many of which are caused by acetaminophen toxicity.[54] ALF is associated with a high risk of mortality in the absence of liver transplantation. Any patient suspected of having ALF should be emergently referred to a transplant center for evaluation. The urgency of transplant in these patients is to prevent irreversible cerebral edema associated with ALF; once significant cerebral edema leading to intracranial hypertension has occurred, death is imminent and transplantation is contraindicated. Outcomes after transplant for ALF are comparable to those performed for other indications with a 1-year survival rate of 80%.[55]

IMMUNOSUPPRESSION

Immunosuppression after transplant requires a balance between prevention of graft rejection and minimization of the side effects of immunosuppressive drugs. At most centers, the combination of a calcineurin inhibitor (CNI), steroids, and an antiproliferative drug are used in the immediate posttransplant period (**Box 5**). This triple regimen has

---

Box 5
Common immunosuppressive agents used after transplant

Steroids

Calcineurin inhibitors

    Tacrolimus

    Cyclosporin

Purine analogue or inhibitor of purine salvage pathway

    Mycophenolate mofetil

    Azathioprine

Mammalian targets of rapamycin inhibitors

    Sirolimus

    Everolimus

been found to have superior rates of patient and graft survival compared with dual-agent immunosuppression with CNI and steroids.[56] Over the next several months, steroids are weaned off first but remain the mainstay therapy for the treatment of any acute cellular rejection. Steroid-free immunosuppression is used in some centers with good results. Maintenance immunosuppressive therapy in the long term primarily often consists of CNI monotherapy, although newer potent immunosuppressants, such as sirolimus and everolimus, are being studied as alternatives to spare the side effects of CNI.[57,58]

Box 6
Posttransplant complications and monitoring

Early complications

Hemorrhage

Primary graft nonfunction

Hepatic artery thrombosis

Portal vein, hepatic vein thrombosis

Biliary leak

Biliary stricture

Acute cellular rejection

Infections (bacterial, viral, fungal)

Late complications

Chronic rejection

Recurrent liver disease

   HCV

   HBV

   Autoimmune diseases (primary biliary cirrhosis, primary sclerosing cholangitis, autoimmune hepatitis)

HCC

Long-term monitoring

Obesity

Hypertension

Hyperlipidemia

Cardiovascular disease

Renal insufficiency

Osteoporosis

Secondary malignancies

   Posttransplant lymphoproliferative disorder

   Nonmelanoma skin cancer

   Head and neck cancer

   Lymphoma

   Kaposi's sarcoma

   Colorectal cancer

POSTTRANSPLANT COMPLICATIONS

Complications after LT can be divided into those that occur in the early stages, which are often caused by the surgical complexity of transplantation, and those that occur in later stages, which are related to graft rejection, recurrence of primary liver disease, and management of chronic medical conditions (**Box 6**). Two serious early complications require prompt recognition, as they may necessitate emergent retransplant: hepatic artery thrombosis (HAT) and primary graft nonfunction. The incidence of HAT is 4.4%, and it is associated with a high overall mortality rate of 33%.[59] Early detection of this complication when the patient is still asymptomatic is critical, so revascularization can be attempted to salvage the graft.[60] Despite attempts at revascularization, the rate of retransplant for HAT is still 53%.[59] Primary liver graft nonfunction is also a rare but life-threatening condition characterized by acute hepatic failure with rapidly rising transaminases, absent bile production, marked coagulopathy, encephalopathy, and hemodynamic instability and is usually fatal without retransplant. Fortunately, the survival rates after retransplant for primary graft nonfunction is not significantly different than those for other indications of retransplant.[61] Both of these early complications of transplant are indications for UNOS status 1A listing for retransplant because of the high risk of mortality.

As the results after LT continued to improve over the last few decades, increasing attention has been directed toward management of preexisting or de novo chronic medical conditions and some unique long-term complications of LT. LT recipients are known to have an increased risk of metabolic syndrome including obesity, diabetes, hypertension, hyperlipidemia, and cardiovascular disease.[62–65] Management of these chronic medical conditions and their risk factor modification are critical to ensure continued excellent graft function and overall survival of the recipient decades after transplant. Additionally, LT recipients are at increased risk for a variety of de novo malignancies owing to long-term immunosuppression as well as recurrence of any primary hepatic malignancy in the posttransplant setting (see **Box 6**). Transplant recipients should continue to receive all routine age-appropriate cancer screening and targeted evaluation of specific malignancies if symptoms arise. Lastly, recurrence of the primary hepatic disease can occur for all autoimmune-based liver diseases and viral hepatitis, with the most challenging problem being recurrent HCV, as discussed previously. With newer direct-acting antiviral agents being developed, we should be optimistic that successful treatment of recurrent HCV with interferon-free regimens will be accessible and feasible in the near future.

REFERENCES

1. Organ procurement and Transplantation Network data as of July 8, 2014. Available at: http://optn.transplant.hrsa.gov. Accessed July 19, 2014.
2. Saunders JB, Walters JR, Davies P, et al. A 20-year prospective study of cirrhosis. Br Med J (Clin Res Ed) 1981;282:263–6.
3. Gines P, Quintero E, Arroyo V. Compensated cirrhosis: natural history and prognosis. Hepatology 1987;7:122–8.
4. Kamath PS, Wiesner RH, Malinchoc M, et al. A model to predict survival in patients with end-stage liver disease. Hepatology 2001;33:464–70.
5. Malinchoc M, Kamath PS, Gordon FD, et al. A model to predict poor survival in patients undergoing transjugular intrahepatic portosystemic shunts. Hepatology 2000;31:864–71.

6. Freeman RB, Gish RG, Harper A, et al. Model for end-stage liver disease (MELD) exception guidelines: results and recommendations from the MELD Exception Study Group and Conference (MESSAGE) for the approval of patients who need liver transplantation with diseases not considered by the standard MELD formula. Liver Transpl 2006;12:S128–36.

7. Nair S, Verma S, Thuluvath PJ. Obesity and its effect on survival in patients undergoing orthotopic liver transplantation in the United States. Hepatology 2002;35: 105–9.

8. Martin R, DiMartini A, Feng S, et al. AASLD practice guidelines: evaluation for liver transplantation in adults. Hepatology 2014;59:1144–65.

9. Swanson KL, Wiesner RH, Nyberg SL, et al. Survival in portopulmonary hypertension: Mayo Clinic experience categorized by treatment subgroups. Am J Transplant 2008;8:2445–53.

10. Arguedas MR, Abrams GA, Krowka MJ, et al. Prospective evaluation of outcomes and predictors of mortality in patients with hepatopulmonary syndrome undergoing liver transplantation. Hepatology 2003;37:192–7.

11. Cameron AM, Ghobrial RM, Yersiz H, et al. Optimal utilization of donor grafts with extended criteria: a single- center experience in over 1000 liver transplants. Ann Surg 2006;243:748–53.

12. Merion RM, Rush SH, Dykstra DM, et al. Predicted lifetimes for adult and pediatric split liver versus adult whole liver transplant recipients. Am J Transplant 2004;4:1792–7.

13. Pichlmayr R, Ringe B, Gubernatis G, et al. Transplantation of a donor liver to 2 recipients (splitting transplantation)–a new method in the further development of segmental liver transplantation. Langenbecks Arch Chir 1988;373:127–30 [in German].

14. Cauley RP, Vakili K, Fullington N, et al. Deceased-donor split-liver transplantation in adult recipients: is the learning curve over? J Am Coll Surg 2013;217:672–84.e1.

15. Doyle MB, Maynard E, Lin Y, et al. Outcomes with split liver transplantation are equivalent to those with whole organ transplantation. J Am Coll Surg 2013;217: 102–12 [discussion: 113].

16. Abt P, Crawford M, Desai N, et al. Liver transplantation from controlled non-heart-beating donors: an increased incidence of biliary complications. Transplantation 2003;75:1659–63.

17. Foley DP, Fernandez LA, Laverson G, et al. Donation after cardiac death: the University of Wisconsin experience with liver transplantation. Ann Surg 2005;242: 724–31.

18. Berg CL, Gillespie BW, Merion RM, et al. Improvement in survival associated with adult-to-adult living donor liver transplantation. Gastroenterology 2007;133: 1806–13.

19. Freise CE, Gillespie BW, Koffron AJ, et al. Recipient morbidity after living and deceased donor liver transplantation: findings from the A2ALL Retrospective Cohort Study. Am J Transplant 2008;8:2569–79.

20. Ghobrial RM, Freise CE, Trotter JF, et al. Donor morbidity after living donation for liver transplantation. Gastroenterology 2006;135:468–76.

21. Trotter JF, Adam R, Lo CM, et al. Documented deaths of hepatic lobe donors for living donor liver transplantation. Liver Transpl 2006;12:1485–8.

22. Lim JK, Keeffe EB. Liver transplantation for alcoholic liver disease: current concepts and length of sobriety. Liver Transpl 2004;10:S31–8.

23. Everhart JE, Beresford TP. Liver transplantation for alcoholic liver disease: a survey of transplantation programs in the United States. Liver Transpl Surg 1997;3: 220–6.

24. Cuadrado A, Fabrega E, Casafont F, et al. Alcohol recidivism impairs long-term patient survival after orthotopic liver transplantation for alcoholic liver disease. Liver Transpl 2005;11:420–6.

25. Pageaux GP, Bismuth M, Penny P, et al. Alcohol relapse after liver transplantation for alcoholic liver disease: does it matter? J Hepatol 2003;38:629–34.

26. Garcia-Retortillo M, Forns X, Feliu A, et al. Hepatitis C kinetics during and immediately after transplantation. Hepatology 2002;35:680–7.

27. Everson GT, Trotter J, Forman L, et al. Treatment of advanced hepatitis C with a low accelerating dosage regimen of antiviral therapy. Hepatology 2005;42:255–62.

28. Forman LM, Lewis JD, Berlin JA, et al. The association between hepatitis C infection and survival after orthotopic liver transplantation. Gastroenterology 2002;122:889–96.

29. Berenguer M. Natural history of recurrent hepatitis C. Liver Transpl 2002;8:S14–8.

30. Gane EJ. The natural history of recurrent hepatitis C and what influences this. Liver Transpl 2008;14(Suppl 2):S36–44.

31. Berenguer M, Prieto M, Rayón JM, et al. Natural history of clinically compensated hepatitis C virus-related graft cirrhosis after liver trans- plantation. Hepatology 2000;32:852–8.

32. McCashland T, Watt K, Lyden E, et al. Retransplantation for HCV: results of a US multicenter transplant study. Liver Transpl 2007;12:1246–53.

33. Fontana RJ, Hughes EA, Bifano M, et al. Sofosbuvir and daclatasvir combination therapy in a liver transplant recipient with severe recurrent cholestatic hepatitis c. Am J Transplant 2013;13:1601–5.

34. Kim WR, Poterucha JJ, Kremers WK, et al. Outcome of liver transplantation for hepatitis B in the United States. Liver Transpl 2004;10:968–74.

35. Todo S, Demetris AJ, Van Thiel D, et al. Orthotopic liver transplantation for patients with hepatitis B virus-related liver disease. Hepatology 1991;13:619–26.

36. Angus PW, McCaughan GW, Gane EJ, et al. Combination low-dose hepatitis B immune globulin and lamivudine therapy provides effective prophylaxis against posttransplantation hepatitis B. Liver Transpl 2000;6:429–33.

37. Gane EJ, Angus PW, Strasser S, et al. Lamivudine plus low-dose hepatitis B immunoglobulin to prevent recurrent hepatitis B following liver transplantation. Gastroenterology 2007;132:931–7.

38. Wadhawan MG, Vij V, Goyal N, et al. Living related liver transplant (LRLT) in HBV DNA negative cirrhosis without hepatitis B immune globulin (HBIG). Hepatol Int 2011;5:38 [50].

39. Fung J, Cheung C, Chan SC, et al. Entecavir monotherapy is effective in suppressing hepatitis B virus after liver transplantation. Gastroenterology 2011;141:1212–9.

40. Yao FY, Ferrell L, Bass NM, et al. Liver transplantation for hepatocellular carcinoma: expansion of the tumor size limits does not adversely impact survival. Hepatology 2001;33:1394–403.

41. Duffy JP, Vardanian A, Benjamin E, et al. Liver transplantation criteria for hepatocellular carcinoma should be expanded: a 22-year experience with 467 patients at UCLA. Ann Surg 2007;246:502–11.

42. Kobayashi A, Miwa S, Nakata T, et al. Disease recurrence patterns after R0 resection of hilar cholangiocarcinoma. Br J Surg 2010;97:56–64.

43. Washburn WK, Lewis WD, Jenkins RL. Aggressive surgical resection for cholangiocarcinoma. Arch Surg 1995;130:270–6.

44. Heimbach JK, Gores GJ, Haddock MG, et al. Liver transplantation for unresectable perihilar cholangiocarcinoma. Semin Liver Dis 2004;24:201–7.

45. Gores GJ, Gish RG, Sudan D, et al. Model for end-stage liver disease (MELD) exception for cholangiocarcinoma or biliary dysplasia. Liver Transpl 2006;12: S95–7.

46. Murad DS, Kim WR, Harnois DM, et al. Efficacy of neoadjuvant chemoradiation followed by liver transplantation, for perihilar cholangiocarcinoma at 12 US centers. Gastroenterology 2012;143:88–98.

47. Ragni MV, Belle SH. Impact of human immunodeficiency virus infection on progression to end-stage liver disease in individuals with hemophilia and hepatitis C virus infection. J Infect Dis 2001;183:1112–5.

48. Soriano V, Barreiro P, Nunez M. Management of chronic hepatitis B and C in HIV-coinfected patients. J Antimicrob Chemother 2006;57:815–8.

49. Fauci AS, Schnittman SM, Poli G, et al. Immunopathogenetic mechanisms in human immunodeficiency virus (HIV) infection. Ann Intern Med 1991;114: 678–93.

50. Miro JM, Laguno M, Moreno A, et al, Hospital Clinic OLT in HIV Working Group. Management of end stage liver disease (ESLD): what is the current role of orthotopic liver transplantation (OLT)? J Hepatol 2006;44(1 Suppl):S140–5.

51. Mindikoglu AL, Regev A, Magder LS. Impact of human immunodeficiency virus on survival after liver transplantation: analysis of United Network for Organ Sharing database. Transplantation 2008;85:359–68.

52. Miro JM, Montejo M, Castells L, et al. Outcome of HCV/HIV-coinfected liver transplant recipients: a prospective and multicenter cohort study. Am J Transplant 2012;12:1866–76.

53. Trey C, Davidson CS. The management of fulminant hepatic failure. In: Popper H, Schaffner F, editors. Progress in liver diseases. New York: Grune & Stratton; 1970. p. 282–98.

54. Polson J, Lee WM, American Association for the Study of Liver Disease. AASLD position paper: the management of acute liver failure. Hepatology 2005;41:1179–97.

55. Larson AM, Polson J, Fontana RJ, et al. Acetaminophen-induced acute liver failure: results of a United States multicenter, prospective study. Hepatology 2005; 42:1364–72.

56. Wiesner RH, Shorr JS, Steffen BJ, et al. Mycophenolate mofetil combination therapy improves long-term outcomes after liver transplantation in patients with and without hepatitis C. Liver Transpl 2005;11:750.

57. Levy G, Schmidli H, Punch J, et al. Safety, tolerability, and efficacy of everolimus in de novo liver transplant recipients: 12- and 36-month results. Liver Transpl 2006;12:1640–8.

58. Zaghla H, Selby RR, Chan LS, et al. A comparison of sirolimus vs. calcineurin inhibitor-based immunosuppressive therapies in liver transplantation. Aliment Pharmacol Ther 2006;23:513–20.

59. Bekker J, Ploem S, de Jong KP. Early hepatic artery thrombosis after liver transplantation: a systematic review of the incidence, outcomes and risk factors. Am J Transplant 2009;9:746–57.

60. Duffy JP, Hong JC, Farmer DG, et al. Vascular complications of orthotopic liver transplantation: experience in more than 4,200 patients. J Am Coll Surg 2009; 208:896–903 [discussion: 903].

61. Uemura T, Randall HB, Sanchez EQ, et al. Liver retransplantation for primary nonfunction: analysis of a 20-year single-center experience. Liver Transpl 2007;13: 227–33.

62. Richards J, Gunson B, Johnson J, et al. Weight gain and obesity after liver transplantation. Transpl Int 2005;18:461–6.

63. Akarsu M, Bakir Y, Karademir S, et al. Prevalence and risk factors for obesity after liver transplantation: a single-center experience. Hepat Mon 2013;13:e7569.
64. Baid S, Cosimi AB, Farrell ML, et al. Posttransplant diabetes mellitus in liver transplant recipients: risk factors, temporal relationship with hepatitis C virus allograft hepatitis, and impact on mortality. Transplantation 2001;72:1066–72.
65. Johnston SD, Morris JK, Cramb R, et al. Cardiovascular morbidity and mortality after orthotopic liver transplantation. Transplantation 2002;73:901–6.

Assessment of Jaundice in the Hospitalized Patient

 CrossMark

Priya Kathpalia, MD[a], Joseph Ahn, MD, MS[b],*

KEYWORDS

- Jaundice • Cholestasis • Hyperbilirubinemia • Benign postoperative jaundice
- Cholestasis of sepsis

KEY POINTS

- Jaundice signifies a disorder in bilirubin metabolism.
- A thorough assessment of the clinical history and physical exam findings together with laboratory analysis and imaging studies are required to determine the cause of jaundice.
- The clinician must be able to recognize which conditions associated with jaundice warrant urgent endoscopy or evaluation for liver transplantation.

OVERVIEW

Jaundice originates from the Latin word "galbinus," which describes a yellow-green color. Icterus comes from the Greek word "ikteros," which meant both yellow bird and jaundice; historically, yellow birds were used as a "cure" for jaundice.[1] However, it has since come to be understood that jaundice is not a disease but rather a feature of disordered bilirubin metabolism that often signifies liver dysfunction. In general, the yellow discoloration occurs as a result of bilirubin deposition in the sclerae, mucosa, and skin when levels rise higher than 3 mg/dL.[2] Management is aimed at identifying and addressing the cause of the dysregulation in bilirubin metabolism.

Jaundice in the hospitalized patient is not an uncommon consultation for the general gastroenterologist. The National Hospital Ambulatory Medical Care Survey analyzed more than 1 billion emergency department visits from 1995 to 2004 and found that 400,000 patients had a diagnosis of jaundice. Nearly 50% of these were older than age 15; certainly the frequency and cause of jaundice depends on the patient population being studied.[3]

Disclosures: None.
[a] Division of Gastroenterology and Hepatology, University of California, San Francisco, 513 Parnassus Avenue, Med Sci Room S-356, San Francisco, CA 94143, USA; [b] Division of Gastroenterology and Hepatology, Oregon Health & Science University, 3181 Southwest Sam Jackson Park Road, Portland, OR 97239–3098, USA
* Corresponding author.
E-mail address: ahnj@ohsu.edu

Clin Liver Dis 19 (2015) 155–170
http://dx.doi.org/10.1016/j.cld.2014.09.009
1089-3261/15/$ – see front matter © 2015 Elsevier Inc. All rights reserved.

This article provides a systematic approach to evaluating jaundice in adult patients with a focus on conditions that require urgent endoscopic intervention or evaluation for liver transplantation.

PATHOGENESIS

More than 75% of bilirubin is made from senescent red blood cell (RBC) breakdown in the reticuloendothelial system, with the remaining coming from ineffective RBC production or heme proteins, such as myoglobin and cytochrome enzymes.[2,4] Hepatocytes take up and conjugate this bilirubin within the sinusoids before excretion in the biliary tree.

Unconjugated bilirubin is fat-soluble, allowing it to cross the blood-brain barrier. In the newborn, it is this unconjugated hyperbilirubinemia that can lead to kernicterus. Unconjugated bilirubin becomes conjugated via the glucuronosyltransferase enzyme; in this form, the bilirubin becomes soluble in bile. Conjugated bilirubin can then be transported to the gallbladder where it is stored, transported to the duodenum to be excreted in stool, or converted into urobilinogen and excreted via the kidney (**Fig. 1**). The components of bile are integral for fat metabolism, absorption of fat-soluble vitamins, and excretion of bilirubin and its waste products.

It is postulated that bile flow can be altered by specific cytokines (tumor necrosis factor-α, interleukin-1 and -6) by upregulating expression of intercellular adhesion molecules, which in turn alters bile flow.[5] Bile flow can also be affected by endotoxins and exotoxins that are associated with infections or inflammatory states. Thus it is not surprising that common causes of hyperbilirubinemia encompass various viral and bacterial infectious etiologies.

Highlights:
- Bilirubin is produced by senescent RBC breakdown, ineffective RBC production, and heme proteins
- The enzyme glucuronosyltransferase conjugates bilirubin, which is then converted to urobilinogen in the liver before being stored or excreted in the bile ducts
- Bile flow can be altered by cytokines in inflammatory states

DIFFERENTIAL DIAGNOSIS

Rather than providing an exhaustive differential, this article focuses on the most common conditions and those diagnoses that should not be missed.

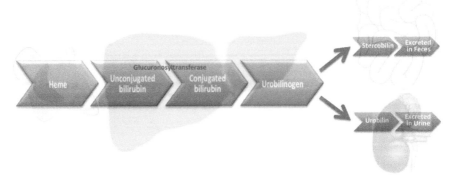

Fig. 1. Overview of bilirubin metabolism.

Isolated Disorders of Bilirubin Metabolism

Jaundice may be a result of a primarily nonhepatic cause that results in dysregulation of bilirubin metabolism (**Fig. 2**). Conditions that result in an increased heme load, such as hemolytic anemias, resorption of hematomas, excessive blood transfusions, and ineffective erythropoiesis (ie, from thalassemias), increase unconjugated bilirubin production. A genetic condition, Gilbert syndrome, affects 3% to 7% of the population and leads to isolated unconjugated hyperbilirubinemia.[6,7] In this entirely benign condition, the glucuronosyltransferase enzyme is impaired, especially in situations of stress, such as after surgery, pain, or fasting with a resultant elevation of total bilirubin as high as 5.3 mg/dL reported in some studies.[8]

Major Points:
- Conditions that increase heme protein load can result in unconjugated hyperbilirubinemia
- Gilbert syndrome, a benign genetic condition, can also lead to impaired bilirubin conjugation

Extrahepatic Disease Processes

Certain extrahepatic diseases can also lead to jaundice and must be considered in the differential, especially if patients present with isolated bilirubin elevation. The most common cause of extrahepatic biliary obstruction is choledocholithiasis, which can lead to hyperbilirubinemia with associated elevations in aspartate aminotransferase, alanine aminotransferase, and alkaline phosphatase. Superimposed infections in patients with choledocholithiasis can result in acute cholangitis (discussed later).

Choledocholithiasis is often associated with concurrent abdominal pain but can also be asymptomatic. Biliary obstruction can also be caused by strictures related to cholangiocarcinoma; pancreatic cancer; metastatic disease to adjacent lymph nodes; postoperative strictures (after cholecystectomy or liver transplantation); or external compression of the common bile duct by a cystic duct stone or stone in the neck of the gallbladder, known as Mirizzi syndrome. Primary sclerosing cholangitis often occurs in the setting of inflammatory bowel disease (primarily ulcerative colitis) and can lead to tight strictures that impair bile flow. Large pancreatic cysts or pseudocysts, especially at the head of the pancreas, can also lead to similar compression. In addition, abscesses or larger fluid collections can also cause external compression

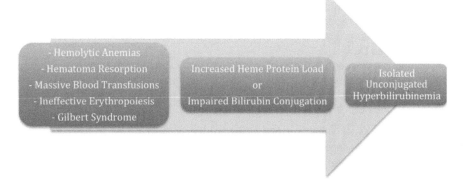

Fig. 2. Disease states leading to isolated unconjugated hyperbilirubinemia.

of the biliary tree. Bilomas may develop after cholecystectomy or other intra-abdominal procedures and can result in external compression of the biliary tree.[9]

Major Points:
- Choledocholithiasis and biliary strictures can lead to extrahepatic cholestasis

Intrahepatic Disease Processes

Intrahepatic disease processes that cause jaundice involve a mixed hepatocellular and cholestatic process, generally involving pathology that affects the parenchyma and bile ducts. Thus the differential for hepatocellular jaundice is broad, ranging from (1) acute liver injury or acute liver failure, (2) chronic liver diseases with predominant hepatocellular injury, and (3) infiltrative diseases with more prominent cholestasis than hepatocellular injury.

Acute liver injury or acute liver failure

Jaundice is often the presenting sign in patients with no previous liver disease who develop acute liver injury or failure. Acute liver injury and acute liver failure involve elevated serum aminotransferases with a new coagulopathy (international normalized ratio ≥ 1.5). In the latter, hepatic encephalopathy is also present distinguishing between the two entities and signifying a worse prognosis. Known causes include toxin or drug-induced liver injury (DILI), autoimmune hepatitis, ischemic hepatitis, and viral hepatitis. Viral hepatitis must be excluded with diagnostic testing for hepatitis A, B, and C. Hepatitis D must be considered in patients with underlying chronic hepatitis B, or in those with risk factors for parenteral transmission of viral hepatitis. Hepatitis E should be considered in the immunosuppressed patient and in those with exposure risk factors. Although rare, Wilson disease can also present as acute liver failure; this diagnosis should be considered and not missed, especially in young patients.[10]

DILI is one of the more common causes of acute liver injury that can present as jaundice within days or weeks of starting a new medication. Zimmerman[11,12] reported that a three-fold elevation of transaminases and a two-fold increase in total bilirubin without overt symptoms of cholestasis, in the absence of other causes of acute liver injury, portended worse outcomes with a mortality of 10% to 50%. Given the potential for significant severity and high mortality of DILI, clinicians should have a high suspicion for DILI in patients presenting with jaundice after starting on antibiotics or other new medications.[5,11–14] Various medications have been known to cause DILI (**Box 1**). Antibiotics including penicillin derivatives, erythromycin, antituberculosis drugs (ethambutol, isoniazid), nitrofurantoin, and antifungals have all been cited as causes.[11,12,14–16] Aside from antibiotics, however, various antihypertensive agents, including the commonly prescribed β-blockers and angiotensin-converting enzyme inhibitors, have been reported as being associated with DILI. In addition, antiepileptics and mood-stabilizing agents including valproic acid and phenytoin have also been known to cause DILI.

In addition, a thorough history should be obtained to exclude the use of any herbal or nonprescribed supplements or over-the-counter medications. Various weight loss and body building supplements, in addition to herbal remedies targeted as joint pain remedies, have been implicated in DILI.[17]

Chronic liver diseases

Patients with underlying chronic liver disease can present with hyperbilirubinemia as their initial presentation. Thus, underlying viral hepatitis, alcoholic liver disease, hemochromatosis, α_1-antitrypsin deficiency, nonalcoholic steatohepatitis, primary biliary cirrhosis, and autoimmune hepatitis should be considered because they can lead to

---

Box 1
Various medications known to cause drug-induced liver injury

Analgesics: Nonsteroidal anti-inflammatory drugs, gold salts

Antibiotics: Amoxicillin-clavulanic acid, flucloxacillin, erythromycin, ethambutol, fluconazole, isoniazid, nitrofurantoin, rifampin, sulfamethoxazole, terbinafine

Anticonvulsants: Phenytoin, valproic acid

Antihypertensives: Angiotensin-converting enzyme inhibitors, β-blockers, methyldopa

Hormonal agents: Androgens, estrogens, oral contraceptives, tamoxifen

Immunosuppresants: Azathioprine, cyclosporine

Psychotropic medications: Benzodiazepines, tricyclic antidepressants

Herbal remedies: Hydroxycut, green tea, anabolic steroids, kava, glucosamine

---

fibrosis and cirrhosis. Patients with new-onset jaundice with underlying chronic liver disease should be evaluated as to the cause of their decompensation, such as infection, development of hepatocellular carcinoma, or cholangiocarcinoma, in addition to the common causes of acute liver injury described previously. In addition, DILI portends a worse prognosis in patients with underlying chronic liver disease.

Infiltrative diseases
Although these conditions can also become chronic, they present with more of a cholestatic process than hepatocellular injury; the first clinical symptom is often jaundice. Malignancies (primarily lymphomas), amyloidosis, tuberculosis, various vasculitides, sarcoidosis, granulomatous hepatitis, and stricturing biliary diseases are among those diseases known to infiltrate the liver that must be considered in patients presenting with jaundice.

Major Points:
- Acute liver failure entails acute liver injury with signs of coagulopathy
- DILI is one of the more common causes of acute liver injury. Several medications have been implicated (see **Box 1**)
- Chronic and infiltrative liver diseases can lead to jaundice depending on the extent and severity of underlying condition

Entities Not to Be Missed

Acute cholangitis
Patients can develop acute ascending cholangitis when there is an obstruction of the bile duct with a superimposed bacterial infection. Although underlying choledocholithiasis is the most common cause of cholangitis, primary sclerosing cholangitis with severe stricturing disease and malignancies causing alteration of bile have also been known to be causes of cholangitis.

In addition to sudden-onset jaundice, up to 75% of patients with acute cholangitis present with concurrent right upper quadrant pain and fever, collectively known as Charcot triad.[18] Given the pathology, these patients often have hyperbilirubinemia and elevated alkaline phosphatase, although early in the course of the disease it is not uncommon to have a disproportionate elevated serum aminotransferases that can mimic viral hepatitis.[18,19] Diagnosis is generally made based on the clinical presentation, although imaging studies can help confirm the diagnosis; ultrasound often reveals the presence of gallstones, whereas computed tomography (CT) of the abdomen better delineates the biliary tree and can identify ductal dilatation.

Once diagnosis is suspected, aggressive intravenous hydration and broad-spectrum antibiotics should be initiated. Endoscopic retrograde cholangiopancreatography (ERCP) allows for diagnostic and therapeutic intervention (biliary stent placement, stone removal, sphincterotomy, and so forth) and should be performed urgently, or emergently if the patient is in septic shock.[20]

Benign postoperative jaundice

Before 1990, posttransfusion hepatitis was a significant concern in patients presenting with jaundice in the immediate postoperative period. However, with improvements in screening methods before transfusion, this is no longer a significant issue. There are a variety of scenarios that can cause postoperative jaundice (**Box 2**). One must consider Gilbert syndrome that may have gone unrecognized before surgery but becomes apparent because of the stress of surgery. Another entity is directly related to the amount of blood transfusions required during prolonged operations; these patients can experience isolated, mainly indirect hyperbilirubinemia within 2 to 4 days after surgery because of the excessive heme load from the blood transfusions.

In addition, depending on the anesthetics or induction drugs used, and their modes of excretion, in combination with the degree of ischemia and hypoperfusion experienced intraoperatively, isolated hyperbilirubinemia and transient jaundice are not uncommon.[21]

Patients undergoing any degree of liver resection can experience jaundice as a result of hepatic insufficiency. In these patients, jaundice can persist for weeks to months until the liver regenerates.[22]

Despite notable jaundice and bilirubin reaching as high as 40 mg/dL, synthetic liver functioning is generally preserved in these patients; therefore, the clinician can distinguish this condition from acute liver injury or acute liver failure.[23]

Cholestasis of sepsis

Cholestasis of sepsis was first described in 1836 after a patient with sepsis related to lobar pneumonia presented with jaundice.[24] Since then, it has become a well-recognized condition thought to occur secondary to abnormalities in the breakdown of bilirubin itself caused by hepatocyte dysfunction or from an excess of bilirubin production (**Box 3**). In the patient with sepsis, excess bilirubin production may be secondary to cholestasis, ischemia from prolonged hypotension or hypoxia, or direct hepatocellular injury. Depending on the antibiotics used for management of sepsis, superimposed DILI is not uncommon and can potentiate hepatic injury. Sulfa drugs, penicillin derivatives, and cephalosporins in particular have been implicated in this setting.[16]

Box 2
Questions for the clinician to consider in patients with postoperative jaundice

Does the patient have underlying Gilbert syndrome?

Did the patient receive significant blood transfusions intraoperatively?

Were hepatically metabolized anesthetics used at time of induction?

Did the patient experience hypotension intraoperatively?

Did the patient undergo some degree of liver resection?

Box 3
Mechanisms leading to cholestasis of sepsis

1. Ischemia/hypoperfusion
2. Hepatocellular injury
3. Drug-induced liver injury
4. Hemolysis, toxin production

Hemolysis, either intravascular or extravascular, can also lead to increased bilirubin production. Prior studies, dating back to the 1980s, have suggested that toxin production itself during septic states can lead to profound hemolysis and even shock. For example, 52 patients with toxic shock syndrome caused by *Staphylococcus aureus*–related infections related to tampon use were studied in one case series; at least 50% of these patients had hyperbilirubinemia and transamintis thought to be related to the bacterial exotoxin production.[25,26] Aside from *S aureus*, exotoxin from *Clostridium perfringens* has been found to cause massive hemolytic anemia that can lead to hyperbilirubinemia and jaundice, and endotoxin produced by *Salmonella typhi* causes direct necrosis of the hepatocytes. Sepsis itself, a profound inflammatory state, can lead to massive cytokine production that can contribute to cholestasis and even direct hepatocyte injury as seen in severe cases of *Salmonella* infection.[16] Although cholestasis and elevated serum aminotransferases in these patients can be severe, studies have shown that these findings are not necessarily related to the severity of the infection and generally improve rapidly with resolution of the underlying sepsis.[27]

Intrahepatic cholestasis of pregnancy

As of 2010, the prevalence of intrahepatic cholestasis of pregnancy (ICP) was reported to be 0.001% to 0.32% in the United States, and 2% to 4% in Scandinavia and Chile. The Hispanic population within the United States has been noted to have an especially high predilection possibly because of genetic predisposition, hormonal variations, and nutritional differences.[28,29] Although a relatively rare diagnosis, ICP is the most common reason for consultation for liver abnormalities in the pregnant patient.[30] The clinician must be able to distinguish jaundice caused by ICP from acute fatty liver of pregnancy (often associated with multiorgan impairment, disseminated intravascular coagulation, or preeclampsia) and other causes of hepatitis.

ICP is generally a result of a genetic mutation in the transporter responsible for the excretion of bile salts; the defect is more prominent with increased levels of estrogen, as in pregnancy or with oral contraceptive use.[31] Interestingly, multiparity is considered a risk factor for cholestasis of pregnancy because of the higher estrogen levels. Symptoms often occur late in the second or early in the third trimester of pregnancy when estrogen levels are at their highest. Aside from being jaundiced, these pregnant patients often complain of extreme pruritus in the limbs, hands, and feet. Laboratory testing reveals an increase in serum total bile salts, serum bilirubin (rarely higher than 5–6 mg/dL), and alkaline phosphatase levels, produced by the bile canaliculi and the placenta.[32,33] Although predominantly a cholestatic process, this diagnosis may also be associated with mild elevated serum aminotransferases, with aspartate aminotransferase and alanine aminotransferase levels rarely exceeding 200 IU/L.[34] If clinical suspicion is high, and other etiologies have been excluded, there is no need to perform liver biopsy in these patients.

Prognosis is excellent for the mother without associated mortality, although the pruritus can be especially burdensome closer to term.[35] Ursodeoxycholic acid is a pregnancy category B drug, and is widely used to ameliorate the symptoms of pruritus. Cholestyramine and antihistamines, such as hydroxyzine, must be used with caution because they are pregnancy category C drugs and may lead to vitamin K malabsorption and neonatal withdrawal syndrome, respectively. However, fetal demise has been reported at 11% in some studies and is thought to be caused by cardiac conduction abnormalities and arrythmias that may occur as unexcreted bile salts cross the placenta.[28,36,37] Thus, fetal monitoring is often performed more frequently in the last trimester in this patient population and labor is often induced at the first sign of fetal distress or by 37 weeks.[32,38]

Post–bone marrow transplant syndromes

Despite strides made in the treatment of hematologic malignancies, the liver can become affected by the side effects of induction therapies, such as high-dose chemotherapy and radiation used before allogeneic hematopoietic stem cell transplantation (HSCT). Veno-occlusive disease (VOD) is thought to occur about 20 to 30 days after HSCT and has an incidence of 10% to 60% depending on the type and dosage of conditioning regimen.[39]

Although the exact inciting event that leads to VOD is unclear, some degree of damage occurs in the hepatic venules that eventually leads to obliteration and necrosis of the centrilobular zones of the liver. Because the sinusoidal endothelial cells are more often affected than hepatic venules, it was proposed that the name be changed from VOD to sinusoidal obstruction syndrome (SOS); hence, these two terms are often used interchangeably.[40]

Patients who have had prior HSCT, who received abdominal irradiation or conditioning regimens with busulfan/melphalan, or who have known underlying liver diseases are more likely to develop VOD/SOS complications post-HSCT. These patients generally present with jaundice, abdominal pain from capsular stretching caused by hepatomegaly, and fluid retention or ascites as outflow obstruction ensues.[41] Bilirubin levels are generally greater than 2 mg/dL. Diagnosis is generally made clinically and generally liver biopsy is unnecessary. Treatment is supportive and aimed at symptom control: diuretics and salt restriction and removal of any potential hepatotoxic agents are key.

VOD/SOS can be difficult to distinguish from acute graft-versus-host disease (GVHD) that generally occurs 3 weeks post-HSCT as engraftment ensues. In addition to cholestasis, GVHD patients generally have hepatocellular injury as evidenced by elevated serum aminotransferases. Unlike VOD/SOS, GVHD rarely causes liver injury alone and causes more systemic symptoms; these patients often have intestinal or skin manifestations that can help to distinguish this condition.[42] Transjugular liver biopsy may be useful to distinguish VOD/SOS from GVHD if the diagnosis is unclear because the treatment of the latter involves more aggressive immunosuppressive regimens that would be ineffective for the former diagnosis.[43]

Major Points:
- Acute cholangitis: Underlying choledocholithiasis, stricturing disease, or malignancies altering bile flow can lead to cholangitis and often require emergent ERCP
- Benign postoperative jaundice: Gilbert syndrome, liver hypoperfusion intraoperatively, massive blood transfusions perioperatively, and various anesthetics can lead to isolated hyperbilirubinemia

- Cholestasis of sepsis: Cytokines released during infectious states, particularly during sepsis, can lead to ischemia, direct hepatocellular injury, or hemolysis that leads to cholestasis
- ICP: Genetic mutations can result in ICP in the pregnant patient during the late second or early third trimester and can be fatal to the fetus
- Post–bone marrow transplant syndromes: SOS must be distinguished from acute GVHD

DIAGNOSTIC APPROACH

A careful history with a thorough review of systems and physical examination help aid in the diagnosis of jaundice in the hospitalized patient. Chopra and Griffin[44] reported, "The diagnosis of jaundiced caused by extrahepatic biliary obstruction can be made with 90% accuracy from results of only the medical history, physical examination, and routine laboratory tests." Pasanen and coworkers[45] studied 220 patients with jaundice and created a diagnostic scoring system (using duration of jaundice, serum protein levels, age, and presence of fevers) to help compare the sensitivity and specificity of clinical evaluation and imaging modalities; clinical evaluation alone had a sensitivity of 86% without adding any other studies to help aid in the diagnosis. Although clinical history and examination plays a large role in diagnosing the cause of the jaundice, laboratory markers and imaging studies can provide further insight on the underlying pathology.

History

The clinical presentation of jaundice can vary from being an incidental finding with mild scleral icterus to overt discoloration throughout the body. When evaluating a patient with jaundice, the timing of symptoms and the rate of development of jaundice can be essential in making the diagnosis. The presence of abdominal pain or symptoms may point toward choledocholithiasis.

In addition, the clinician should ask in detail about alcohol and drug use, the route of drug administration, use of any over-the-counter medications or herbal remedies, sexual and travel histories, tattoos and in what type of setting they were placed, history of prior blood transfusions, prior surgeries, presence of similar symptoms previously, and any significant family history. It is important to assess for underlying chronic liver disease and/or occult cirrhosis and the possibility of undiagnosed congenital liver diseases.

A thorough review of symptoms with special consideration to constitutional symptoms, color of urine and stool, weight loss, pruritus, abdominal pain, and associated arthralgias and malaise can help provide clues to distinguishing between the possible etiologies of the jaundice (**Box 4**).

Major Points:
- It is essential to understand the rate of development of jaundice and timing of symptoms to help establish the underlying diagnosis
- A detailed social and medication history can help provide clues as to the diagnosis

---

Box 4
Key findings in the history that may point toward a certain diagnosis

Infectious etiology: Fevers, chills, fatigue, nausea and vomiting, acute-onset jaundice

Noninfectious etiology: Pruritus, weight loss, abdominal pain

Autoimmune etiology: Arthralgias, malaise, fatigue, slow-onset jaundice

Physical Examination

Certain findings on the physical examination alone can help determine the severity and cause of the underlying liver disease. For example, the clinician may perform a more extensive work-up for chronic liver disease if spider angiomata, palmar erythema, Dupuytren contractures, ascites, caput medusa, or clubbing are observed on examination. If Wilson disease is suspected, an ophthalmologic consultation should be obtained to look for Kayser-Fleischer rings or sunflower cataracts. Hyperpigmentation of the skin and metacarpal changes together with signs of cardiomyopathy (jugular venous distention or extra S3 or S4 heart sounds) point the clinician to consider the diagnosis of hereditary hemochromatosis.

Major Points:
- A thorough physical examination can help identify signs of end-stage liver disease
- Wilson disease and hemochromatosis have particular physical examination findings that are highly specific for those diseases

Laboratory Findings

Laboratory testing may help the clinician determine whether the jaundice is caused by obstruction alone or if there is a concurrent mixed obstructive process. It is ideal to obtain prior laboratory testing, if available, to help serve as a baseline and comparison. In addition, historical laboratory findings can also allow for an assessment of the rate of development of jaundice and can help the clinician correlate the new clinical symptoms with recent events (ie, surgical procedures, new medications, toxin exposures, trauma, and so forth).

The initial laboratory work-up should include a complete blood count with peripheral smear (to look for signs of hemolysis) along with a complete metabolic panel (**Box 5**). If there is a mild elevation in the liver function tests and bilirubin, but the patient is asymptomatic, the blood work should simply be repeated. Alkaline phosphatase is present in the bile canaliculi and can serve as a direct marker for biliary obstruction. However, it can also be produced by bone, placenta, and the kidney. Thus, if the alkaline phosphatase alone is elevated, γ-glutamyltranspeptidase, found in the biliary epithelium, can help distinguish biliary from nonbiliary causes of alkaline phosphatase

---

Box 5
Overview of basic laboratory studies and their significance in the work-up of jaundice

Complete blood count: To check hemoglobin; peripheral smear to look for signs of hemolysis (schistocytes) especially if liver function tests normal

Alanine aminotransferase: Primarily cytosolic enzyme, more specific for liver injury

Aspartate aminotransferase: Cytosolic and mitochondrial enzyme; less sensitive and specific compared with alanine aminotransferase

Bilirubin: Total and fractionated can help determine intrahepatic versus extrahepatic cause

Alkaline phosphatase: Primarily found in bile canaliculi of the liver, but also produced by bone, placenta, and kidney

γ-Glutamyltranspeptidase: Found in biliary epithelium, poor specificity

5-Nucleotidase: Confirmatory test along with alkaline phosphatase and γ-glutamyltranspeptidase to suggest hepatobiliary process

International normalized ratio: Marker of synthetic liver functioning

despite its limited specificity. Another serum marker, 5-nucleotidase, often a send-out test in most institutions, can help confirm a hepatobiliary process as the cause of the alkaline phosphatase elevation.[4] Bilirubin should be fractionated to help distinguish intrahepatic versus extrahepatic causes. Coagulation studies can aid in the assessment of the degree of hepatic dysfunction.

After the basic work-up is completed, further laboratory studies can be ordered based on the clinician's suspicion for the underlying cause of jaundice (**Box 6**). For example, autoimmune markers may be helpful in a young woman with constitutional symptoms or arthralgias. Primary biliary cirrhosis may be considered in an elderly woman with pruritus and jaundice, whereas primary sclerosing cholangitis should be prominent on the differential in a young patient with inflammatory bowel disease and new onset of jaundice. Serologic markers for viral hepatitis should be ordered based on the patient's risk factors and travel history. Wilson disease and hereditary hemochromatosis might be considered in younger patients especially with family history of liver disease.

Major Points:
- A basic laboratory work-up including complete blood count, complete metabolic panel, and coagulation studies should be performed on all patients with new-onset jaundice
- Once this basic work-up is completed, further autoimmune markers, viral serologies, or other disease-specific laboratory findings can be ordered at the clinician's discretion

Imaging Studies

There are a variety of imaging studies of varying diagnostic value in the work-up for jaundice (**Table 1**). Ultrasound is considered first-line therapy in the assessment of jaundice because of its cost-effectiveness and lack of radiation exposure. Studies suggest increased sensitivity in nonobese patients with higher bilirubin concentrations and prolonged duration of jaundice.[47] Ultrasound can provide direct visualization of

---

Box 6
Laboratory markers that may aid in understanding the cause of the jaundice

Autoimmune markers

    Autoimmune hepatitis: ANA, ASMA, anti-LKM1

    Primary biliary cirrhosis: AMA

    Primary sclerosing cholangitis: p-ANCA

Viral hepatitis serologies

Other viral serologies: CMV, VZV, EBV, HSV, HIV

Wilson disease: Urinary copper, serum ceruloplasmin

Hemochromatosis: Iron saturation, ferritin, HFE gene testing

α_1-Antitrypsin deficiency: Measurement of enzyme activity or serum protein electrophoresis[46]

Malignancy: Tumor markers AFP, CEA, CA19-9

Abbreviations: AFP, alpha-fetoprotein; AMA, anti mitochondrial antibody; ANA, antinuclear antibody; anti-LKM1, liver kidney microsomal type 1 antibody; ASMA, anti smooth muscle antibody; CA19-9, carbohydrate antigen 19-9; CEA, carcinoembryonic antigen; CMV, cytomegalovirus; EBV, Epstein-Barr virus; HFE, hemochromatosis; HIV, human Immunodeficiency virus; HSV, herpes simplex virus; p-ANCA, perinuclear antineutrophil cytoplasmic antibodies; VZV, varicella zoster virus.

Table 1
Diagnostic modalities (from least to most invasive) to consider ordering in the patient with jaundice

Type of Study	Advantages/Disadvantages
Ultrasound	Can assess for biliary dilatation, gallstones, venous flow Is cheap, has low radiation
MRI/CT scan	Can identify obstructive masses, features of cirrhosis Has more radiation than ultrasound
Percutaneous transhepatic cholangiography	Useful for higher biliary obstructions, ductal malignancies Allows for stent placement
ERCP	Identifies extrahepatic biliary disease causing jaundice Allows for removal of stones, biliary stent placement
Liver biopsy	Helps to distinguish hepatocellular injury from obstructive process Can measure hepatic venous pressure gradient (HVPG) via transjugular approach

the biliary dilatation, presence of gallstones, and if performed with Doppler can assess the patency of the portal and hepatic veins and the hepatic artery. However, ultrasound has limitations in obese patients and is an operator-dependent test.

Based on institutional availability and the findings on ultrasound, MRI or CT scans are generally obtained next and can more precisely identify obstructive masses, parenchymal liver disease, and features of cirrhosis.[2] However, cholesterol stones can be missed on CT because they are isodense with bile, which is why ultrasound is considered the gold standard for cholelithiasis.[48]

Next, imaging studies that allow for direct therapeutic intervention can be performed. Assy and colleagues[5] found that "percutaneous transhepatic cholangiography (PTC) and ERCP have in common 99% sensitivity and specificity for the diagnosis of biliary obstruction, and both are capable of demonstrating the site and the nature of the obstruction in more than 90% of patients."[49] Both PTC and ERCP not only aid in diagnosis by direct visualization of the obstruction, but these tests also allow for direct therapeutic intervention whether it be stone removal, sphincterotomy, stent placement, or drainage maneuvers if necessary. PTC is preferred for higher biliary obstructions (eg, at the bifurcation of the hepatic ducts), whereas endoscopic ultrasound and ERCP remain the gold standard for extrahepatic biliary disease causing jaundice. Magnetic resonance cholangiopancreatography is a useful test in the patient with low pretest probability of finding an obstructive lesion that would require therapeutic intervention or in the patient with multiple comorbidities where diagnosis should be fully confirmed before proceeding with the more invasive ERCP. In the event of an obstructive lesion, magnetic resonance cholangiopancreatography may help guide planning between ERCP and PTC.[50]

Major Points:
- Ultrasound is the most cost-effective and safe imaging study to perform in the work-up for jaundice
- PTC and ERCP allow for direct visualization of the biliary tree with the ability to provide therapeutic interventions concurrently if necessary

Other Diagnostic Modalities

Hepatobiliary Iminodiacetic Acid (HIDA) Scan scans may be helpful if ultrasound is equivocal but there is still a high clinical suspicion of biliary obstruction. However, this is a nuclear medicine test and thus can be more time consuming than other imaging modalities.[51]

Liver biopsy is considered the gold standard diagnostic modality but given possible morbidity, is not considered a first-line diagnostic test. The experienced clinician reaches for the liver biopsy at the appropriate time, generally when the patient continues to have abnormal liver function tests with jaundice without definitive signs of obstruction on imaging or endoscopic studies. The transjugular approach, often done in the interventional radiology suite, is associated with reduced bleeding complications and is preferred, especially if the patient has a degree of coagulopathy. Transjugular liver biopsies also allow for measurement of the hepatic venous pressure gradient that can assess for underlying portal hypertension in the patient with jaundice. Biopsy can guide not only therapy but also provide prognostic information based on the degree of liver injury.[4]

Major Points:

- HIDA scans are useful if there is a high suspicion of biliary obstruction
- Liver biopsy, although the gold standard diagnostic modality for evaluating jaundice, is infrequently obtained, especially if a diagnosis can be made clinically

PROGNOSIS

In most cases of jaundice, the underlying cause is often multifactorial (ie, an elderly patient started on antibiotics for septic shock from an acute abdomen, in the intensive care unit with hypotension requiring pressors, and now with persistent jaundice). However, if triggers are identified and addressed, most patients without underlying chronic liver disease recover with time. Prompt diagnosis and treatment of the triggers that led to the jaundice in the first place is key to reducing morbidity and mortality.

Major Points:

- Generally, prognosis is favorable if the underlying cause of jaundice is determined and the patient has no prior chronic liver disease

WHAT NOT TO MISS

Given the high mortality with acute liver failure if left untreated, the jaundiced patient presenting with altered mental status and coagulopathy without pre-existing liver disease requires special attention. In addition, those diseases, such as obstructive cholangitis, that have potential therapeutic interventions (ie, ERCP) should not be missed. Those diseases with genetic predisposition, such as Wilson disease, hereditary hemochromatosis, and α_1-antitrypsin deficiency, must not be missed because early diagnosis allows for possible medical therapy and genetic screening and earlier intervention for family members.

Major Points:

- It is especially important for the clinician to diagnose acute liver failure given the high associated morbidity

WHEN TO REFER TO A TRANSPLANT CENTER

Patients with acute liver failure should be referred emergently to determine candidacy for liver transplant.

Aside from the more acute presentation, those jaundiced patients with known complications of end-stage liver disease (including hepatic encephalopathy, ascites, spontaneous bacterial peritonitis, and variceal bleeding) who are otherwise transplant candidates should be referred for assessment of suitability as candidates for transplant.

If clinical history and examination findings, laboratory testing, and imaging modalities still do not provide guidance on the underlying diagnosis, these patients should be referred to a gastroenterologist or hepatologist for further work-up. Similarly, patients with a known trigger who have persistent liver enzyme abnormalities with clinical symptoms should be referred for closer monitoring; if their clinical status worsens and they require emergent transplantation, it is helpful for these patients to have already established care at a liver transplant center.

Major Points:
- Patients with acute liver failure should be referred to a liver transplant center to determine suitability for transplantation
- Patients with cirrhosis should be closely followed by a gastroenterologist or hepatologist to monitor and treat associated complications of end-stage liver disease and assess the potential need and candidacy for transplant

FUTURE DIRECTION

Currently, few studies have assessed the outcomes of patients with jaundice because of the heterogeneity of causes and multiple confounding of variables that can lead to jaundice. Further data on the outcomes of jaundice are needed and may be obtained with multicenter registries and insurance and closed system data set analysis. Such studies are eagerly awaited.

Major Points:
- Multicenter registries may provide outcome-based data on jaundice to guide future diagnostic and therapeutic interventions

ACKNOWLEDGMENTS

The authors thank Dr Anjana Pillai of Emory University and Dr Brintha Enestvedt and Dr Sharlene D'Souza of OHSU for their helpful comments and review of the article.

REFERENCES

1. Habib HA, Saunders M. The yellow bird of jaundice: recognizing biliary obstruction. Nursing 2011;41(10):28–35.
2. Roche SP, Kobos R. Jaundice in the adult patient. Am Fam Physician 2004;69(2): 299–304.
3. Wheatley M, Heilpern K. Jaundice: an emergency department approach to diagnosis and management. Emerg Med Pract 2008;10(3):1–24.
4. Winger J, Michelfelder A. Diagnostic approach to the patient with jaundice. Prim Care 2011;38:469–82.
5. Assy N, Jacob G, Spira G, et al. Diagnostic approach to patient with cholestatic jaundice. World J Gastroenterol 1999;5(3):252–62.
6. Mousavi S, Malek M, Babaei M. Role of overnight rifampin test in diagnosing Gilbert's syndrome. Indian J Gastroenterol 2005;24:108–10.
7. Horsfall LJ, Nazareth I, Pereira SP, et al. Gilbert's syndrome and the risk of a death: a population-based cohort study. J Gastroenterol Hepatol 2013;28(10): 1643–7.

8. Bosma PJ, Chowdhury JR, Bakker C, et al. The genetic basis of the reduced expression of bilirubin UDP-glucuronosyltransferase 1 in Gilbert's syndrome. N Engl J Med 1995;333(18):1171–5.
9. Dasgupta TK, Sharma V. Intrahepatic bilomas: a possible complication of cholecystectomy? Br J Clin Pract 1992;46(4):272–3.
10. Polson J, Lee WM. AASLD position paper: the management of acute liver failure. Hepatology 2005;41(5):1179–97.
11. Zimmerman HJ. Drug-induced liver disease. Clin Liver Dis 2000;4:73–96.
12. Zimmerman HJ. Drug-induced liver disease. In: Schiff ER, Sorrell MF, Maddrey WC, editors. Schiff's diseases of the liver. 8th edition. Philadelphia: Lippincott-Raven Publishers; 1999. p. 973–1064.
13. Bjornsson E, Olsson R. Outcome and prognostic markers in severe drug-induced liver disease. Hepatology 2005;42(2):481–9.
14. Senior JR. Regulatory perspectives. In: Kaplowitz N, DeLeve LD, editors. Drug-induced liver disease. New York: Marcel Dekker; 2003. p. 739–54.
15. Fairley C, McNeil J, Desmond P, et al. Risk factors for development of flucloxacillin associated jaundice. BMJ 1993;306:233–5.
16. Chand N, Sanyal AJ. Sepsis induced cholestasis. Hepatology 2007;45(1): 230–41.
17. Rossi S, Navarro V. Herbs and liver injury: a clinical perspective. Clin Gastroenterol Hepatol 2014;12:1069–76.
18. Kinney T. Management of ascending cholangitis. Gastrointest Endosc Clin N Am 2007;17:289–306.
19. van Erpecum K. Complications of bile-duct stones: acute cholangitis and pancreatitis. Best Pract Res Clin Gastroenterol 2006;20(6):1139–52.
20. Attasaranya S, Fogel E, Lehman G. Choledocholithiasis, ascending cholangitis, and gallstone pancreatitis. Med Clin North Am 2008;92(4):925–60.
21. Faust TW, Reddy KR. Postoperative jaundice. Clin Liver Dis 2004;8(1):151–66.
22. Fevery J. Bilirubin in clinical practice: a review. Liver Int 2008;28(5):592–605.
23. Molina E, Raddy R. Postoperative jaundice. Clin Liver Dis 1999;3(3):477–88.
24. Garvin IP. Remarks on pneumonia biliosa. South Med Surg J 1837;1:536–44.
25. Shands K, Schmid G, Dan B, et al. Toxic-shock syndrome in menstruating women. Association with tampon use and Staphylococcus aureus, and clinical features in 52 cases. N Engl J Med 1980;303:1436–42.
26. Banks J, Foulis AK, Ledingham I, et al. Liver function in septic shock. J Clin Pathol 1982;35:1249–52.
27. Pirovino M, Meister F, Rubli E, et al. Preserved cytosolic and synthetic liver function in jaundice of severe extrahepatic infection. Gastroenterology 1989;96:1589–95.
28. Pathak B, Sheibani L, Lee R. Cholestasis of pregnancy. Obstet Gynecol Clin North Am 2010;37(2):269–82.
29. Lee RH, Goodwin TM, Greenspoon J, et al. The prevalence of intrahepatic cholestasis of pregnancy in a primarily Latina Los Angeles population. J Perinatol 2006;26:527–32.
30. Williamson C, Geenes V. Intrahepatic cholestasis of pregnancy. Obstet Gynecol 2014;124:120–33.
31. Keitel V, Vogt C, Häussinger D, et al. Combined mutations of canalicular transporter proteins cause severe intrahepatic cholestasis of pregnancy. Gastroenterology 2006;131(2):624–9.
32. Davies MH, da Silva RC, Jones SR, et al. Fetal mortality associated with cholestasis of pregnancy and the potential benefit of therapy with ursodeoxycholic acid. Gut 1995;37:580–4.

33. Glantz A, Marschall HU, Mattsson LA. Intrahepatic cholestasis of pregnancy: relationships between bile acid levels and fetal complications rates. Hepatology 2004;40(2):467–74.
34. Hay JE. Liver disease in pregnancy. Hepatology 2008;47(3):1067–76.
35. Matin A, Sass DA. Liver disease in pregnancy. Gastroenterol Clin North Am 2011; 40(2):335–53.
36. Mays JK. The active management of intrahepatic cholestasis of pregnancy. Curr Opin Obstet Gynecol 2010;22(2):100–3.
37. Williamson C, Gorelik J, Eaton BM, et al. The bile acid taurocholate impairs rat cardiomyocyte function: a proposed mechanism for intra-uterine fetal death in obstetric cholestasis. Clin Sci (Lond) 2001;100:363–9.
38. Geenes V, Chappell LC, Seed PT, et al. Association of severe intrahepatic cholestasis of pregnancy with adverse pregnancy outcomes: a prospective population-based case-control study. Hepatology 2014;59:1482–91.
39. Qi K, Li H, An L, et al. The correlation between platelet activation and liver injury by conditioning and bone marrow transplantation. Transplant Proc 2014;46: 1523–30.
40. DeLeve LD, Shulman HM, McDonald GB. Toxic injury to hepatic sinusoids: sinusoidal obstruction syndrome (veno-occlusive disease). Semin Liver Dis 2002; 22(1):27–42.
41. Baron F, Deprez M, Beguin Y. The veno-occlusive disease of the liver. Haematologica 1997;82(6):718–25.
42. Sinicrope F. Gastrointestinal complications: Hepatic Complications of Bone Marrow Transplantation. In: Kufe DW, Pollock RE, Weichselbaum RR, et al, editors. Holland-Frei Cancer Medicine, 6th edition. Chapter 155. Hamilton (ON): BC Deckerl; 2003. Available at: http://www.ncbi.nlm.nih.gov/books/NBK13099/.
43. McDonald GB, Shulman HM, Wolford JL, et al. Liver disease after human marrow transplantation. Semin Liver Dis 1987;7:210–29.
44. Chopra S, Griffin PH. Laboratory tests and diagnostic procedures in evaluation of liver disease. Am J Med 1985;79(221):230.
45. Pasanen PA, Pikkarainen P, Alhava E, et al. Evaluation of a computer-based diagnostic score system in the diagnosis of jaundice and cholestasis. Scand J Gastroenterol 1993;28(8):732–6.
46. Limdi JK, Hyde GM. Evaluation of abnormal liver function tests. Postgrad Med J 2003;79:307–12.
47. Gold RP, Casarella WJ, Stern G, et al. Transhepatic cholangiography: the radiological method of choice in suspected obstructive jaundice. Radiology 1979; 133(1):39–44.
48. Malhotra A, Rabouhans J. Computer tomography in emergency radiology. In: Chan O, editor. ABC of Emergency Radiology. Malden (MA): Blackwell Publishing/BMJ Books; 2007. p. 35–151.
49. Khan MA, Khan AA, Shafqat F. Comparison of ultrasonography and cholangiography (ERCP/PTC) in the differential diagnosis of obstructive jaundice. J Pak Med Assoc 1996;46:188–90.
50. Gentile N, Greenlund A. 66-year-old woman with painless jaundice. Mayo Clin Proc 2012;87(10):1021–4.
51. Kim EE, Moon TY, Delpassand ES. Nuclear hepatobiliary imaging. Radiol Clin North Am 1993;31(4):923–33.

Liver Disease in the Adolescent

Alisha M. Mavis, MD, Estella M. Alonso, MD*

KEYWORDS

• Adolescent • Liver disease • Nonalcoholic fatty liver disease • Hepatitis

KEY POINTS

- There are challenges that must be addressed to effectively care for, not only liver disease in the adolescent but also the patient as a whole.
- Evaluation of an adolescent with new-onset liver enzyme abnormalities should be individualized based on the patient's history and physical exam, but there are a few diseases that need to be ruled out for any adolescent with elevated liver enzymes.
- Due to the development changes occurring in adolescence, monitoring for adherence, risk-taking behaviors, and signs of psychological diseases, such as anxiety and depression, is imperative when caring for an adolescent with liver disease.
- Transition of care to adult-centered care is a continuous process throughout adolescence and should incorporate interventions to promote self-management skills and adherence.

CARING FOR ADOLESCENTS WITH LIVER DISEASE

Adolescence is a unique and sometimes challenging time in a young person's life. This time marks the transition from childhood into adulthood and is exemplified by cognitive, psychosocial, and emotional development, as well as physical and pubertal growth. Furthermore, adolescents are trying to gain independence and create a secure identity during this critical time.[1] However, unparalleled growth of physical, cognitive, and psychosocial development may limit the adolescent's ability to perceive or judge risk appropriately. **Fig. 1** depicts the interdependence between the developmental achievements in adolescence.

Cognitive development during adolescence not only includes the development of more advanced reasoning skills and the ability to think abstractly but also the capacity to think about how others perceive them. As a result of this formal operational thought

Disclosure: None.
Department of Pediatrics, Northwestern University, Feinberg School of Medicine, Siragusa Transplantation Center, Ann & Robert H. Lurie Children's Hospital, 225 East Chicago Avenue, Chicago, IL 60611, USA
* Corresponding author.
E-mail address: e-alonso@northwestern.edu

Clin Liver Dis 19 (2015) 171–185
http://dx.doi.org/10.1016/j.cld.2014.09.010
1089-3261/15/$ – see front matter © 2015 Elsevier Inc. All rights reserved.

liver.theclinics.com

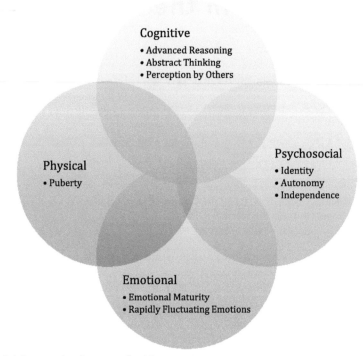

Fig. 1. Adolescent developmental achievements.

process combined with rapid emotional and physical changes during puberty, many youth start to think that everyone is thinking about them, so as to develop an imaginary audience. This thinking can be harmful to an adolescent with a chronic illness or new-onset illness, especially liver disease. A young person may try to deny or hide their illness because they fear the imaginary audience (peers) may find out about their illness, or the adolescent may try to prove the condition does not exist.[2] Because the audience is very real to the adolescent, the clinician must be sympathetic and find solutions to not only address the health care needs of the patient, but also the social needs.

The psychosocial development that occurs during adolescence includes establishing an identity and developing autonomy. As an adolescent explores their identity they may experiment with a variety of behaviors, activities, and peer groups, including risk-taking and dangerous behaviors.[3] For a patient with liver disease, some of these risk-taking behaviors may involve an increased risk because of the underlying disease. It is also during this period that patients may start presenting signs and symptoms of psychological diseases, such as anxiety and depression. Adolescents put such an emphasis on relating to and fitting in a peer group, that having a chronic liver disease and being different may cause symptoms of anxiety or depression. Therefore, it is essential for every adolescent with liver disease to have an established medical home that not only provides anticipatory guidance and health advice to the parents and patient, but also interventions as needed and an open dialogue with the adolescent.[4]

The development of independence is a gradual process for a young person and a time when the peer group influence grows stronger and they are less interested in parental advice. However, the development of self-management for adolescents with chronic health needs usually lags behind their psychosocial development. One study looking at independent health care behaviors in adolescents with inflammatory bowel disease, reported that many patients 18 years and older were still assisted by parents.[5] There are similar studies in the pediatric liver transplant population reporting that patients diagnosed and/or transplanted at a younger age have increased difficulty in obtaining independence regarding self-management care.[1,6,7] It is imperative for the clinician to foster and encourage the young person's motivation to develop self-management skills throughout adolescence.

Caring for adolescents with liver disease is a gratifying experience. However, these are just a few of the challenges that must be addressed to effectively care for not only the disease but also the patient as a whole.

EVALUATION OF THE ADOLESCENT WITH NEW-ONSET LIVER ENZYME ELEVATION

Up to 9% of asymptomatic people can have elevated liver enzymes including aminotransferases (alanine aminotransferase [ALT] and aspartate aminotransferase [AST]), γ-glutamyltransferase (GGT), and/or alkaline phosphatase.[8] An extensive evaluation of all abnormal test results would expose many patients to unnecessary risks and expense; however, failure to evaluate even minor liver enzyme elevations that persist beyond 8 to 12 weeks may mean missing the early diagnosis of a potentially treatable disease. By understanding the pattern of biochemical markers of liver injury, one can further categorize the differential diagnoses for an adolescent patient with new-onset liver laboratory abnormalities.

Elevated ALT and AST suggests liver cell injury and does not evaluate the function of the liver. ALT mainly exists in the liver but can be found in very low concentrations in other tissues. However, AST is found in multiple tissues including liver, cardiac, skeletal muscle, kidney, brain, pancreas, lung, leukocyte, and erthrocyte.[9] Because AST is found in several other tissues, ALT is considered the more liver-specific enzyme. In addition, it has been suggested that ALT correlates with the degree of abdominal adiposity.[10]

Aminotransferase activity may be elevated because of a variety of reasons. **Box 1** reviews potential causes for abnormal aminotransferase activity. Nonalcoholic fatty liver disease (NAFLD) is currently one of the most common causes of aminotransferase elevation in adolescents and adults. Infectious causes of elevated ALT and AST levels must be excluded, including viral hepatitis (A, B, C, E); other viral infections (cytomegalovirus [CMV], Epstein-Barr virus [EBV], herpes simplex virus, varicella zoster virus); and bacteria, fungal, and parasitic infections. Metabolic causes of elevated aminotransferases in the adolescent are Wilson disease, α_1-antitrypsin (A1AT) deficiency, hemochromatosis, and cystic fibrosis (CF). Immunologic causes include autoimmune hepatitis (AIH), acute fatty liver of pregnancy, and HELLP syndrome. Medication- and toxin-induced liver injury is not uncommon in adolescence and can usually be elicited in the history and confirmed by demonstration of a pattern of injury characteristic for the suspected agent on liver biopsy. Other causes of elevated aminotransferase activity include vascular disease, such as Budd-Chiari syndrome, ischemic hepatitis, sinusoidal obstruction syndrome, and infiltrative liver diseases, such as sarcoidosis and amyloidosis. Nonhepatic causes of abnormal aminotransferase levels include cardiac disease, thyroid disease, celiac disease, anorexia nervosa, adrenal insufficiency, myopathy, and strenuous exercise. The clinician should not overlook the possibility of alcoholic liver disease when evaluating the adolescent with elevated liver enzymes, because drinking alcohol is a risk-taking activity that

---

Box 1
Causes of elevated aminotransferases

Nonalcoholic fatty liver disease	Biliary tract
Infectious	Primary sclerosing cholangitis
Viral hepatitis (A, B, C, D, E)	Alagille syndrome
Epstein-Barr virus	Progressive familial intrahepatic cholestasis
Cytomegalovirus	Biliary atresia
Herpes simplex virus	Primary biliary cirrhosis
Bacterial	Vascular
Fungal	Ischemic hepatitis
Parasitic	Sinusoidal obstruction syndrome
Severe acute respiratory syndrome	Budd-Chiari syndrome
Metabolic	Infiltrative
α_1-Antitrypsin deficiency	Sarcoidosis
Wilson disease	Amyloidosis
Hemochromatosis	Nonhepatic
Cystic fibrosis	Cardiac disease
Immunologic	Celiac disease
Autoimmune hepatitis	Thyroid disease
Acute fatty liver of pregnancy	Myopathy
HELLP syndrome	Malnutrition
Toxin/medication	Anorexia nervosa
Alcohol	Adrenal insufficiency
Allergic reaction	Strenuous exercise
Hepatotoxic medication	Macro AST

---

many young adults partake in with peers or in isolation but do not eagerly discuss with an adult.

Alkaline phosphatase predominately originates from bone and liver, but is also present in the small intestine, kidneys, and placenta. An elevation may suggest biliary obstruction, bile duct epithelium injury, or cholestasis. However, an isolated alkaline phosphatase elevation without a GGT elevation may be caused by bone disease or a time of increased bone growth, as in children and adolescents. Alkaline phosphatase can be fractionated to determine if it is originating from bone or liver. An elevated alkaline phosphatase is usually from the liver if there is simultaneous elevation of other measures of cholestasis. Biliary causes of alkaline phosphatase elevation include cholelithiasis, drug hepatotoxicity, primary sclerosing cholangitis (PSC), and primary biliary cirrhosis. In addition, there are rare cases of benign familial intestinal alkaline phosphatase elevation.

GGT is present in hepatocytes and biliary epithelial cells, and kidney, pancreas, spleen, heart, brain, and seminal vesicles. GGT is the most sensitive marker for biliary tract disease but is not very specific. It is elevated up to six or seven times the upper limit of normal for the adult reference range in normal, full-term neonates but usually decreases to a normal reference range level by about 6 months of age. Alcohol and drugs, including phenytoin and phenobarbital, may cause GGT elevation.

Prothrombin time/international normalized ratio, glucose, and serum albumin are tests used to evaluate the synthetic function of the liver. These laboratory tests should be evaluated for any patient with new-onset liver enzyme elevations.

The first step in evaluation of a patient with new-onset liver enzyme elevations is a detailed and comprehensive history to identify potential risk factors for liver disease and a thorough physical examination to look for signs of chronic liver disease. The work-up for elevated liver enzymes in an adolescent should be individualized based on the patient's history and physical examination. However, there are a few diseases that need to be ruled out for any adolescent with elevated liver enzymes (**Table 1**). Depending on the acuity of the illness and enzyme elevations, infectious causes must be evaluated. EBV and hepatitis A usually cause a symptomatic, acute self-limited hepatitis. However, hepatitis B and hepatitis C may be diagnosed in an asymptomatic patient, and should always be assessed. Autoimmune hepatitis, A1AT deficiency, and Wilson disease are a few diseases that need to be ruled in or out in all adolescents with elevated liver enzymes despite symptoms. NAFLD may be suspected based on the patient's growth chart and examination. The clinician should ask about any recent illnesses or exposure to people with an illness. Many viruses can cause an acute hepatitis that is self-limited and resolves without sequela. If drug-induced liver injury is high on the differential based on the patient's

Table 1
Evaluation of an adolescent with elevated liver enzymes

Disease	Testing
Hepatitis A	Hepatitis A antibody
Hepatitis B	Hepatitis B surface antibody Hepatitis B surface antigen Hepatitis B core antibody
Hepatitis C	Hepatitis C antibody
Hepatitis E	Hepatitis BE antibody Hepatitis BE surface antigen
EBV	EBV IgM antibody EBV polymerase chain reaction
CMV	CMV IgM antibody CMV polymerase chain reaction
Autoimmune hepatitis	Autoantibodies to nuclei Smooth muscle antibody Liver/kidney microsome antibody Total IgG
α_1-Antitrypsin deficiency	α_1-Antitrypsin phenotype
Wilson disease	Ceruloplasmin serum 24-h urinary copper
Hemochromatosis	Complete blood count Total iron Total iron-binding capacity Transferrin saturation Ferritin

history, the drug in question should be discontinued immediately. Patients that have elevated GGT, alkaline phosphatase, or bilirubin should also have a liver ultrasound to evaluate for any anatomic abnormalities, such as bile duct dilatation, gallstones, or a liver mass.

COMMON LIVER DISEASES IN THE ADOLESCENT
Nonalcoholic Fatty Liver Disease

The prevalence of NAFLD varies widely depending on the population; however, world-wide prevalence of NAFLD is estimated between 6% and 30% with a median of 20% in the general adult population.[11] It is estimated to be about 30% in the United States.[12] Obesity is a common and well-documented risk factor for NAFLD. With the rise in obesity rates in the United States, there is also an increase in the diagnosis of NAFLD, which can lead to nonalcoholic steatohepatitis and cirrhosis. Age, gender, and ethnicity are all associated with the varying prevalence of NAFLD. Fatty liver disease increases with age, and the possibility of disease progression to advance fibrosis increases in older patients. Many studies report male gender as a risk factor for NAFLD.[11] Hispanic individuals also have a significantly higher prevalence of fatty liver disease compared with non-Hispanic whites. Non-Hispanic blacks have a much lower prevalence of NAFLD.[12,13] There is a higher prevalence in patients with metabolic syndrome, type 2 diabetes mellitus, and dyslipidemia.

Patients with NAFLD are usually asymptomatic, but they may have right upper quadrant pain, hepatomegaly, or several nonspecific symptoms including weakness, fatigue, or abdominal discomfort. Mild elevation of aminotransferase activity or hepatomegaly may be the only finding in patients with NAFLD. NAFLD may be suspected based on history and physical examination, but the diagnostic gold standard is still a liver biopsy. Several noninvasive methods for diagnosing NAFLD are being evaluated and may be clinically useful in the future. The only treatment of NAFLD at this time is lifestyle modification with weight loss and increased physical activity, which helps to reduce hepatic steatosis but does not reverse fibrotic changes. Loss of at least 3% to 5% of total body weight is needed to improve steatosis, but weight loss up to 10% may be required to improve necroinflammation.[14,15] A practical approach to a patient suspected of having fatty liver disease based on history and elevated aminotransferases for at least 1 month is to draw laboratory studies to rule out other diseases, such as AIH, A1AT deficiency, Wilson disease, hemochromatosis, and thyroid disease. It is also important to obtain laboratory studies to evaluate for metabolic syndrome because of the high prevalence of metabolic syndrome in patients with NAFLD. If the laboratory results do not point to a specific disease, it is reasonable to defer the liver biopsy for 6 to 12 months to allow the patient time to lose weight and possibly show improvement in the aminotransferases.[16]

Autoimmune Hepatitis

AIH is a chronic hepatitis caused by nonresolving inflammation of the liver of unknown cause. It is characterized by immunologic features and circulating autoantibodies. The onset is usually insidious with many nonspecific symptoms including fatigue, nausea, abdominal pain, joint pain, and jaundice. However, the clinical spectrum is broad and ranges from an asymptomatic presentation to presenting in acute liver failure. AIH is usually suspected and typed based on circulating autoantibodies to nuclei and/or smooth muscle or to liver/kidney microsomes and/or liver cytosol antigen. Patients with AIH may also have high serum globulin concentrations including a high IgG, elevated aminotransferases, GGT, alkaline phosphatase, and/ or bilirubin. Women are affected more frequently (gender ratio, 3.6:1), but it is seen at all ages and in all ethnic groups.[17] Children with AIH may have autoimmune PSC even without inflammatory bowel disease, so it is important to evaluate for PSC in all children with AIH. GGT may be a better indicator of biliary disease in adolescents and children because alkaline phosphatase can be elevated due to bone activity in growing children. Liver biopsy is recommended to establish the diagnosis of AIH and help guide treatment. Interface hepatitis is the most common histologic sign of AIH, but there may also be plasma cell infiltration, lobular inflammation, fibrosis, and rarely granulomas.[18]

Treatment is similar in children and adults. However, all children diagnosed with AIH should be started on treatment at the time of diagnosis regardless of the severity of disease activity because children seem to present with a more severe disease process.[17] Standard therapy for AIH in adolescents usually consists of prednisone with or without azathioprine. The prednisone is typically tapered to a low mainte-nance dose during the first few months of treatment provided there is prompt response in liver enzymes. There are many side effects related to the use of predni-sone, including weight gain, higher body mass index, stunted linear growth, and pu-bertal delay, which are important to consider when treating adolescents with AIH. Budesonide, a topical steroid, with azathioprine is a reasonable alternative treatment with fewer side effects, including less weight gain and lower body mass index, which may be used to maintain remission in adolescents with steroid-related side effects. Azathioprine is also used as maintenance therapy alone.[19] Some patients are able to completely stop therapy with close serologic monitoring and after 2 to 3 years of biochemical remission and histologic resolution.[20] About 20% of children with type 1 AIH are able to permanently discontinue immunosuppressive therapy without disease recurrence, but this rarely is the case in children with type 2 AIH.[21] Disease refractory to standard therapy typically progresses to cirrhosis and may necessitate liver transplant.

Viral Hepatitis

There are numerous infections, bacterial and viral, that can cause an acute hepatitis that resolves with the infection and does not cause long-term damage. Viral hepatitis including hepatitis A, B, C, and E viruses may cause elevated aminotransferases. Hep-atitis A and E cause an acute, self-limited infection and are spread via fecal-oral route. Hepatitis A vaccination is recommended for individuals at risk or traveling. There is currently no vaccination against hepatitis E. Conversely, hepatitis B and C usually pre-sent in adolescence as a chronic infection. Aminotransferase activity is typically elevated with acute viral hepatitis, but may be closer to normal in chronic hepatitis, especially hepatitis C. Hepatitis B virus (HBV) may be vertically transmitted from mother to baby or through contact with the blood or other body fluids of an infected person. HBV may cause symptomatic acute hepatitis within the first 6 months of infec-tion, but many individuals are completely asymptomatic and clear the virus within 6 months of contracting. Up to 50% of children who contract the virus before 6 years of age develop chronic hepatitis, and the risk of chronic infection in patients with verti-cally acquired hepatitis B approaches 90%.[22]

There is no treatment available for acute hepatitis B, but there are treatment regi-mens for chronic HBV. Vaccination against hepatitis B is the mainstay of hepatitis B prevention. Hepatitis D can cause an acute or chronic infection, but can only replicate in patients with HBV infection. Hepatitis C virus (HCV) is a bloodborne virus that can cause an acute or chronic infection and may also be vertically transmitted. Up to

85% of patients infected with hepatitis C develop chronic HCV. There is not a hepatitis C vaccine, but there are multiple treatments available. Most adolescent patients with HBV and HCV acquired the virus via vertical transmission. However, because of the high-risk behaviors that young adults participate in, it is important to test for HBV and HCV when evaluating an adolescent with elevated liver enzymes even if they have tested negative in the past.

Systemic viral infections can also cause abnormal aminotransferase levels. Elevated ALT and AST caused by EBV is frequently seen in conjunction with acute mononucleosis and a positive monospot test and is usually self-limited. However, EBV serology may need to be evaluated if the monospot test is negative because it does not have a high sensitivity and may be negative early in the course of EBV infection. Jaundice occurs in less than 10% of children with EBV infection.[23] CMV infection in the immune-competent patient generally presents as a subclinical case and is self-resolving. Disseminated CMV infection in the immune-compromised patient may cause severe organ damage or mortality. Herpes simplex virus is predominantly diagnosed in neonatal, pregnant, and immune-compromised patients and presents with fulminant hepatitis and high mortality.

Metabolic Disease

Wilson disease

Wilson disease is an inherited autosomal-recessive metabolic disease that leads to the impairment of cellular copper transport. ATP7B, the defective gene, encodes a hepatic copper-transporting protein that plays a key role in human copper metabolism. This defect results in decreased copper transport from the liver into bile causing excess copper accumulation in several organs but most notably in the liver, brain, cornea, and kidney. The excess hepatic copper leads to hepatocyte damage. The worldwide prevalence of Wilson disease is approximately 1 in 30,000 live births with a slight male predominance.[24,25] Most patients with Wilson disease are diagnosed between the ages of 5 and 35 years and may present with hepatic, neurologic, and/or psychiatric symptoms. Children usually present with liver disease between the ages of 9 and 13 years.[26] The hepatic manifestations of Wilson disease vary greatly and consist of asymptomatic laboratory abnormalities and steatosis, acute hepatitis and acute liver failure with an associated Coombs-negative hemolytic anemia, chronic hepatitis, and cirrhosis. Biochemical abnormalities may include elevated aminotransferases, low serum ceruloplasmin, elevated 24-hour urinary copper, Coombs-negative hemolytic anemia, thrombocytopenia, or coagulopathy. Additional signs and symptoms associated with hepatic Wilson disease are Kayser-Fleischer rings (50% patients with hepatic disease and diagnosed on slit-lamp examination), abdominal pain, hepatomegaly, jaundice, splenomegaly, ascites, upper gastrointestinal bleeding, or mental status changes caused by hepatic encephalopathy.[24] Liver biopsy shows a high hepatic copper concentration.

Treatment of Wilson disease is life long and involves removing the tissue copper that has accumulated and preventing reaccumulation of excess copper. Potent copper chelators (trientene and D-penicillamine) at moderate doses are used to treat copper overload, whereas low doses are used to help prevent copper accumulation. Patients are also maintained on a low-copper diet and avoid copper-rich foods (chocolate, shellfish, nuts, mushrooms, unprocessed wheat). Dietary copper intake in a general diet is about 1 to 5 mg per day and the recommended daily copper intake is 0.9 mg per day for a healthy individual. Patients who present with acute liver failure may require a liver transplant. First-degree relatives of any patient newly diagnosed with Wilson disease need to be screened for Wilson disease.

α_1-antitrypsin deficiency

A1AT deficiency is an underrecognized disorder affecting the lung, liver, and rarely skin. It is the most common known genetic cause of liver disease leading to pediatric liver transplantation. A1AT is a serum glycoprotein synthesized mainly in the liver in large quantities and secreted into the serum. Its physiologic function is to inhibit neutrophil proteases released during periods of inflammation to protect host tissue from nonspecific injury. There are many known mutations of the A1AT gene but most patients with liver disease are homozygous for the Z mutant allele (Pi*ZZ). This occurs approximately 1 in 2000 to 5000 births in North American and European populations.[27] The A1AT mutant Z gene directs the synthesis of a mutant protein that is abnormally folded and retained intracellularly within the hepatocyte rather than being excreted. The accumulation of the mutant protein within hepatocytes triggers a cascade of chronic hepatocellular apoptosis, regeneration, and end-organ injury, which leads to liver injury, cirrhosis, and hepatocelllular carcinoma given the right environmental triggers.[28,29] Patients may present with neonatal hepatitis and cholestasis or as an adolescent with elevated aminotransferases, elevated GGT, and hepatomegaly. Mild liver disease at diagnosis can continue to progress to advanced liver disease. There is currently no medical treatment of A1AT, but liver transplant may be used to treat patients with end-stage liver disease.

Biliary Atresia

Biliary atresia (BA) is an idiopathic, progressive obliterative disease of the extrahepatic biliary tree that presents in neonates with biliary obstruction. It is the most common indication for liver transplant in children. The overall incidence is 1 in 8000 to 19,000 live births and there are 250 to 400 new cases per year in the United States. Once diagnosed with BA a Kasai procedure is promptly performed to enhance the flow of bile. Less than half of patients with BA make it into adolescence with their native liver. The outcomes for adults with BA with their native liver at 20 years are promising with all of them having normal pubertal development and greater than 75% achieving a normal average height. In addition, 60% participate in standard daily activities including 33% holding down employment, 27% being enrolled in school, and 32% being married. Even with all the positive outcomes, 10% report depression and about 5% are heavy drinkers.[30] The hepatic complications associated with BA post-Kasai include portal hypertension (PTN), cirrhosis, gastrointestinal bleeding, late bacterial cholangitis, coagulopathy, and pruritis. PTN and recurrent cholangitis are frequent complications with high morbidity and mortality that necessitate the need for liver transplant. PTN may occur in up to two-thirds of long-term survivor patients with BA and their native liver. It is often defined by complications of PTN, such as gastrointestinal bleed or by endoscopic findings (varices). Some noninvasive markers of PTN include splenomegaly, thrombocytopenia, and low albumin.

There are a few endoscopic therapies available for patients with variceal bleeding including banding and sclerotherapy. Octreotide is usually effective for immediate medical management but is not a long-term therapy. Patients with low bilirubin and variceal hemorrhage have a better prognosis than patients with higher bilirubin levels and variceal bleed.[31] In select patients with compensated liver disease and variceal bleeding refractory to medical and endoscopic therapies, a transjugular intrahepatic portosystemic shunt maybe a viable alternative as a bridge to liver transplant.[32] Cholangitis is another common complication defined as fever, acholic stools, and elevated liver enzymes. It is not uncommon for a patient with suspected cholangitis to have a negative blood culture. Most cholangitis is caused by enteric pathogens including *Escherichia coli*, *Enterobacter*, and *Klebsiella* and treated effectively with cephalosporins, aminoglycosides, or levofloxacin. However, recurrent cholangitis increases the risk of variceal hemorrhage and thus the need for evaluation for liver transplant. Most adolescent patients with BA and their native liver eventually need a liver transplant.

Cystic Fibrosis

CF is a common disease with an incidence of 1 in 3000 live births and a current life expectancy of 40 years. Less than one-third of patients with CF have clinically significant liver disease. There is a male predominance in patients with CF and liver disease. About 50% of patients with CF and liver disease are noted to have steatosis, whereas up to 12% have cholithiasis, and roughly 5% to 7% have focal to multilobular biliary cirrhosis.[33] CF liver disease is primarily diagnosed in patients with severe CF transmembrane regulator mutations. Absence of CF transmembrane regulator function causes dehydration, concentration, and decreased alkalinization of duct contents producing precipitation of biliary secretions, which leads to biliary obstruction and inflammation causing biliary cirrhosis. Liver enzymes are not a good indicator of hepatic injury because up to 50% of patients with CF liver disease only have intermittently abnormal laboratory studies including elevated aminotransferases and GGT.[34] Elevated bilirubin is uncommon. There are minimal treatment options for CF liver disease. Ursodeoxycholic acid may improve bile flow and liver enzymes and it is postulated that it may have a cytoprotective effect. Some patients have progression of their biliary cirrhosis to multilobular cirrhosis with PTN, but few overall develop ascites and varices. Transjugular intrahepatic portosystemic shunt and banding are effective therapies for PTN secondary to CF liver disease. β-Blockers may cause bronchospasm so they are not a good treatment choice. Liver transplant is reserved for patients with severe synthetic liver dysfunction. Patients with CF also have an increased risk of gastrointestinal tract malignancies with a third of them being hepatic or biliary tract in origin. This risk increases with age and peaks after the third decade.[35]

Primary Sclerosing Cholangitis

PSC is a chronic, progressive cholestatic liver disease of unknown cause characterized by inflammation and fibrosis of intrahepatic and extrahepatic bile ducts leading to the formation of multifocal bile duct strictures. Up to 90% of patients with PSC have underlying ulcerative colitis; however, only about 5% of patients with ulcerative colitis have PSC.[36] Many of the patients that present with PSC during childhood and adolescence do not develop symptoms suggestive of ulcerative colitis until later in life. There is a slight male predominance. About half of patients are asymptomatic at the time of presentation, or they may have nonspecific symptoms, such as fatigue and pruritus. Biochemical abnormalities include an elevated alkaline phosphatase with mildly elevated aminotransferases, and physical examination may reveal jaundice, hepatomegaly, splenomegaly, or excoriations. PSC is diagnosed by cholangiography and a liver biopsy is not always required. There is no proved treatment that slows the progression of the disease, but there are many medical and surgical therapies to treat the pruritus, strictures, and complications of PSC. Liver transplant may be considered in patients with advanced disease.

Inherited Disorders of Cholestasis

Alagille syndrome

Alagille syndrome is an autosomal-dominant inherited disease of cholestasis and is the most common disorder associated with bile duct paucity. The incidence is 1 in 100,000 live births with more than half of patients having a de novo mutation on the

JAG1 or NOTCH 2 genes.[37] There is variable penetrance and phenotypic expression. Patients are usually diagnosed as an infant when they are noted to have a direct hyperbilirubinemia, elevated aminotransferases, and a disproportionally elevated GGT. The common clinical features include chronic cholestasis; cardiac anomalies; butterfly vertebrae; posterior embryotoxon of the eye; and dysmorphic facies consisting of a triangular facies, deep-set eyes, and a broad nasal bridge. These patients may also have renal disease, pancreatic insufficiency, developmental delay, short stature, or intracranial hemorrhage. Vascular anomalies in multiple organs, including the central nervous system, are common. There is a 10% to 15% risk of intracranial hemorrhage with an associated 30% mortality. These bleeds respond well to surgical clip ligation.[38] Treatment of Alagille syndrome involves managing the different diseases in each affected organ system.

Progressive familial intrahepatic cholestasis

Progressive familial intrahepatic cholestasis (PFIC) is a heterogenous group of disorders defined by defective secretion of bile acids or other components of bile. These disorders usually present during infancy with cholestasis, coagulopathy caused by vitamin K malabsorption, elevated aminotransferases, and a normal or nearly normal GGT in PFIC 1 and PFIC 2. PFIC is associated with growth failure and progressive liver disease. PFIC 1 is autosomal-recessive and is distinguished by missense mutations in the ATP8B1 gene. Patients with PFIC 1 usually present within the first year of life, have a low or normal GGT, and have intense pruritus. The progression to biliary cirrhosis is variable but they may respond to a biliary diversion with some improvement in pruritus and a slowing of the progression of liver disease.[39]

PFIC 2 is caused by a defect in the ABCB11 gene that encodes BSEP, an ATP-dependent bile acid transporter. BSEP actively transports bile acids across the canalicular membrane into bile. Absence of BSEP function leads to a low serum GGT, low cholesterol, and chronic intrahepatic cholestasis with progression to cirrhosis usually in the first 5 to 10 years of life. Patients with PFIC 2 have about a 15% increased risk of cancer. Hepatocellular carcinoma is the most common form, but cholangiocarcinoma and pancreatic adenocarcinoma may also occur.[40]

PFIC 3 involves a mutation in the ABCB4 gene, which encodes MDR3. Absence of MDR3 results in failure of phospholipid transport into bile. Patients with PFIC 3 are noted to have a high GGT and liver biopsy shows ductal proliferation. Depending on the mutation, patients may present with clinical cholestasis in early childhood or they may present with a milder form of the disease at an older age. Pruritus is usually milder in PFIC 3, but the disease can still progress to end-stage liver disease. Treatment of patients with PFIC involves addressing nutritional deficiencies, including fat-soluble vitamin supplementation, and pruritus. Ursodeoxycholic acid might improve mild pruritus; however, severe pruritis is often refractory to medical therapy and requires surgery for biliary diversion. Biliary diversion may help the pruritus, but it might also improve biochemical abnormalities and slow the progression of liver disease. Liver transplant is a feasible option for patients with end-stage liver disease or pruritus refractory to all medical and surgical therapies.

Benign recurrent intrahepatic cholestasis is on the opposite end of the spectrum of PFIC but is caused by a mutation on the ATP8B1 gene, the same gene that causes PFIC 1. Benign recurrent intrahepatic cholestasis is an autosomal-recessive disease and is defined as intermittent episodes of cholestasis. Patients may present at any age, including adolescence, and the frequency of episodes is widely variable. During an episode, patients present with conjugated hyperbilirubinemia, pruritus, anorexia, and malaise. Each episode may last for weeks to months with a complete clinical, biochemical, and histologic normalization. There is no treatment of benign recurrent intrahepatic cholestasis and the frequency of episodes seems to decrease with age.[39]

MANAGEMENT APPROACH TO THE ADOLESCENT WITH LIVER DISEASE

Caring for adolescents with liver disease can be far more challenging than any other age group. The clinician must juggle management of what are complex liver diseases while fully considering the patient's psychosocial health. Young people are undergoing major changes in their psychosocial and physical development while at the same time trying to gain independence during adolescence. Unfortunately, the progress in self-management skills usually lags behind psychosocial development and pediatric clinicians and parents are not always tuned in to the need to guide the adolescent's development of self-management skills. Self-management skills include adhering to the treatment regimen, taking responsibility for medications, getting required blood tests in a timely manner, scheduling and attending appointments, and recognizing signs and symptoms suggesting a change in their health status. Typically, chronologic age is frequently used as the criteria to determine the patient's readiness for a somewhat abrupt transition from child-centered health care to adult-centered health care. However, studies have shown that when responsibilities for health-related tasks are gradually shifted throughout adolescence in a developmentally appropriate manner, the adolescent gains the skills, knowledge, and experience necessary to master self-management skills and the independence required to be successful in the adult health care system.[41]

Adherence is a key component in developing self-management skills and is a universal concern when caring for adolescents. There is considerable literature discussing the psychosocial factors that predict nonadherence. Some of these factors include family interactions, psychological symptoms in the patient, barriers to adherent behavior, the disease process, level of self-management skills, care patterns including timing and frequency of medications and clinic appointments, and socioeconomic status.[42,43] However, there are strategies for improving adherence consisting of simplifying the treatment regimen; assessing and addressing common risk factors and obstacles to adherence; leveraging electronic devices to provide reminders, such as text messaging and alarms for medications; and remaining connected to the patients through more frequent follow-up.[44]

Appropriate psychosocial support is essential for any patient and family diagnosed with a liver disease, especially chronic liver disease. There is an increasing body of literature reporting symptoms of anxiety, significant stress, and posttraumatic stress disorder in patients and parents diagnosed with a perceived or actual life-threatening illness. In addition, the number of complications associated with the disease does not correlate with psychological symptoms.[45] One study reports that children with NAFLD have higher levels of depression compared with obese control subjects and the depression does not necessarily improve with standard of care measures, such as lifestyle changes and weight loss.[46] It has also been reported that chronic illnesses in childhood impact cognition and is associated with limitations in school and increased missed school days.[47] Thus, providers should consider scheduling routine follow-up for adolescents at times that do not interfere with school attendance.

Transition from pediatric-centered health care to adult-centered health care is part of a developmental process for patients with chronic childhood illnesses and requires a multidisciplinary approach. Transition of care is not the same as transfer of care, because transfer of care is only one small step in the transition of care to the adult health care system and does not mark the end of the transition process. Transition of care should begin around 10 to 12 years depending on the developmental maturity of the patient and is a multifaceted process that addresses the medical, psychosocial, and educational needs of the adolescent as they prepare to move from pediatric-centered health care to adult-centered health care.[48] Before transfer of care to the adult health care system, the patient must achieve transfer readiness, which includes understanding the illness, self-management skills, and the ability to assume responsibility of his or her health care. In addition, it is helpful to identify an adult health care provider or group at least 6 to 12 months before the transfer and work closely with them during the transfer. This may include joint clinic appointments or scheduled appointments with the adult care provider to become familiar with the practice and expectations of the adult health care system while still following with the pediatric health care provider. Transition preparation is a continuous process and should incorporate interventions to promote self-management skills and adherence as pediatric patients prepare to move from child-centered care to adult-centered care to ensure a successful transfer of care.

REFERENCES

1. Kaufman M, Shemes E, Benton T. The adolescent transplant recipient. Pediatr Clin North Am 2010;57:575–92.
2. Sanders RA. Adolescent psychosocial, social, and cognitive development. Pediatr Rev 2013;34:354–8.
3. Bernheim A, Halfon O, Boutrel B. Controversies about the enhanced vulnerability of the adolescent brain to develop addiction. Front Pharmacol 2013;4:118.
4. Levy S, Williams JF. Adolescent substance use: the role of the medical home. Adolesc Med State Art Rev 2014;25:1–14.
5. van Groningen J, Ziniel S, Arnold J, et al. When independent healthcare behaviors develop in adolescents with inflammatory bowel disease. Inflamm Bowel Dis 2012;18:2310–4.
6. Aujoulat I, Janssen M, Libion F, et al. Internalizing motivation to self-care: a multifaceted challenge for young liver transplant recipients. Qual Health Res 2014;24:357–65.
7. Piering K, Arnon R, Miloh TA, et al. Developmental and disease-related influences on self-management acquisition among pediatric liver transplant recipients. Pediatr Transpl 2011;15:819–26.
8. Ioanou GN, Boyko EJ, Lee SP. The prevalence and predictors of elevated serum aminotransferase activity in the United States in 1999-2002. Am J Gastroenterol 2006;101:76–82.
9. Lee TH, Kim WR, Poterucha JJ. Evaluation of elevated liver enzymes. Clin Liver Dis 2012;16:183–98.
10. Ruhl CE, Everhart JE. Trunk fat is associated with increased serum levels of alanine aminotransferase in the United States. Gastroenterology 2010;138:1346–56.
11. Vernon G, Baranova A, Younossi ZM. Systematic review: the epidemiology and natural history of non-alcoholic fatty liver disease and non-alcoholic steatohepatitis in adults. Aliment Pharmacol Ther 2011;34:274–85.
12. Browning JD, Szczepaniak LS, Dobbins R, et al. Prevelance of hepatic steatosis in an urban population in the United States: impact of ethnicity. Hepatology 2004;40:1387–95.
13. Wagenknecht LE, Scherzinger AL, Stamm ER, et al. Correlates and heritability of nonalcoholic fatty liver disease in a minority cohort. Obesity (Silver Spring) 2009;17:1240–6.

14. Harrison SA, Fecht W, Brunt EM, et al. Orlistat for overweight subjects with nonalcoholic steatohepatitis: a randomized prospective trial. Hepatology 2009;49: 80–6.
15. Promrat K, Kleiner DE, Niemeier HM, et al. Randomized controlled trial testing the effects of weight loss on nonalcoholic steatohepatitis. Hepatology 2010;51: 121–9.
16. Chalasani N, Younossi Z, Lavine JE, et al. The diagnosis and management of non-alcoholic fatty liver disease: practice guideline by the American Gastroenterological Association, American Association for the Study of Liver Diseases, and American College of Gastroenterology. Gastroenterology 2012;142:1592–609.
17. Manns MP, Czaja AJ, Gorham JE, et al. Diagnosis and management of autoimmune hepatitis. Hepatology 2010;51:2193–213.
18. Dienes HP, Popper H, Manns M, et al. Histological features in autoimmune hepatitis. Gastroenterol 1989;27:327–30.
19. Woynarowski M, Nemeth A, Baruch Y, et al. Budesonide versus prednisone with azathioprine for the treatment of autoimmune hepatitis in children and adolescents. J Pediatr 2013;163:1347–53.
20. Della Corte C, Sartorelli MR, Sindoni CD, et al. Autoimmune hepatitis in children: an overview of the disease focusing on current therapies. Eur J Gastroenterol Hepatol 2012;24:739–46.
21. Gregorio GV, Portmann B, Reid F, et al. Autoimmune hepatitis in childhood: a 20-year experience. Hepatology 1997;25:541–7.
22. Borgia G, Carleo MA, Gaeta GB, et al. Hepatitis B in pregnancy. World J Gastroenterol 2012;18:4677–83.
23. Yang SI, Geong JH, Kim JY. Clinical characteristics of primary Epstein Barr virus hepatitis with elevation of alkaline phosphatase and γ-glutamyltransferase in children. Yonsei Med J 2014;55:107–12.
24. Huster D. Wilson disease. Best Pract Res Clin Gastroenterol 2010;24:531–9.
25. Litwin T, Gromadzka G, Czlonkowska A. Gender differences in Wilson's disease. J Neurol Sci 2012;312:31–5.
26. European Association for Study of Liver. EASL clinical practice guidelines: Wilson's disease. J Hepatol 2012;56:671–85.
27. de Serres FJ, Blanco I, Fernandez-Bustillo E. Genetic epidemiology of alpha-1 antitrypsin deficiency in North America and Australia/New Zealand: Australia, Canada, New Zealand and the United States of America. Clin Genet 2003;64: 382–97.
28. Schilsky M, Oikonomou I. Inherited metabolic liver disease. Curr Opin Gastroenterol 2005;21:275–82.
29. Teckman JH. Liver disease in alpha-1 antitrypsin deficiency: current understanding and future therapy. COPD 2013;10(Suppl 1):35–43.
30. Lykavieris P, Chardot C, Sokhn M, et al. Outcome in adulthood of biliary atresia: a study of 63 patients who survived for over 20 years with their native liver. Hepatology 2005;41:366–71.
31. Shneider BL, Abel B, Haber B, et al. Portal hypertension in children and young adults with biliary atresia. J Pediatr Gastroenterol Nutr 2012;55:567–73.
32. Emre S, Dugan C, Frankenberg T, et al. Surgical portosystemic shunts and the Rex bypass in children: a single-centre experience. HPB (Oxford) 2009;11:252–7.
33. Yankaskas JR, Marshall BC, Sufian B, et al. Cystic fibrosis adult care: consensus conference report. Chest 2004;125(1 Suppl):1S–39S.
34. Wilschanski M, Durie PR. Patterns of GI disease in adulthood associated with mutations in the CFTR gene. Gut 2007;56:1153–63.

35. Neglia JP, FitzSimmons SC, Maisonneuve P, et al. The risk of cancer among patients with cystic fibrosis. Cystic Fibrosis and Cancer Study Group. N Engl J Med 1995;332:494–9.
36. Rojas-Feria M, Castro M, Suárez E, et al. Hepatobiliary manifestations in inflammatory bowel disease: the gut, the drugs and the liver. World J Gastroenterol 2013;19:7327–40.
37. Nguyen KD, Sundaram V, Ayoub WS. Atypical causes of cholestasis. World J Gastroenterol 2014;20:9418–26.
38. Tumialán LM, Dhall SS, Tomak PR, et al. Alagille syndrome and aneurysmal subarachnoid hemorrhage. Case report and review of the literature. Pediatr Neurosurg 2006;42:57–61.
39. Strubbe B, Geerts A, Van Vlierberghe H, et al. Progressive familial intrahepatic cholestasis and benign recurrent intrahepatic cholestasis: a review. Acta Gastroenterol Belg 2012;75:405–10.
40. Strautnieks SS, Byrne JA, Pawlikowska L, et al. Severe bile salt export pump deficiency: 82 different ABCB11 mutations in 109 families. Gastroenterology 2008; 134:1203–14.
41. McDonagh JE. Growing up and moving on: transition from pediatric to adult care. Pediatr Transplant 2005;9:364–72.
42. Shemesh E. Psychosocial adaptation and adherence. In: Fine RN, Webber SA, Olthoff KM, et al, editors. Pediatric solid organ transplantation. 2nd edition. Malden (MA): Blackwell; 2007. p. 418–24.
43. Bender B, Milgrom H, Apter A. Adherence intervention research: what have we learned and what do we do next? J Allergy Clin Immunol 2003;112:489–94.
44. Smith BA, Shuchman M. Problem of nonadherence in chronically ill adolescents: strategies for assessment and intervention. Curr Opin Pediatr 2005;17:613–8.
45. Mintzer LL, Stuber ML, Seacord D, et al. Traumatic stress symptoms in adolescent organ transplant recipients. Pediatrics 2005;115:1640–4.
46. Kerkar N, D'Urso C, Van Nostrand K, et al. Psychosocial outcomes for children with nonalcoholic fatty liver disease over time and compared with obese controls. J Pediatr Gastroenterol Nutr 2013;56:77–82.
47. Moser JJ, Veale PM, McAllister DL, et al. A systematic review and qualitative analysis of neurocognitive outcomes in children with four chronic illnesses. Paediatr Anaesth 2013;23:1084–96.
48. Blum RW, Garell D, Hodgman CH, et al. Transition from child-centered to adult health-care systems for adolescents with chronic conditions. A position paper of the Society for Adolescent Medicine. J Adolesc Health 1993;14:570–6.

Diagnosis and Management of Hereditary Hemochromatosis

Reena J. Salgia, MD*, Kimberly Brown, MD

KEYWORDS

- Hemochromatosis • Iron saturation • Ferritin • Cirrhosis • Liver transplant

KEY POINTS

- Hereditary hemochromatosis (HH) is a diagnosis most commonly made in patients with elevated iron indices (transferrin saturation and ferritin), and *HFE* genetic mutation testing showing C282Y homozygosity.
- The HFE mutation is believed to result in clinical iron overload through altering hepcidin levels resulting in increased iron absorption.
- The most common clinical complications of HH include cirrhosis, diabetes, nonischemic cardiomyopathy, and hepatocellular carcinoma.
- Liver biopsy should be performed in patients with HH if the liver enzymes are elevated or serum ferritin is greater than 1000 µg/L. This is useful to determine the degree of iron overload and stage the fibrosis.
- Treatment of HH with clinical iron overload involves a combination of phlebotomy and/or chelation therapy. Liver transplantation should be considered for patients with HH-related decompensated cirrhosis.

INTRODUCTION

Although hereditary hemochromatosis (HH) is a less common cause of cirrhosis than chronic viral hepatitis, it remains the most commonly identified genetic disorder in the white population. The prevalence of HH varies worldwide, with the highest frequency of disease occurring among those of northern European ancestry.[1] Since this disease was first described by Trousseau in 1865, many studies have led to a greater understanding of the underlying pathophysiology. HH was initially noted to be associated with increased iron deposition in organ tissue, leading to cirrhosis, heart failure, diabetes, arthritis, and a high risk for hepatocellular carcinoma (HCC).[2] Then a seminal

Disclosures: The authors have no relevant affiliations or financial involvement.
Division of Gastroenterology and Hepatology, Henry Ford Hospital, 2799 West Grand Boulevard, Detroit, MI 48202, USA
* Corresponding author.
E-mail address: rsalgia1@hfhs.org

Clin Liver Dis 19 (2015) 187–198
http://dx.doi.org/10.1016/j.cld.2014.09.011
1089-3261/15/$ – see front matter © 2015 Elsevier Inc. All rights reserved.
liver.theclinics.com

paper in 1996 revealed the *HFE* gene mutation, which causes a substitution of tyrosine for cysteine at the amino acid 282 position (C282Y).[3] Subsequently two additional mutations were noted, aspartate for histidine (H63D), and cysteine for serine (S65C). The most common form of *HFE*-related HH is associated with the C282Y homozygous mutation, and less commonly compound heterozygotes with either C282Y/H63D or C282Y/S65C.[4] Non-*HFE* associated hemochromatosis is rare, accounting for less than 15% of inherited iron overload.[5] This article provides a brief overview of the pathophysiology of hemochromatosis, and an up-to-date summary of the diagnosis and management of HH.

PATHOPHYSIOLOGY

HH is a genetic disorder broadly characterized by excessive total body iron storage.[1,6] Several mechanisms explain this imbalance of iron homeostasis in HH. The initial theory was noted as the "crypt cell hypothesis," reflecting the interplay between the HFE protein and β_2-microglobulin.[7,8] Together these two proteins form a complex with transferrin receptor-1, which is located predominantly in the duodenal crypt enterocytes. There the complex would sense and regulate dietary iron absorption. It is also hypothesized that this complex acts at the level of the hepatocyte membrane to sense iron stores.[9] However, the more recent discovery of hepcidin, a small peptide hormone that is encoded by a gene expressed in the liver, has altered the predominant theory of iron overload associated with HH. Hepcidin controls iron absorption in the duodenum. The levels of circulating hepcidin vary based on systemic iron stores.[10] The interaction between HFE and the transferrin receptors is paramount to the sensing of iron at the hepatocyte membrane.[11] When iron stores are elevated, hepcidin is released and binds to ferroportin in macrophages and enterocytes. There it blocks the export of iron from macrophages and decreases intestinal iron absorption (**Fig. 1**).[12,13] When the HFE protein is mutated, the expression of hepcidin decreases and intestinal iron absorption increases. Although it remains unclear how the mutated HFE gene controls hepcidin in HH, a decrease in hepcidin results in a rise of iron efflux from macrophages and enterocytes, and increased intestinal iron absorption into organ tissue.[14] Hence the liver is the major regulator of iron metabolism, and in patients with HH this mechanism is altered by abnormally low hepcidin levels.[15]

The presence of elevated iron stores in the liver over time can lead to hepatic fibrosis and cirrhosis. Iron has been shown to cause increased oxidative stress and damage to hepatocytes and mitochondrial function.[16–18] These hepatocytes are injured and release Kupffer cells, which stimulate hepatic stellate cells to increase production of collagen.[19] Over time this process leads to the development of cirrhosis.

DIAGNOSIS
Clinical Presentation

Because of variable penetrance of clinical HH, end-organ damage is noted in less than 10% of patients who are homozygous for the C282Y mutation.[20] The clinical phenotype is expressed in 24% to 43% of males and 1% to 14% of females.[21] Clinical disease is noted even less frequently in patients who are compound heterozygotes (C282Y/H63D positive), who account for approximately 5% of cases of HH.[4,22] Women also present with clinical features later in life, largely related to monthly menstruation resulting in iron loss and having a protective effect. However, the disease prevalence is similar between men and women, resulting from earlier recognition and screening for this disease.[23,24]

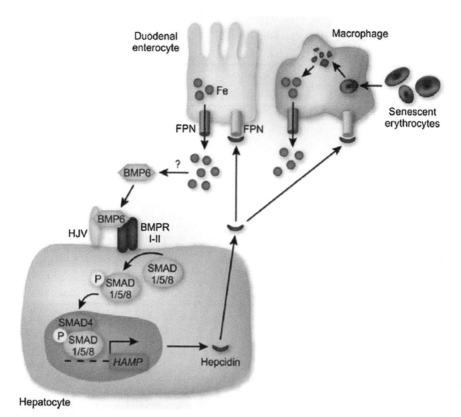

Fig. 1. Iron homeostasis as regulated by hepcidin. BMPR, bone morphogenetic protein receptor; FPN, ferroportin; HJV, hemojuvelin; SMAD, Sma and Mad related protein. (*From* Camaschella C. BMP 6 orchestrates iron metabolism. Nat Genet 2009;41(4):386–8; with permission.)

The clinical features of HH are highly variable, with signs and symptoms that can involve multiple organ systems. Aside from liver involvement leading to cirrhosis, iron overload from HH can involve the heart, pancreas, skin, pituitary gland, gonads, and joints (**Table 1**).[1,4] Multiple studies have found that the predominant clinical features in patients with HH include (from most common to least common) cirrhosis, lethargy, hyperpigmentation of the skin, loss of libido, testicular atrophy, diabetes, abdominal pain, and arthralgias.[25–27]

Laboratory Testing

The initial suspicion for HH is largely made based on clinical features, biochemical abnormalities, and genetic testing, with liver biopsy less commonly needed to make an initial diagnosis. Elevated serum ferritin (SF) levels and transferrin-iron saturation (TS) are readily available serum markers that help to identify patients with HH. These tests should be performed on patients with chronically elevated liver enzymes.[1] Ferritin levels greater than 200 µg/L for females and greater than 300 µg/L for males are considered abnormal.[23,28] Ferritin is known to be elevated in the absence of elevated iron stores. For example, the presence of viral hepatitis, nonalcoholic fatty liver disease, or alcoholic liver disease and other chronic inflammatory conditions can all cause elevations in SF levels.[1] The TS is calculated based on total body iron divided

Table 1
Signs, symptoms, and clinical presentation of HH

Organ System	Sign/Symptom	Physical Examination
General	Weakness, fatigue, lethargy Weight loss Apathy	
Liver	Abdominal pain	Hepatomegaly Splenomegaly Cutaneous stigmata (spider angiomata, palmar erythema) Gynecomastia
Cardiac	Heart failure Arrhythmia	Cardiomegaly Elevated JVP
Pancreas	Hyperglycemia from diabetes	
Skin		Hyperpigmentation, "bronze skin" Porphyria cutanea tarda
Endocrine	Loss of libido Hypothyroidism	Testicular atrophy
Joints	Arthralgias	Arthritis (second and third MCP) Joint swelling

Abbreviations: JVP, jugular venous pressure; MCP, metacarpophalangeal joint.

by total iron-binding capacity. A saturation level higher than 45% again raises suspicion for HH.[23,28] If either the SF or TS is abnormal, then the HFE genetic mutation analysis should be performed.[1] A result of C282Y homozygous genotype is consistent with a diagnosis of HH in the setting of iron overload.[29] It is less common for C282Y/H63D compound heterozygous genotype or H63D homozygous genotype to develop clinically significant iron overload; however, it has been described.[22,30] The Hemochromatosis and Iron Overload Screening study screened 99,711 North American patients and found that SF was elevated (>200 µg/L in women and >300 µg/L in men) in 57% of female and 88% of male C282Y homozygotes.[23] Multiple studies have shown that marked elevations in SF to values greater than 1000 µg/L are a stronger predictor of advanced hepatic fibrosis and cirrhosis in patients with documented HH.[29,31–33] When an elevated ferritin greater than 1000 µg/L is combined with elevated transaminases and platelet count less than $200 \times 10(9)/L$, the positive predictive value for cirrhosis is 80% in patients with C282Y homozygosity.[34] These findings have also been shown to increase the mortality risk associated with HH.[35] Patients with C282Y homozygosity who have normal iron studies should have an annual measurement of their ferritin level.[4]

Screening for Hereditary Hemochromatosis

Screening for HH should also be performed in patients with a family history of HH or a suspicion based on suspected organ involvement of elevated iron stores.[1,23] **Fig. 2** is a diagnostic algorithm for screening patients at-risk for HH. It is recommended that all first-degree relatives of a patient with HH should undergo family screening. Screening can be performed with SF, TS, and HFE mutation testing. The inheritance pattern is autosomal-recessive with mutations in the HFE gene on chromosome 6.[3,36] Children of an affected parent can be tested or alternatively the other parent can be tested.[37] It is generally recommended that if children are going to be screened, testing should be

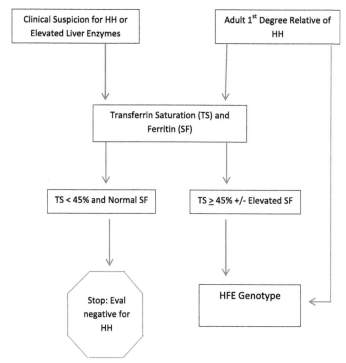

Fig. 2. Diagnostic algorithm for HH. Elevated SF is greater than 200 µg/L in females and greater than 300 µg/L in males.

done once they reach adulthood.[38] There is a negligible risk of developing clinical HH before the age of 18.

Histology

The main purpose of liver biopsy in the diagnosis of HH is to stage the degree of fibrosis. It is important to determine if patients have cirrhosis for prognosis and to initiate surveillance for HCC and esophageal varices.[39] SF is valuable to discriminate which patients should proceed with a biopsy. Specifically, ferritin greater than 1000 µg/L in C282Y homozygotes has been shown in several studies to be predictive of cirrhosis, with a prevalence of 20% to 45%.[32,34] Ferritin levels less than 1000 µg/L in the same population is associated with a low prevalence of 2% for determining cirrhosis. However, this does not apply in patients with a coexisting cause for liver disease, such as chronic viral hepatitis, alcoholic liver disease, or nonalcoholic fatty liver disease.[29,31,32,34] Additionally, liver biopsy should be performed in patients with elevated iron studies, elevated liver enzymes, and non-C282Y genotypes of HH. This can exclude the presence of a coexisting cause of liver injury.[1]

Liver biopsy specimens should be processed using standard hematoxylin-eosin stain, Masson trichrome stain, and an additional Perl Prussian blue stain. The Prussian blue stain helps to capture the distribution of hepatic iron (**Fig. 3**).[40] A quantitative assessment of hepatic iron stores can also be performed. This measurement, the hepatic iron concentration or similarly the hepatic iron index, is abnormal at levels higher than 36 µmol/g and 1.9, respectively.[41–44] In the clinical setting, hepatic iron concentration is more commonly used, with hepatic iron index reserved more for the research

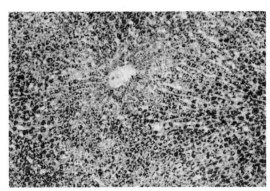

Fig. 3. Perl Prussian blue stain on a liver biopsy in hemochromatosis. (*Reproduced from* University of Utah WebPath slide set; with permission.)

setting. Hepatic iron concentration has been shown to correlate well with a noninvasive method of estimating hepatic iron stores using T2-weighted MRI.[45,46] Additionally, another noninvasive method of determining cirrhosis that is gaining popularity is use of transient elastography. These methods reduce the need for performing liver biopsy as frequently.

Non-HFE Hereditary Hemochromatosis

There are other inherited forms of HH that are less common, and non–HFE-related. These account for less than 5% of cases of inherited HH. Examples include juvenile hemochromatosis, mutation in the transferrin receptor 2 gene, and a mutation in the ferroportin (SLC40A1) gene.[5] The most common of these is juvenile hemochromatosis, which has two potential genetic mutations.[47] Most common is type 2a HH, which is caused by a mutation in the hemojuvelin gene on chromosome 1q.[48] Less common is type 2b HH, caused by a mutation in the hepcidin gene. The presence of this mutation results in upregulation of iron absorption.[47] A mutation in the transferrin receptor 2 gene results in abnormal sensing of iron stores by hepatocytes. In turn this leads to an autosomal-recessive form of HH, also known as type 3 HH.[49] The excess iron is deposited in the hepatocytes, as is similar to HFE-related HH. A rare cause of HH results from mutations in the SLC40A1 gene, responsible for the iron transporter protein, ferroportin. Mutations in this gene result in impaired iron export, with deposition of iron noted in the hepatocytes and in reticuloendothelial cells.[50] The inheritance pattern is autosomal-dominant, and also known as type 4 HH.[51] Genetic testing for all of these mutations is often unavailable in the clinical setting, particularly for the SLC40A1 gene mutation. Liver biopsy can be a useful diagnostic tool in patients with non-HFE HH to determine the extent of iron overload and the distribution.[5,52] Presently, there are no recommendations to screen patients for non–HFE-related HH.[1]

MANAGEMENT AND TREATMENT
Goals of Management

Early identification and treatment of patients with HH with clinical iron overload can improve their morbidity and mortality. The mainstay of treatment has been through phlebotomy. Although no randomized controlled trial has been performed comparing phlebotomy with no phlebotomy for these patients, there is evidence of improvement in certain clinical features with treatment.[53,54] Phlebotomy in patients with liver disease can slow the progression to cirrhosis, and also reduces the risk of developing HCC. HCC is rare in patients with HH in the absence of cirrhosis.[55] However, patients with HH-related cirrhosis are at an elevated risk of developing HCC, with 30% of disease-related deaths noted to be from the development of liver cancer.[54,56] Tissue iron overload has in fact been shown to increase the likelihood of a variety of cancers, not just HCC.[57] In early stages of hepatic fibrosis, reversal of fibrosis can be noted in some patients with reduction of tissue iron stores, and can also normalize liver enzymes. Once cirrhosis is established, improvement in fibrosis is not expected with phlebotomy.[58] Phlebotomy can also improve diabetes management and control, decrease fatigue, improve cardiac function, reduce skin hyperpigmentation, and improve abdominal pain. Patients with arthropathy or hypogonadism rarely see improvement in symptoms with phlebotomy.[58–61]

Phlebotomy

The initial goal of therapeutic phlebotomy is to decrease the SF level to between 50 and 100 µg/L to assume that the excess iron stores have been depleted.[1] Each unit of blood removed is 400 to 500 mL of whole blood and contains approximately 200 to 250 mg of iron. Phlebotomy should be initiated once weekly, depending on the baseline hemoglobin. The hemoglobin needs to be monitored closely, ensuring that this does not decrease to less than 80% of the baseline value.[1] During the first year of phlebotomy, it is recommended that a hemoglobin is checked before each phlebotomy, and that ferritin levels are monitored with every 10 to 12 phlebotomies. TS usually does not decrease until iron stores are depleted, so it is more accurate to initially monitor the ferritin.[1] Once the ferritin is reduced to 50 to 100 µg/L, testing should be done more frequently so as to avoid iron deficiency, and maintenance phlebotomy can be scheduled. The frequency of maintenance is variable, ranging for some patients every 4 weeks to yearly or even less often for others.[1] During the maintenance phase, a ferritin level up to 100 µg/L is tolerated, because prior recommendations to aggressively keep the ferritin levels very low (<50 µg/L) may paradoxically decrease hepcidin stores and then promote reaccumulation of iron.[1] Presently, there are insufficient data to support phlebotomy for asymptomatic patients with HH who do not have elevated iron stores.

Iron Chelators and Dietary Modification

Few patients with HH are intolerant of phlebotomy because of baseline anemia or hematologic disorders. These patients should be considered for iron chelation therapy, such as deferoxamine or deferasirox.[62,63] Dietary changes have not been shown to be necessary for patients undergoing treatment, except in the setting of patients who may eat diets very rich in iron. Pharmacologic iron supplementation is advised against.[4] Vitamin C can interfere with the mobilization of iron stores by saturating transferrin. This results in increased free radical activity.[64] Most commonly this is seen with pharmacologic doses of vitamin C, which is also not recommended in patients undergoing treatment of HH.

Cirrhosis Management

Progression to advanced cirrhosis or decompensated cirrhosis is not reversed with phlebotomy. Patients who have developed decompensation of their liver disease should be considered for orthotopic liver transplantation. Over the past few decades, the outcome of patients transplanted for HH-related cirrhosis has improved, with posttransplant survival now similar to other patients post–orthotopic liver transplantation. A recent study showed post–liver transplant survival for patients with HH to be

83% at 1 year and 67% at 5 years.[65,66] The most likely explanation for this is because of earlier identification of the disease, instituting early treatment and adequate removal of iron excess before transplant. This has decreased the likelihood of perioperative mortality associated with cardiac disease and infection, and posttransplant malignancy.[67]

Similar to other patients with cirrhosis, the American Association for the Study of Liver Diseases guidelines recommends that all patients with cirrhosis from HH undergo surveillance for HCC. Patients with HH have an annual incidence of HCC of 3% to 4% in the setting of underlying cirrhosis.[68] This risk remains elevated despite adequate phlebotomy and removal of excess tissue iron, although long-term studies are needed.[55] Screening and surveillance is recommended with a combination of abdominal ultrasound ± alpha fetoprotein every 6 to 12 months.[68]

SURVIVAL AND PROGNOSIS

Overall, the survival of patients with HFE-related HH is affected by their clinical phenotype; the presence or absence of cirrhosis; and other HH-related comorbidities, such as diabetes and cardiac disease. Patients who express the clinical phenotype and have untreated disease have a higher mortality risk than the general population.[27,54] Patients without the clinical phenotype have a similar overall survival to the general population.[27] In the setting of cirrhosis, patients with HH have a higher risk of death regardless of their treatment status.[27] There has been no prospective study comparing phlebotomy with placebo. This is unlikely to occur because it would be deemed unethical given the effectiveness and safety profile of phlebotomy. However, phlebotomy seems to improve survival, likely because of slowing the rate of clinical progression and associated comorbid conditions. Patients with decompensated cirrhosis from HH who undergo a liver transplant have overall comparable survival outcomes with other transplant recipients, and have a normalization of their hepcidin levels after transplantation.[66] This prevents the development of iron overload from HH in the graft.

SUMMARY

Because of a greater understanding of the genetic factors causing HH, there is an earlier recognition and diagnosis of patients with HH. The clinical phenotype of iron overload associated with HH remains a rare liver disease in comparison with viral hepatitis or fatty liver disease. However, it can have important clinical consequences that affect multiple organ systems including the liver, heart, skin, joints, and endocrine function if not recognized and managed at an early stage. HFE-associated hemochromatosis is responsible for most cases of HH. Liver biopsy is performed in select cases to stage the degree of hepatic fibrosis and/or quantify hepatic iron content. Patients with biochemical evidence of iron overload and clinical features of hemochromatosis should be managed ideally with phlebotomy. Patients with advanced cirrhosis and decompensation should be considered for liver transplantation, and should undergo regular surveillance for HCC. In the future, clinicians will likely continue to better understand the central mechanism underlying iron metabolism in HH. Although genetic testing for the HFE genetic mutation is now commonly available, gene testing for rarer causes of HH can be difficult to perform in the clinical setting. Given the infrequent presentation of these disorders, it is unclear if this testing will become commercially available in the near future. Overall the future for patients undergoing liver transplantation for HH remains bright, with comparable posttransplant outcomes with other liver transplant recipients.

REFERENCES

1. Bacon BR, Adams PC, Kowdley KV, et al. Diagnosis and management of hemo-chromatosis: 2011 practice guideline by the American Association for the Study of Liver Diseases. Hepatology 2011;54(1):328–43.
2. Simon M, Bourel M, Genetet B, et al. Idiopathic hemochromatosis. Demonstration of recessive transmission and early detection by family HLA typing. N Engl J Med 1977;297(19):1017–21.
3. Feder JN, Gnirke A, Thomas W, et al. A novel MHC class I-like gene is mutated in patients with hereditary haemochromatosis. Nat Genet 1996;13(4):399–408.
4. European Association for the Study of the Liver. EASL clinical practice guidelines for HFE hemochromatosis. J Hepatol 2010;53(1):3–22.
5. Pietrangelo A. Non-HFE hemochromatosis. Semin Liver Dis 2005;25(4):450–60.
6. Parkkila S, Niemela O, Britton RS, et al. Molecular aspects of iron absorption and HFE expression. Gastroenterology 2001;121(6):1489–96.
7. Fleming RE, Britton RS, Waheed A, et al. Pathogenesis of hereditary hemochro-matosis. Clin Liver Dis 2004;8(4):755–73, vii.
8. Parkkila S, Waheed A, Britton RS, et al. Immunohistochemistry of HLA-H, the pro-tein defective in patients with hereditary hemochromatosis, reveals unique pattern of expression in gastrointestinal tract. Proc Natl Acad Sci U S A 1997; 94(6):2534–9.
9. Waheed A, Parkkila S, Saarnio J, et al. Association of HFE protein with transferrin receptor in crypt enterocytes of human duodenum. Proc Natl Acad Sci U S A 1999;96(4):1579–84.
10. Nemeth E, Ganz T. The role of hepcidin in iron metabolism. Acta Haematol 2009; 122(2–3):78–86.
11. D'Alessio F, Hentze MW, Muckenthaler MU. The hemochromatosis proteins HFE, TfR2, and HJV form a membrane-associated protein complex for hepcidin regu-lation. J Hepatol 2012;57(5):1052–60.
12. Nemeth E, Tuttle MS, Powelson J, et al. Hepcidin regulates cellular iron efflux by bind-ing to ferroportin and inducing its internalization. Science 2004;306(5704):2090–3.
13. Camaschella C. BMP6 orchestrates iron metabolism. Nat Genet 2009;41(4): 386–8.
14. Pietrangelo A. Hereditary hemochromatosis: pathogenesis, diagnosis, and treat-ment. Gastroenterology 2010;139(2):393–408, 408.e1–2.
15. van Dijk BA, Laarakkers CM, Klaver SM, et al. Serum hepcidin levels are innately low in HFE-related haemochromatosis but differ between C282Y-homozygotes with elevated and normal ferritin levels. Br J Haematol 2008;142(6):979–85.
16. Philippe MA, Ruddell RG, Ramm GA. Role of iron in hepatic fibrosis: one piece in the puzzle. World J Gastroenterol 2007;13(35):4746–54.
17. Bacon BR, Tavill AS, Brittenham GM, et al. Hepatic lipid peroxidation in vivo in rats with chronic iron overload. J Clin Invest 1983;71(3):429–39.
18. Bacon BR, Britton RS. The pathology of hepatic iron overload: a free radical–mediated process? Hepatology 1990;11(1):127–37.
19. Olynyk JK, Britton RS, Stephenson AH, et al. An in vitro model for the study of phagocytosis of damaged hepatocytes by rat Kupffer cells. Liver 1999;19(5): 418–22.
20. Beutler E, Felitti VJ, Koziol JA, et al. Penetrance of 845G–> A (C282Y) HFE hered-itary haemochromatosis mutation in the USA. Lancet 2002;359(9302):211–8.
21. Rossi E, Olynyk JK, Jeffrey GP. Clinical penetrance of C282Y homozygous HFE hemochromatosis. Expert Rev Hematol 2008;1(2):205–16.

22. Cheng R, Barton JC, Morrison ED, et al. Differences in hepatic phenotype between hemochromatosis patients with HFE C282Y homozygosity and other HFE genotypes. J Clin Gastroenterol 2009;43(6):569–73.
23. Adams PC, Reboussin DM, Barton JC, et al. Hemochromatosis and iron-overload screening in a racially diverse population. N Engl J Med 2005;352(17):1769–78.
24. Allen KJ, Gurrin LC, Constantine CC, et al. Iron-overload-related disease in HFE hereditary hemochromatosis. N Engl J Med 2008;358(3):221–30.
25. Edwards CQ, Cartwright GE, Skolnick MH, et al. Homozygosity for hemochromatosis: clinical manifestations. Ann Intern Med 1980;93(4):519–25.
26. Milder MS, Cook JD, Stray S, et al. Idiopathic hemochromatosis, an interim report. Medicine 1980;59(1):34–49.
27. Niederau C, Fischer R, Sonnenberg A, et al. Survival and causes of death in cirrhotic and in noncirrhotic patients with primary hemochromatosis. N Engl J Med 1985;313(20):1256–62.
28. Bassett ML, Halliday JW, Ferris RA, et al. Diagnosis of hemochromatosis in young subjects: predictive accuracy of biochemical screening tests. Gastroenterology 1984;87(3):628–33.
29. Bacon BR, Olynyk JK, Brunt EM, et al. HFE genotype in patients with hemochromatosis and other liver diseases. Ann Intern Med 1999;130(12):953–62.
30. Gochee PA, Powell LW, Cullen DJ, et al. A population-based study of the biochemical and clinical expression of the H63D hemochromatosis mutation. Gastroenterology 2002;122(3):646–51.
31. Guyader D, Jacquelinet C, Moirand R, et al. Noninvasive prediction of fibrosis in C282Y homozygous hemochromatosis. Gastroenterology 1998;115(4):929–36.
32. Morrison ED, Brandhagen DJ, Phatak PD, et al. Serum ferritin level predicts advanced hepatic fibrosis among U.S. patients with phenotypic hemochromatosis. Ann Intern Med 2003;138(8):627–33.
33. Allen KJ, Bertalli NA, Osborne NJ, et al. HFE Cys282Tyr homozygotes with serum ferritin concentrations below 1000 microg/L are at low risk of hemochromatosis. Hepatology 2010;52(3):925–33.
34. Beaton M, Guyader D, Deugnier Y, et al. Noninvasive prediction of cirrhosis in C282Y-linked hemochromatosis. Hepatology 2002;36(3):673–8.
35. Barton JC, Barton JC, Acton RT, et al. Increased risk of death from iron overload among 422 treated probands with HFE hemochromatosis and serum levels of ferritin greater than 1000 mug/L at diagnosis. Clin Gastroenterol Hepatol 2012;10(4):412–6.
36. Edwards CQ, Cartwright GE, Skolnick MH, et al. Genetic mapping of the hemochromatosis locus on chromosome six. Hum Immunol 1980;1(1):19–22.
37. Adams PC. Implications of genotyping of spouses to limit investigation of children in genetic hemochromatosis. Clin Genet 1998;53(3):176–8.
38. Kanwar P, Kowdley KV. Diagnosis and treatment of hereditary hemochromatosis: an update. Expert Rev Gastroenterol Hepatol 2013;7(6):517–30.
39. Garcia-Tsao G, Sanyal AJ, Grace ND, et al. Prevention and management of gastroesophageal varices and variceal hemorrhage in cirrhosis. Hepatology 2007;46(3):922–38.
40. Deugnier Y, Turlin B. Pathology of hepatic iron overload. Semin Liver Dis 2011;31(3):260–71.
41. Bassett ML, Halliday JW, Powell LW. Value of hepatic iron measurements in early hemochromatosis and determination of the critical iron level associated with fibrosis. Hepatology 1986;6(1):24–9.

42. Kowdley KV, Trainer TD, Saltzman JR, et al. Utility of hepatic iron index in American patients with hereditary hemochromatosis: a multicenter study. Gastroenterology 1997;113(4):1270–7.
43. Summers KM, Halliday JW, Powell LW. Identification of homozygous hemochromatosis subjects by measurement of hepatic iron index. Hepatology 1990; 12(1):20–5.
44. Sallie RW, Reed WD, Shilkin KB. Confirmation of the efficacy of hepatic tissue iron index in differentiating genetic haemochromatosis from alcoholic liver disease complicated by alcoholic haemosiderosis. Gut 1991;32(2):207–10.
45. St Pierre TG, Clark PR, Chua-anusorn W, et al. Noninvasive measurement and imaging of liver iron concentrations using proton magnetic resonance. Blood 2005; 105(2):855–61.
46. Emond MJ, Bronner MP, Carlson TH, et al. Quantitative study of the variability of hepatic iron concentrations. Clin Chem 1999;45(3):340–6.
47. Pietrangelo A. Juvenile hemochromatosis. J Hepatol 2006;45(6):892–4.
48. Papanikolaou G, Samuels ME, Ludwig EH, et al. Mutations in HFE2 cause iron overload in chromosome 1q-linked juvenile hemochromatosis. Nat Genet 2004; 36(1):77–82.
49. Camaschella C, Roetto A, Cali A, et al. The gene TFR2 is mutated in a new type of haemochromatosis mapping to 7q22. Nat Genet 2000;25(1):14–5.
50. Olynyk JK, Trinder D, Ramm GA, et al. Hereditary hemochromatosis in the post-HFE era. Hepatology 2008;48(3):991–1001.
51. Pietrangelo A, Caleffi A, Corradini E. Non-HFE hepatic iron overload. Semin Liver Dis 2011;31(3):302–18.
52. Brunt EM. Pathology of hepatic iron overload. Semin Liver Dis 2005;25(4): 392–401.
53. Adams PC, Speechley M, Kertesz AE. Long-term survival analysis in hereditary hemochromatosis. Gastroenterology 1991;101(2):368–72.
54. Niederau C, Fischer R, Purschel A, et al. Long-term survival in patients with hereditary hemochromatosis. Gastroenterology 1996;110(4):1107–19.
55. Kowdley KV. Iron, hemochromatosis, and hepatocellular carcinoma. Gastroenterology 2004;127(5 Suppl 1):S79–86.
56. Adams PC, Deugnier Y, Moirand R, et al. The relationship between iron overload, clinical symptoms, and age in 410 patients with genetic hemochromatosis. Hepatology 1997;25(1):162–6.
57. Ko C, Siddaiah N, Berger J, et al. Prevalence of hepatic iron overload and association with hepatocellular cancer in end-stage liver disease: results from the National Hemochromatosis Transplant Registry. Liver Int 2007;27(10):1394–401.
58. Falize L, Guillygomarc'h A, Perrin M, et al. Reversibility of hepatic fibrosis in treated genetic hemochromatosis: a study of 36 cases. Hepatology 2006;44(2): 472–7.
59. Bomford A, Williams R. Long term results of venesection therapy in idiopathic haemochromatosis. Q J Med 1976;45(180):611–23.
60. Kelly TM, Edwards CQ, Meikle AW, et al. Hypogonadism in hemochromatosis: reversal with iron depletion. Ann Intern Med 1984;101(5):629–32.
61. Cundy T, Butler J, Bomford A, et al. Reversibility of hypogonadotrophic hypogonadism associated with genetic haemochromatosis. Clin Endocrinol 1993;38(6): 617–20.
62. Phatak P, Brissot P, Wurster M, et al. A phase 1/2, dose-escalation trial of deferasirox for the treatment of iron overload in HFE-related hereditary hemochromatosis. Hepatology 2010;52(5):1671–779.

63. Brittenham GM, Griffith PM, Nienhuis AW, et al. Efficacy of deferoxamine in preventing complications of iron overload in patients with thalassemia major. N Engl J Med 1994;331(9):567–73.

64. Lynch SR, Cook JD. Interaction of vitamin C and iron. Ann N Y Acad Sci 1980;355: 32–44.

65. Yu L, Ioannou GN. Survival of liver transplant recipients with hemochromatosis in the United States. Gastroenterology 2007;133(2):489–95.

66. Bardou-Jacquet E, Philip J, Lorho R, et al. Liver transplantation normalizes serum hepcidin level and cures iron metabolism alterations in HFE hemochromatosis. Hepatology 2014;59(3):839–47.

67. Farrell FJ, Nguyen M, Woodley S, et al. Outcome of liver transplantation in patients with hemochromatosis. Hepatology 1994;20(2):404–10.

68. Bruix J, Sherman M. Management of hepatocellular carcinoma. Hepatology 2005; 42(5):1208–36.

Portal Vein Thrombosis

 CrossMark

Syed Abdul Basit, MD[a], Christian D. Stone, MD, MPH[a],
Robert Gish, MD[b,*]

KEYWORDS

- Thrombosis • Cirrhosis • Portal vein • Anticoagulation • Thrombophilia
- Thromboelastography • Malignancy

KEY POINTS

- Portal vein thrombosis (PVT) is most commonly found in cirrhosis and often diagnosed incidentally by imaging studies.
- There are 3 important complications of PVT: Portal hypertension with gastrointestinal bleeding, small bowel ischemia, and acute ischemic hepatitis.
- Acute PVT is associated with symptoms of abdominal pain and/or acute ascites, and chronic PVT is characterized by the presence of collateral veins and risk of gastrointestinal bleeding.
- Treatment to prevent clot extension and possibly help to recanalize the portal vein is generally recommended for PVT in the absence of contraindications for anticoagulation.
- PVT may obviate liver transplantation owing to a lack of adequate vasculature for organ/vessel anastomoses.

INTRODUCTION
Definition

Portal vein thrombosis (PVT) is defined as a partial or complete occlusion of the lumen of the portal vein or its tributaries by thrombus formation. Diagnosis of PVT is occurring more frequently, oftentimes found incidentally, owing to the increasing use of abdominal imaging (Doppler ultrasonography, most commonly) performed in the course of routine patient evaluations and surveillance for liver cancer. There are 3 important clinical complications of PVT:

- Small bowel ischemia: PVT may extend hepatofugal, causing thrombosis of the mesenteric venous arch and resultant small intestinal ischemia, which has a mortality rate as high as 50% and may require small bowel or multivisceral transplant if the patient survives.[1]

[a] Section of Gastroenterology and Hepatology, University of Nevada School of Medicine, 2040 West Charleston Boulevard, Suite 300, Las Vegas, NV 89102, USA; [b] Division of Gastroenterology and Hepatology, Department of Medicine, Stanford University School of Medicine, Alway Building, Room M211, 300 Pasteur Drive, MC: 5187 Stanford, CA 94305-5187, USA
* Corresponding author. 6022 La Jolla Mesa Drive, La Jolla, CA 92037.
E-mail address: rgish@robertgish.com

Clin Liver Dis 19 (2015) 199–221
http://dx.doi.org/10.1016/j.cld.2014.09.012
1089-3261/15/$ – see front matter © 2015 Elsevier Inc. All rights reserved.

- Ischemic hepatitis: Because the portal vein accounts for 75%[2] of the blood supply to the liver and 40% of the oxygen to the liver, acute PVT nullifies the liver's ability to resist ischemia owing to its dual blood supply. In acute complete PVT, any hypotensive episode may precipitate or worsen ischemic hepatitis and acute liver failure.
- Gastrointestinal bleeding: PVT may cause acute portal hypertension with subsequent variceal bleeding.

Types

Acute versus chronic

1. Acute PVT. The American Association for the Study of Liver Diseases (AASLD) describes acute PVT as "the sudden formation of a thrombus within the portal vein." The thrombus can variably involve portions of the mesenteric and/or splenic vein.[3] PVT associated with symptoms is commonly classified as acute.
2. Chronic PVT. Also known as portal cavernoma, chronic PVT occurs when the obstructed portal vein is replaced by a network of hepatopetal collateral veins bypassing the thrombosed portion of the vein.[3] A finding of portoportal collaterals or periportal varices which develop over 1 to 3 months typically represents chronic PVT.[4]

Complete versus incomplete

1. Complete PVT is defined by complete obstruction of the portal vein lumen by thrombus. This usually results in hepatofugal venous flow within the mesenteric and splenic vessels.
2. Incomplete PVT thrombosis refers to partial obstruction of the portal vein in which there is still residual hepatopetal flow. This finding might represent either a recanalization of complete PVT or persistent incomplete PVT.

Infected versus noninfected portal vein thrombosis

1. Local inflammation and infection impart a risk for PVT by increasing the local prothrombotic condition and can also result in pylephlebitis (infected, suppurative thrombosis of the portal vein). Common conditions include diverticulitis, appendicitis, and cholecystitis.[5–7] Rarely, in Mirrizi syndrome, in addition to obstructive jaundice, a gallstone in the cystic duct may obstruct the portal vein causing PVT with or without infection.
2. Noninfected thrombus.

Anatomic classification

The anatomic classification of PVT is based on the extent of thrombosis (**Table 1**).[8]

Table 1	
Anatomic classification of PVT	

Class	Anatomic Extent of Thrombosis
1	Thrombosis confined to the portal vein beyond the confluence of the splenic and SMV
2	Extension of thrombus into the SMV, but with patent mesenteric vessels
3	Diffuse thrombosis of splanchnic venous system, but with large collaterals
4	Extensive splanchnic venous thrombosis, but with only fine collaterals

Abbreviations: PVT, portal vein thrombosis; SMV, superior mesenteric vein.

Data from Jamieson NV. Changing perspectives in portal vein thrombosis and liver transplantation. Transplantation 2000;69(9):1772–4.

Malignancy-associated portal vein thrombosis versus bland thrombosis

This type of PVT is based on the underlying malignancy, which is the source of thrombosis. The most common tumor causing tumorous PVT is hepatocellular carcinoma. Other causes can include pancreatic, biliary, islet cell, and metastatic cancers (**Table 2**).

Incidence and Prevalence

The prevalence of PVT in the general population is about 1%, although it varies widely among patient populations based on the underlying pathophysiology and etiology.[9] Cirrhosis and hepatocellular carcinoma have the highest risk of PVT (odds ratio, 17).[9] In cirrhosis, the risk of PVT increases with worsening liver disease (more advanced portal hypertension) with a reported incidence of 11% to 17% overall,[10–12] 14% to 39% in orthotopic liver transplantation, and 13% to 44% with hepatoma (**Table 3**).[12–15] Based on the authors' clinical observations, chronic PVT occurs most commonly in the setting of cirrhosis and is often diagnosed incidentally by imaging studies. The current literature does not demonstrate this definitively because most studies do not distinguish between acute and chronic PVT. Large-scale epidemiologic studies that combine autopsy and clinical data are needed to refine this point further. In most noncirrhotic, non–hepatocellular carcinoma patients, acute PVT is related to more than 1 systemic and local risk factor, with myeloproliferative disorder as the most prevalent cause overall.[3,16] The risk factors and etiologic causes for chronic and acute PVT are the same in noncirrhotic, non–hepatocellular carcinoma patients.[17]

Pathophysiology and Etiology

PVT results from a combination of local (tumor, infection, constriction)[1,3,16,18] and systemic[2,3,16,18–24] risk factors that can be identified in 30% and 70% of patients, respectively (see **Table 2**).[3] Myeloproliferative disorders frequently present with PVT, with an incidence of 30% to 40% in this population.[3] The relative risks and comparison of thrombophilic conditions are shown in **Table 4**.[25] PVT generally occurs in the presence of multiple risk factors. The following pathophysiologic mechanisms encompass the basis of thrombus development and propagation.

Cirrhosis as a hypercoagulable state

- Decrease in procoagulants except factor VIII and von Willebrand factor
- Decrease in anticoagulants
- Platelet-related alterations
- Hyperfibrinolysis
- Altered blood flow

In normal individuals, thrombomodulin and thrombin activate protein C (PC) are part of the balance between the procoagulant and anticoagulant state. Factor VIII is one of the primary procoagulants of the coagulation cascade and levels generally decline with worsening liver function, but can be high representing an acute phase reactant. Activated PC along with cofactors protein S and factor V cause factor VIII inhibition and thus a decreased tendency for thrombus formation when deficient regardless of the actual factor VIII level.[26] Normally, the addition of thrombomodulin to individual plasma specimens decreases thrombus formation, but this is not true in patients with cirrhosis.[27] This phenomenon reflects partial resistance of PC to thrombomodulin and is directly proportional to the degree of liver dysfunction. The prothrombotic tendency in liver disease is thus directly proportional to the level of factor VIII and inversely proportional to the PC level. Thus, the factor VIII:PC ratio can be considered an index of procoagulant imbalance in advanced liver disease. Similarly, antithrombotic protein

Table 2
Risk factors for portal vein thrombosis (PVT)

Local Risk Factors	Systemic Risk Factors
Cirrhosis	Thrombophilia
Liver synthetic function preserved but there is an inciting event	Myeloproliferative disorders
Splenectomy	Polycythemia vera
Surgical portosystemic shunting	Essential thrombocythemia
TIPS dysfunction	Unclassified myeloproliferative
Thrombophilia	Antiphospholipid syndrome
Advanced liver disease w/synthetic dysfunction but absence of obvious precipitating factors:	Paroxysmal nocturnal hemoglobinuria
	Factor V Leiden mutation
	Factor II mutation
Portal hypertension: reduced hepatopetal flow	Protein C deficiency
	Protein S deficiency
Cirrhosis as a hypercoagulable state	Antithrombin III deficiency
Noncirrhosis	Plasminogen deficiency
Malignant (solid tumors)	Hyperhomocysteinemia
Hepatocellular carcinoma	MTHFR homozygote mutation TT677
Cholangiocarcinoma	Sickle cell disease
Gallbladder cancer	Nephrotic syndrome
Metastatic disease of the hepatobiliary tree	Thrombasthenia thrombocystosis
Gastric cancer	Autoimmune and rheumatologic disorders
Pancreatic cancer	Autoimmune hepatitis
Lymphoma	Primary biliary cirrhosis
Nonmalignant	Systemic lupus erythematosus
Gastrointestinal infections	Rheumatoid arthritis
Cholecystitis	Wegener's granulomatosis
Cholangitis	Mixed connective tissue disease
Appendicitis	Behçet syndrome
Diverticulitis	Others
Acute or chronic pancreatitis	Recent pregnancy
Tuberculous lymphadenitis	Recent oral contraceptive use
Inflammatory bowel diseases	Romiplastin in liver cirrhosis
Hepatic hydatid cyst	Eltrombopag in cirrhosis
Pylephlebitis liver abscesses	Interventional treatment of portal hypertension
Duodenal ulcer	
Cytomegalovirus hepatitis	Male sex
Schistosomiasis	Low platelet count
Local cardiovascular risk factors for PVT	
Budd–Chiari syndrome	
Sinusoidal obstruction syndrome	
Constrictive pericarditis	
Tricuspid insufficiency	
Tumor of the right atrium	
Iatrogenic injury to the portal venous system	
Liver and biliary system related procedures	
Endoscopic sclerotherapy of esophageal varices	
Alcoholization/chemoembolization ablation of hepatic tumors	
TIPS/surgical portosystemic shunt	
Hepatectomy or liver transplantation	
Cholecystectomy	
Hepatoportobiliary surgery	
Portography	

General abdominal surgery
   Colectomy
   Splenectomy
   Gastrectomy
   Fundoplication
   Abdominal trauma
Other
   Islet cell injection
   Hemodialysis
Choledochal cyst
Nodular regenerative hyperplasia of the
   liver

Data from Refs.[1–3,16,18–24]

levels decrease in proportion to the severity of the liver disease, representing a forme fruste of liver function tests. Antihemostatic markers such as the D-dimer level are markedly elevated in patients with a Model for End-stage Liver Disease score of greater than 13 owing to decreased liver metabolism of this coagulation breakdown factor.[28]

In patients with cirrhosis, the following platelet-related changes occur[18]:

- Decrease in the absolute number of circulating platelets
- Platelet sequestration in the spleen. Normally, the spleen accommodates one third of the platelet mass, but in cirrhosis, sequestration may rise to 90% of total platelet mass.
- Anti–GPIIb-IIIa antibody, which is found in cirrhotic patients, destroys platelets and lowers the platelet count.[29]
- Levels of disintegrin and metalloprotease with thrombospondin type 1 motif 13 (ADAMTS 13), a naturally occurring plasma metalloproteinase that limits the in vivo function of von Willebrand factor on platelets, are reduced in cirrhosis.[27]
- Platelet plug formation is enhanced owing to elevated von Willebrand factor levels, which are directly proportional to the severity of cirrhosis.

Qualitative defects in platelet function may also predispose to thrombus formation where platelets are actually hyperfunctional for any given platelet level. There are multiple prohemostatic[27,30–35] and antihemostatic[27,32–38] drivers in the different

Table 3
Incidence of portal vein thrombosis (PVT) in different patient cohorts

Associated Pathology	No. of Subjects	Incidence of PVT (%)	Type of Study	Reference
Liver cirrhosis	701	11.2	Doppler ultrasonography	10
	512	16.6	Retrospective	11
Liver carcinoma	435	21.4	Retrospective	13
	101	20	Retrospective	15
	72	44	Autopsy	14
Liver transplant	885	13.8 (no portosystemic shunt)	Cohort study	12
		38.9 (prior portosystemic shunt)		

Table 4
Prevalence and relative risk of portal vein thrombosis (PVT) with prothrombotic condition

Prothrombotic Condition	General Population (%)	Relative Risk
Homozygote factor V Leiden	0.01–0.6 of Caucasians	35–80
Heterozygote FVLM	4–5	10–20
		35 in women using OCP[a]
Heterozygote deficiency of natural anticoagulants		
Protein C[a]	0.2–04	10–20[a]
Protein S[a]	1.3	
Antithrombin III[a]	Up to 0.02	
Prothrombin gene mutation[a]	2–3	4
Hyperhomocystinemia	5	3
Antiphospholipid syndrome	—	8

Abbreviations: FVLM, factor V Leiden mutation; OCP, oral contraceptive pills.
[a] Different authors report different prevalence and relative risk.
Data from Bayraktar Y, Harmanci O. Etiology and consequences of thrombosis in abdominal vessels. World J Gastroenterol 2006;12(8):1165–74.

phases of hemostasis in patients with chronic liver disease as summarized in **Table 5**. Under normal circumstances the coagulation system is balanced in favor of anticoagulation.[39]

- Slow blood flow in the portal venous system increases the propensity to develop thrombi, especially when combined with the hypercoaguable states as defined.[40] The incidence of PVT increases with decreasing velocity through the portal vein, especially with flow velocity of less than 15 cm/s.[28]
- Portal vein flow velocity is inversely related to the severity of the liver disease.[28] According to the location and extension of the PVT, grading systems that can better define PVT extent have been proposed by Nonami and colleagues[12] (**Table 6**) and Yerdel and colleagues[41] (**Table 7**).

Table 5
Patterns of prohemostatic and antihemostatic drivers in the different phases of hemostasis in patients with chronic liver disease

Hemostasis Phase	Prohemostatic Drivers	Antihemostatic Drivers
Primary hemostasis (platelet-vessel wall interactions)	High von Willebrand factor,[30] low ADAMTS 13[31]	Low platelet count[36]
Blood coagulation (thrombin generation and inhibition)	Low anticoagulant factors,[32–34] antithrombin, protein C, high procoagulant factors (factor VIII)[33,34]	Low procoagulant factors[32–34]: Fibrinogen, factors II, V, VII, IX, X, XI
Fibrinolysis (clot dissolution)	Low plasminogen,[35] high PAI[35]	High t-PA,[35] low TAFI,[37,38] low plasmin inhibitor[35]

Abbreviations: ADAMTS 13, a disintegrin and metalloproteinase with a thrombospondin type 1 motif, member 13; PAI, plasminogen activator inhibitor; TAFI, thrombin-activatable fibrinolysis inhibitor; t-PA, tissue plasminogen activator.
From Tripodi A, Mannucci PM. The coagulopathy of chronic liver disease. N Engl J Med 2011;365(2):150; with permission; and Data from Garcia-Pagan JC, Valla DC. Portal vein thrombosis: a predictable milestone in cirrhosis? J Hepatol 2009;51(4):632–4.

Table 6 Proposed grading system for portal vein thrombosis based on location and extent of thrombus	
Grade	**Extent of Thrombosis**
1	Thrombosis of intrahepatic portal vein branches only
2	Thrombosis of first branches of portal vein or at the bifurcation
3	Partial obstruction of the portal vein
4	Complete obstruction of the portal vein trunk

Data from Nonami T, Yokoyama I, Iwatsuki S, et al. The incidence of portal vein thrombosis at liver transplantation. Hepatology 1992;16(5):1195–8.

- Obliterative portal venopathy, a rare cause of PVT, refers to primary occlusion of the intrahepatic portal veins in the absence of cirrhosis, inflammation, or hepatic neoplasia.[42] It is diagnosed by a finding of hepatoportal sclerosis on biopsy and is attributable to an underlying hypercoagulable state in some patients.

Sequential pathophysiologic changes that result from PVT are summarized in **Table 8**.[19,25]

Clinical Presentation

Signs and symptoms of acute portal vein thrombosis[1,3,16]

- Asymptomatic or few symptoms if obstruction is partial.
- Severe colicky pain and nonbloody diarrhea with complete PVT.
- Acute abdominal or lumbar pain with sudden onset or progressive over days to weeks.
- Ileus.
- Abdominal guarding if intra-abdominal infection or intestinal infarction is present.
- Severe pain without peritoneal signs; consider PVT/superior mesenteric vein (SMV) involvement.
- Systemic inflammatory response syndrome in the absence of sepsis.
- Ascites, typically small volume.
- Symptoms of acute PVT are reversible by either recanalization or cavernoma formation.
- Symptoms not resolving in 5 to 7 days or clinical deterioration may reflect mesenteric and arch involvement with complete loss of portal and mesenteric flow.

Table 7 Proposed grading system for portal vein thrombosis (PVT)	
Grade	**Location and Extent of PVT**
1	Minimally or partially thrombosed PV, in which the thrombus is mild or confined to <50% of the lumen with or without minimal extension into the SMV
2	>50% occlusion of the PV, including total occlusion, with or without minimal extension into SMV
3	Complete thrombosis of both PV and proximal SMV (distal SMV open)
4	Complete thrombosis of the PV and both proximal and distal SMV

Abbreviations: PV, portal vein; SMV, superior mesenteric vein.
Data from Yerdel MA, Gunson B, Mirza D, et al. Portal vein thrombosis in adults undergoing liver transplantation: risk factors, screening, management, and outcome. Transplantation 2000;69(9):1873–81.

Table 8
Acute portal vein thrombosis (PVT)-related pathologic changes and compensatory changes

Change Secondary to Acute PVT	Compensatory Mechanism
Compromise of two thirds of liver blood supply	1. Apoptosis of tissue depending on the loss of blood supply 2. Compensatory hypertrophy of tissue with well-preserved blood supply
Increased risk of liver ischemia	Arterial buffer/rescue by arterial vasodilatation
Increase in portal vein pressure	Development of collaterals and portal cavernoma

Mesenteric ischemia/infarction is manifested by persistent pain, bloody diarrhea and ascites, acidosis, renal and respiratory failure. Without treatment, perforation, shock, multiorgan failure, and death are expected.

- Pylephlebitis can manifest with spiking fever, tender liver, and shock.
- Esophageal variceal bleeding.
- Nonvariceal gastrointestinal bleeding, for example, from portal gastropathy or intestinal varices.[43,44] Authors have reported a 39% bleeding risk in PVT with cirrhosis,[44] and 34% gastrointestinal bleeding rate in patients with acute PVT with cirrhosis and hepatocellular carinoma.[9,44] PVT in cirrhosis may be asymptomatic and incidental on imaging studies. However, it should be considered a culprit lesion in cirrhotic patients with new or worsening ascites, gastrointestinal bleeding or hepatic encephalopathy.[14]

Signs and symptoms of chronic portal vein thrombosis[4,21,45–49]

- Asymptomatic in most cases. When discovered incidentally in cirrhotic patients with no symptoms of acute thrombosis, PVT may be assumed to be chronic and should prompt evaluation for a hypercoagulable state.
- Pain only if there is involvement of the mesenteric branch and arch with resultant bowel ischemia.
- Hematemesis and melena are most common owing to the development of portoportal and portosystemic collaterals and hepatic artery dilatation. There is typically minimal change in the hepatic arterial blood supply, but there is always increase in the portal pressure.

Features of portal hypertension

- Gastroesophageal varices with bleeding as the presenting symptom in 20% to 40% of cases. In PVT with cirrhosis, the risk of bleeding increases by 80 to 120 times compared with noncirrhotic patients.
- Portal hypertensive gastropathy.
- Splenomegaly resulting in pancytopenia.
- Ascites.
- Pseudocholangiocarcinoma sign on endoscopic retrograde cholangiopancreatography reflects the presence of dilated collaterals.
- Abnormalities in the extrahepatic biliary tree are found in up to 80% of chronic PVT cases. These findings are mostly asymptomatic but can cause cholestasis, cholangitis, choledocholithiasis.
- Portal biliopathy results from varices or compression of the biliary tree by the venous plexus of Petren. Ischemic injury or infection leads to biliary stricture. Symptoms include pain, recurrent fever, or jaundice.
- Choledocholithiasis with or without cholelithiasis.

Diagnosis

Ultrasonography

Color Doppler ultrasonography (CDUS) is often the first choice of investigation because sensitivity and specificity range from 60% to 100%.[21,50] Ultrasonography without Doppler imaging does not provide information about flow dynamics. Given its high negative predictive value, if CDUS confirms portal vein patency, then no further studies are required.[2,51] The sensitivity of ultrasonography for diagnosis of PVT may depend on the stage of obstruction and has been reported to be 100% in stages 3 and 4.[41]

Ultrasound findings of portal vein thrombosis[16,52,53]

- Echogenic lesion within the lumen of the portal vein. Loss of venous flow.
- Portal cavernoma.
- Inability to identify the portal vein.
- Dilatation of a thrombosed segment of the PVT.

A newer technique, contrast-enhanced ultrasonography,[54] utilizes microbubbles as a contrast medium, is more sensitive than CDUS for characterization of thrombi, and can visualize hypoechoic thrombi. Endoscopic ultrasonography has been reported to be both sensitive and specific and can detect small and nonocclusive thrombi[25]; however, given its more invasive nature, it should be considered only in patients undergoing endoscopy for some other indication.

Computed tomography and MRI

Computed tomography (CT) is the second most common imaging test to identify PVT after ultrasonography and may be the best method to define the anatomy of the vascular changes. Intravenous contrast should be used to increase sensitivity. The key findings of PVT by contrast CT are[3]:

- Lack of luminal enhancement in the portal vein;
- Increased hepatic arterial enhancement in arterial phase films; and
- Decreased venous enhancement in the liver during the portal phase.

CT is also of value for identifying secondary bowel complications, such as bowel infarction, and underlying pathology like a mass or intra-abdominal infection/abscess.[2,25] MRI has comparable sensitivity to CT scan. Magnetic resonance cholangiopancreatography is the investigation of choice for diagnosis of portal biliopathy.

Portal angiography

Angiography is limited to preoperative vascular mapping in patients who are candidates for liver transplantation. PVT is seen as a filling defect of the portal vein trunk or one of its branches. The portal vein may not be visualized in the presence of SMV thrombosis.[51] Angiography is rarely required thanks to widespread use of CT and MRI.

Thromboelastography

Thromboelastography refers to the dynamic assessment of whole blood coagulation and viscoelastic properties of clot formation under low shear conditions. It may be utilized to evaluate the coagulation status in patients with PVT.[55] Traditional clotting parameters like prothrombin time or International Normalized Ratio (INR) and partial thromboplastin time do not accurately reflect the procoagulant and anticoagulant imbalance in patients with cirrhosis[56] and consumptive coagulopathy.[57] Thromboelastography, in contrast, measures vitamin K–dependent cofactors, fibrinogen levels, platelet function, and fibrinolysis in addition to other coagulation factors and their respective functions. It is an emerging tool to describe functional clot formation and clot stability, and to identify a hypercoagulable state in patients with PVT with or without cirrhosis. Bone marrow biopsy or flow studies are supplementary tests utilized to identify an underlying hematologic cause of PVT. Similarly, diagnostic testing for paroxysmal nocturnal hemoglobinuria or other rare conditions may be necessary in cases of PVT without obvious cause. There are other potentially useful or complementary laboratory studies (**Table 9**).[2,3,49]

Stepwise approach to the diagnosis of suspected portal vein thrombosis
American Association for the Study of Liver Diseases 2009 guidelines for the approach to patients with suspected acute portal vein thrombosis[3]

- Consider acute PVT in any patient with abdominal pain of more than 24 hours' duration.
- If acute PVT is suspected, CT scan with and with intravenous contrast or CDUS should be obtained.
- In acute PVT and high fever and chills, septic pylephlebitis should be considered and blood cultures should be obtained routinely.
- In acute PVT, symptoms of pain, ascites, thinning of the intestinal wall, lack of mucosal enhancement of thickened intestinal wall, or the development of multi-organ failure are evidence of intestinal infarction and surgical exploration should be considered.

Proposed approach to patient with chronic portal vein thrombosis

- Consider chronic PVT in any patient with newly diagnosed portal hypertension.
- Obtain CDUS and then either CT or MRI to make a diagnosis of PVT.

Table 9 Potentially useful or complementary laboratory studies during portal vein thrombosis (PVT) evaluation	
Test	**Comment/Associated Disorder**
Liver chemistry	May be normal if no concurrent liver disease; can be abnormal in portal ductopathy/biliopathy
Complete blood count	Leukocytosis may indicate intra-abdominal infection; polycythemia, thrombocytosis may be reflective of myeloproliferative disorders
Thromboelastography JAK2 MPD	
CD55, CD59	Paroxysmal nocturnal hemoglobinuria
Anti-cardiolipin antibody Lupus anticoagulant Anti-Beta2 glycoprotein 1 antibody	Antiphospholipid syndrome
Factor V Leiden	Protein C resistance
Protein C and S level	
Factor II deficiency	G21010 mutation
Anti-thrombin activity	Inherited if test is also positive in first degree relative
Homocysteine level	

Data from Parikh S, Shah R, Kapoor P. Portal vein thrombosis. Am J Med 2010;123(2):111–9; and DeLeve LD, Valla DC, Garcia-Tsao G, et al. Vascular disorders of the liver. Hepatology 2009;49(5):1729–64. 2–3.

- PVT diagnosis is based on the absence of a visible portal vein and its replacement with collateral veins.

A similar approach has been recommended by Plessier and colleagues[16]:

- Consider acute PVT in all patients with:
  - Sudden epigastric or diffuse abdominal pain associated with systemic inflammatory response syndrome; or
  - Known or suspected prothrombotic condition.
- A radiological report assessing PVT will ideally comment on:
  - Presence or absence of a local factor including liver tumor or cirrhosis;
  - Thrombus extension to the mesenteric or splenic vein;
  - Ascites, congestion, or ischemia of the bowel; and
  - Presence of malignant changes in the liver and in the thrombus.

Investigate all patients for a prothrombotic factor regardless of whether a local factor is evident.

MANAGEMENT GOALS
Indications for Treatment of Portal Vein Thrombosis

The overarching initial goal of treatment of acute PVT is to prevent the development of PVT-related complications, namely gastrointestinal bleeding (variceal, portal gastropathic), ascites, ischemic hepatitis, extension of clot to the SMV, and small intestinal ischemia/infarction. With regard to chronic PVT, the goal of treatment is to recanalize the portal vein in addition to preventing the complications as discussed.

PHARMACOLOGIC STRATEGIES
Anticoagulation

Acute portal vein thrombosis in patients with a procoagulant condition
The goal of treatment of acute PVT is to recanalize the obstructed vein. Anticoagulation should be started as early as possible. Six months of treatment can achieve 90% recanalization (50% complete and 40% partial).[3]

Patient subtypes that stand most to benefit from anticoagulant therapy for acute PVT[43,58]:

1. Patients with demonstrated prothrombotic states:
   - With absent or small varices that have never bled; or
   - Without predictable bleeding sites outside the gastrointestinal tract during anticoagulant therapy.
2. Patients with prothrombotic states and esophageal varices that have never bled if adequate prophylaxis for bleeding from portal hypertension has been instituted.

Summary recommendations for treatment of acute portal vein thrombosis in patients with a procoagulant disorder

- Start anticoagulation as early as possible if there is no active gastrointestinal bleeding. Rate of recanalization is 69% if anticoagulation is started in the first week, but 25% if anticoagulation is started in second week.[59]
- Endoscopic treatment for active variceal bleeding; primary or secondary prophylaxis for bleeding with β-blocker.
- If acute PVT, continue anticoagulation for at least 3 months. Reimage and if no recanalization; then continue anticoagulation for an additional 3 months.

- In a permanent, noncorrectable prothrombotic condition, continue lifelong anti-coagulation if there are no contraindications.
- Long-term anticoagulation in patients with SMV involvement, if there are no contraindications

Acute or chronic portal vein thrombosis in noncirrhotic patients

In noncirrhotic patients with acute PVT that is untreated, the most recent comprehensive review of studies reported that the rate of spontaneous recanalization is low (16.7%), although it should be noted that out of 29 studies, only 4 described patients in whom no anticoagulation was given (a total of only 12 cases), so the data are very limited.[60] Anticoagulation should be given for at least 3 months in all patients. When an underlying persistent prothrombotic state has been documented, lifelong anticoagulant therapy is recommended.[61] Current AASLD guidelines for PVT recommend lifelong anticoagulation in the following conditions:[3]

Acute or chronic PVT in noncirrhotic patients with

- Permanent, noncorrectable prothrombotic disorder; and
- Current or previous SMV involvement (after instituting primary or secondary prophylaxis for gastrointestinal bleeding).

When the decision for anticoagulation is made, then heparin or low-molecular-weight (LMW) heparin should be used initially followed by an oral anticoagulant (warfarin) with goal of an INR of 2 to 2.5.[18] An algorithm that has recently been suggested for treatment of noncirrhotic acute PVT[62] is shown in **Fig. 1**.

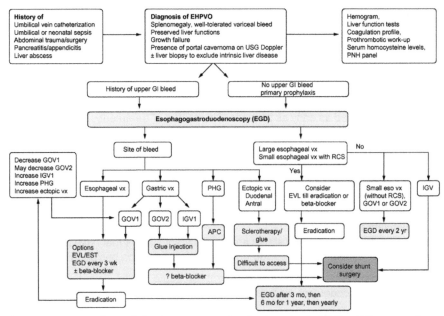

Fig. 1. Treatment of noncirrhotic acute portal vein thrombosis (PVT). APC, argon plasma coagulation; EHPVO, extrahepatic portal vein obstruction; EVL, endoscopic variceal ligation; EST, endoscopic sclerotherapy; GI, gastrointestinal; GOV, gastro-oesophageal varices; IGV, isolated gastric varices; PHG, portal hypertensive gastropathy; PNH, paroxysmal nocturnal hemoglobinuria; RCS, red color signs; USG, ultrasonography; vx, varices. (*From* Khanna R, Sarin SK. Non-cirrhotic portal hypertension - diagnosis and management. J Hepatol 2014; 60(2):421–41; with permission.)

Acute portal vein thrombosis in cirrhotic patients

This scenario poses a challenge in clinical decision making. No consensus exists on the questions of when or if anticoagulation should be instituted, or on choice and duration of anticoagulation. The AASLD guidelines state that a decision regarding anticoagulation should be made on a case-by-case basis in this high-risk patient group.[3] It is reasonable to consider anticoagulation in the setting of a known prothrombotic condition or SMV thrombosis, but only after prophylaxis for gastrointestinal bleeding with endoscopic band ligation (EBL) and/or nonselective β-blocker therapy.

The majority of the patients with cirrhosis and PVT have a complication of decompensated liver disease including 43% with gastrointestinal bleeding.[63] Anticoagulation is recommended for at least 12 months to achieve complete recanalization. Lifelong treatment is used to prevent recurrent thrombosis, which occurs in 27% to 38% of patients.[63,64] As shown in **Fig. 2**, recanalization rates with anticoagulation therapy in cirrhotic patients reported by various studies vary substantially, ranging from 42%[65] to 100%,[66] with most studies reporting rates between those extremes.[63,64,67–72] Lengthier therapy has been shown to improve results, with 33.3% recanalization after 6 months of anticoagulation increasing to 75% after 11 months.[64]

Advantages of low-molecular-weight heparin over vitamin K agonists in the treatment of portal vein thrombosis[70]

- Easily reversible in case of hemorrhagic complication.
- No requirement for INR monitoring, which may be suboptimal in patients with cirrhosis.
- Vitamin K agonists are used in patients with baseline INR greater than 2, but this practice is not validated.

The specific choice of the anticoagulant selected is debatable among experts and options are summarized in **Table 10**. Patients with cirrhosis and PVT should undergo repeated EBL until eradication of varices before starting anticoagulation. Hold

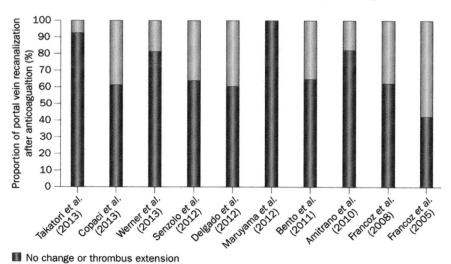

No change or thrombus extension
Complete or partial recanalization

Fig. 2. Outcome of anticoagulation for the treatment of portal vein thrombosis in patients with cirrhosis. (*From* Qi X, Han G, Fan D. Management of portal vein thrombosis in liver cirrhosis. Nat Rev Gastroenterol Hepatol 2014;11(7):435–446. Reprinted by permission from Macmillan Publishers Ltd.)

		PVT, n (Complete/ Partial)	Recanalization, n	Previous GI Bleed, n	Reference

Table 10
Comparison of different anticoagulation therapies for portal vein thrombosis (PVT) in cirrhosis

Anticoagulant	Patients, N	PVT, n (Complete/ Partial)	Recanalization, n	Previous GI Bleed, n	Reference
LMWH/VKA	55	14/41	33	24	63
Enoxaparin	28	5/23	21	—	64
Nadroparin	35	11/24	21	10	70
VKA	19	18/1	8	14	65

Abbreviations: LMWH, low-molecular-weight heparin; VKA, vitamin K agonists.

anticoagulation for 2 weeks after the last ligation owing to the bleeding risk associated with postligation ulceration. β-Blockers could be considered as prophylaxis instead of EBL in patients with medium to large varices and no history of bleed or high risk signs on endoscopy.[73] If warfarin is selected, then a thrombin generation test with or without thrombomodulin is preferred over INR and other tests of anticoagulation such as anti-factor Xa assays.[73]

Summary guidelines for patients with portal vein thrombosis, cirrhosis, and no prothrombotic disorder

- Screening endoscopy to evaluate for varices. If large varices, history of bleeding, or signs of high risk for bleeding, then EBL until eradication. For medium varices with no stigmata of bleeding or active or previous bleeding, then use a nonselective β-blocker.
- Start anticoagulation 2 weeks after last EBL and when variceal eradication is achieved.
- If anticoagulation is considered, start as early as possible because delay has been associated with lower rates of recanalization.
- LMW heparin is the preferred therapy especially if baseline INR of greater than 2.
- If a vitamin K agonist is considered, start initial bridging with heparin or LMW heparin. Thereafter, goal INR is 2 to 3.
- No specific duration of anticoagulation is recommended; however, 6 months or more is associated with an higher rate of recanalization.
- An algorithmic approach suggested by Qi and colleagues[73] is depicted in **Fig. 3**.

Chronic portal vein thrombosis in cirrhosis and noncirrhosis
The AASLD guidelines describe 3 categories of therapy for chronic PVT.[3]

Recommendations for prevention and treatment of bleeding
- Screen for gastroesophageal varices.[74]
- Use β-blockers or EBL for large varices in patients with portal cavernoma for primary or secondary prophylaxis.[75] Avoid endoscopic sclerotherapy because it may induce PVT.
- β-Blockers and EBL have similar efficacy in prevention of variceal bleeding.[76] In patients who fail a single therapy, both should be utilized.[16,45]
- Transjugular intrahepatic portosystemic shunt (TIPS) if endoscopic and β-blocker therapies fail.

Prevention of recurrent thrombosis Only 30% of eligible patients with PVT receive anticoagulant treatment[21] despite the evidence that it can prevent recurrent

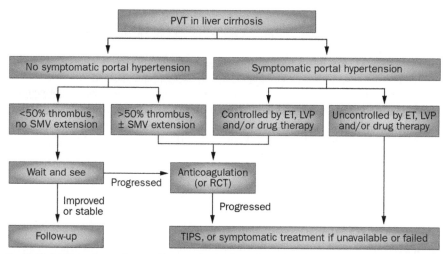

Fig. 3. Guidelines for patients with portal vein thrombosis (PVT), cirrhosis, and no prothrombotic disorder. ET, endoscopic therapy; LVP, large volume paracentesis; RCT, randomized controlled trial; SMV, superior mesenteric vein; TIPS, transjugular intrahepatic portosystemic shunt. (*From* Qi X, Han G, Fan D. Management of portal vein thrombosis in liver cirrhosis. Nat Rev Gastroenterol Hepatol 2014;11(7):435–446. Reprinted by permission from Macmillan Publishers Ltd.)

thrombosis without increasing the risk of gastrointestinal bleeding.[3] Indications for permanent anticoagulation are best individualized. Clinical factors to consider when deciding on anticoagulation include the following[16]:

- Thrombotic potential of the underlying condition may tip the balance toward anticoagulation.[77]
- Personal or family history of venous thromboembolism.
- Recurrent abdominal pain owing to extensive thrombosis in the portovenous system.
- Low bleeding risk despite anticoagulation.
- Extension of thrombus to the SMV.[16]

American Association for the Study of Liver Diseases guidelines for anticoagulation treatment in chronic portal vein thrombosis[3]

- Consider long-term anticoagulation in noncirrhotic patients with chronic PVT and with a permanent risk factor for venous thrombosis, provided there are no major contraindications.
- Always treat or prophylax for gastroesophageal varices before initiating anticoagulation.

Treatment of portal biliopathy Portal biliopathy, also known as portal hypertensive biliopathy or portal ductopathy, refers to intrahepatic and extrahepatic biliary tract, gallbladder, and cystic duct abnormalities that arise secondary to chronic PVT.[49] In chronic PVT, engorged collateral veins (eg, plexus of Petren) cause compression of the biliary tree with resultant structural changes in the intrahepatic and extrahepatic ductal system. Typically, portal biliopathy presents with signs and symptoms of biliary obstruction, including cholangitis.

Treatment recommendations

- Asymptomatic patients with normal liver function tests do not require treatment.[48,49]
- Patients with elevated alkaline phosphatase and bilirubin in the setting of portal hypertension should be investigated for choledocholithiasis.[48,49]
- Patients with symptomatic obstruction or cholangitis caused by portal biliopathy--induced stones or stricture require endoscopic retrograde cholangiopancreatography with stone removal, stricture dilation, or stent insertion.[3]
- An algorithmic approach to a patient with portal biliopathy has been proposed (**Fig. 4**).[48]

Role of Tissue Plasminogen Activator

- Thrombolytics (tissue plasminogen activator) can be infused into the portal vein indirectly by injection into the superior mesenteric artery through the femoral or radical artery. Alternatively, they may be infused directly into the portal vein via a percutaneous transhepatic or transjugular intrahepatic approach.
- In a stable patient with no contraindication, an intraportal thrombolytic should first be infused for 6 to 24 hours. If this fails, then mechanical thrombectomy with stenting can be attempted.[78]
- A transhepatic approach to the portal vein is the preferred means of access in the noncirrhotic patient and can facilitate catheter manipulation and endovascular recanalization.[78]

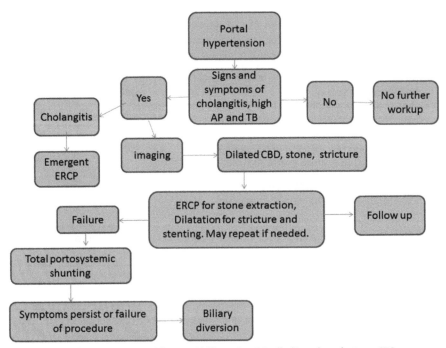

Fig. 4. Approach to a patient with portal biliopathy. AP, alkaline phosphatase; CBD, common bile duct; ERCP, endoscopic retrograde cholangiopancreatography; TB, total bilirubin. (*From* Chandra R, Kapoor D, Tharakan A, et al. Portal biliopathy. J Gastroenterol Hepatol 2001;16(10):1086–92. Reprinted by permission from John Wiley & Sons.)

- Surgical thrombectomy is not recommended owing to the recurrence of thrombosis and associated surgical morbidity and mortality.[50]

NONPHARMACOLOGIC STRATEGIES
Endoscopy

Endoscopic banding, sclerotherapy, and glue injection are therapeutic modalities employed in the treatment of active variceal bleeding or for prophylaxis. As described in various sections of this article, bleeding should be addressed prior to consideration of anticoagulation for PVT.

Transjugular Intrahepatic Portosystemic Shunt

- There are multiple contraindications to TIPS placement, and its feasibility depends on the extent of the PVT.
- TIPS helps to recanalize the portal vein and prevents rethrombosis in patients with PVT and cirrhosis. TIPS insertion and recanalization may be combined with mechanical thrombectomy and/or acute anticoagulation, but does not necessarily prevent progression of clot. Therefore, concurrent chronic anticoagulation should be considered.[79]
- TIPS can halt clot progression and lower the grade of thrombosis.[80]
- TIPS has been used as a primary treatment for PVT in lieu of anticoagulation. In the setting of active or high risk for gastrointestinal bleeding, TIPS placement can permit anticoagulation by reducing the bleeding risk.[80]
- TIPS has been used as rescue treatment for chronic PVT-related complications, including variceal bleed and small bowel infarction.[81]

In general, there are multiple contraindications to TIPS placement, including those that are absolute (primary prevention of variceal bleeding, congestive heart failure, multiple hepatic cysts, uncontrolled systemic infection or sepsis, uncontrolled systemic infection or sepsis, severe pulmonary hypertension) and those that are relative (hepatoma especially if central, obstruction of all hepatic veins, severe coagulopathy [INR > 5], thrombocytopenia of $<20,000/cm^3$, moderate pulmonary hypertension, and possibly PVT).[82] However, depending on the extent of thrombosis, TIPS may be attempted in the following instances:[83]

- Partially occluded main portal vein (MPV).
- Completely occluded MPV in which thrombectomy could be attempted by a combination of transjugular and transhepatic or transsplenic approaches.
- Completely occluded or obliterated MPV with large caliber collaterals.
- Avoid TIPS in patients with a fibrotic cord or MPV obliteration with fine collaterals.
- TIPS should be considered in cases of advanced (grades 2–4) PVT if there is a contraindication to anticoagulation.[77]
- In patients with PVT and existing TIPS, restenting of TIPS can be performed with or without thrombus removal (eg, via balloon or suction embolectomy, basket extraction of clot or mechanical thrombectomy).[77]
- TIPS in combination with portal vein thrombectomy may be performed before and to facilitate liver transplantation.

Direct Intrahepatic Portosystemic Shunt

Direct intrahepatic portosystemic shunt, a percutaneous approach to access the portal system, has indications similar to that of TIPS, but is used when an intrahepatic portal vein branch cannot be visualized during TIPS attempt.

Thrombectomy

Evidence regarding the use of thrombolytics for the treatment of PVT in patients with cirrhosis is very limited and clinical use is rare.[73] Thrombolysis should be used with caution in asymptomatic patients and should be reserved for thrombus extension into the SMV and secondary intestinal ischemia only. Intravascular ultrasonography may be used to assist in the formation of a mesocaval shunt. Direct intrahepatic portosystemic shunt, a percutaneous approach to access the portal system, has indications similar to that of TIPS but is used when an intrahepatic portal vein branch cannot be visualized during TIPS attempt.

SELF-MANAGEMENT STRATEGIES

The importance of patient adherence to treatment principles of chronic liver disease and PVT cannot be overstated. Optimization of liver function and prevention of decompensation may be facilitated by patient compliance with general recommendations including avoidance of alcohol and other drug-induced liver toxicity, prophylaxis against gastrointestinal bleeding, spontaneous bacterial peritonitis, adherence to diuretic therapy, dietary restriction of sodium, and so on.

EVALUATION, ADJUSTMENT, AND RECURRENCE
Pylephlebitis

An infected thrombus of the portal vein is usually a complication of intra-abdominal infection, most commonly appendicitis and diverticulitis. The most likely organisms found in this condition are *Bacteroides* spp and *Escherichia coli*.[5,84,85] Broad spectrum antibiotics should be started quickly. A minimum of 4 weeks of antibiotics is recommended for septic thrombophlebitis and 6 weeks in cases complicated by macroscopic liver abscesses.[86,87] The role of anticoagulation for septic PVT is not completely clear. Early anticoagulation may minimize the risk of bowel ischemia and infarction. Improved outcomes[86] and higher rates of recanalization have been reported with anticoagulation; however, a higher risk of SMV thrombosis was shown in patients on anticoagulation.[85,86] Baril and colleagues[88] recommend anticoagulation in patients with pylephlebitis with neoplasm, hematological disease, hypercoagulable state or involvement of superior and inferior mesenteric vein thrombosis.

Summary: treatment of pylephlebitis

- Start antibiotics early then deescalate according to culture results.
- Continue antibiotics for 4 weeks for septic PVT, and 6 weeks if liver abscesses present.
- Identify source of infection and manage with surgery if indicated.
- Consider anticoagulation if there is no contraindication.
- Reimage at a later time to confirm recanalization and rule out a PVT complication, such as, portal vein hypertension.

Portal Vein Thrombosis in a Pregnant Patient

- Women of childbearing age account for 25% of patients with noncirrhotic PVT. Common risk factors are myeloproliferative disorder and antiphospholipid syndrome.[89]
- The rate of miscarriage is up to 20%.
- Manage gastrointestinal bleeding with prophylaxis or endoscopic therapy.
- Limited data suggest that anticoagulation is safe in pregnant women with PVT and prothrombotic factors and with higher risk of intestinal ischemia.

- Pregnancy is not contraindicated in stable PVT patients.
- Drug of choice is LMW heparin or unfractionated heparin. Warfarin should be avoided in the first trimester.[90]

Portal Vein Thrombosis and Liver Transplantation

- The incidence of PVT in patients awaiting transplant is high[12] and can pose serious consequences in posttransplant patients.[3]
- AASLD recommends pretransplant CDUS on every patient to evaluate for PV patency,[91] and repeated imaging is required during the wait period.[79] In the past, liver transplant was considered technically not feasible in PVT patients.[41]
- PVT incidence increases with worsening liver function in cirrhotic patients. LMW heparin has been used prophylactically to reduce the risk of PVT.[3]
- In trials, vitamin K agonists, and LMW heparin have achieved 40% to 75% complete or partial recanalization.[79]
- Success of recanalization is low in patients with complete thrombosis; anticoagulation may be relegated to preventing thrombus extension in these patients.[79]
- Screening for varices and prophylaxis for variceal bleeding are recommended.

SUMMARY

This article has summarized the multiple etiologic factors that lead to PVT in noncirrhotic patients. It has furthermore highlighted the coagulation derangements that underlie the pathogenesis of PVT in cirrhosis. We have stressed the importance of proper and timely diagnosis of PVT and emphasized the recognition of several life-threatening complications in the hope that more clinicians will offer anticoagulation for PVT which to date remains undertreated in general practice.

REFERENCES

1. Plessier A, Darwish-Murad S, Hernandez-Guerra M, et al. Acute portal vein thrombosis unrelated to cirrhosis: a prospective multicenter follow-up study. Hepatology 2010;51(1):210–8.
2. Parikh S, Shah R, Kapoor P. Portal vein thrombosis. Am J Med 2010;123(2):111–9.
3. DeLeve LD, Valla DC, Garcia-Tsao G, et al. Vascular disorders of the liver. Hepatology 2009;49(5):1729–64.
4. Harmanci O, Bayraktar Y. How can portal vein cavernous transformation cause chronic incomplete biliary obstruction? World J Gastroenterol 2012;18(26):3375–8.
5. Kasper DL, Sahani D, Misdraji J. Case records of the Massachusetts General Hospital. Case 25–2005. A 40-year-old man with prolonged fever and weight loss. N Engl J Med 2005;353(7):713–22.
6. Wong K, Weisman DS, Patrice KA. Pylephlebitis: a rare complication of an intra-abdominal infection. J Community Hosp Intern Med Perspect 2013;3(2).
7. Zimhony O, Katz M. A patient with fever and jaundice. QJM 2012;105(4):381–2.
8. Jamieson NV. Changing perspectives in portal vein thrombosis and liver transplantation. Transplantation 2000;69(9):1772–4.
9. Ogren M, Bergqvist D, Bjorck M, et al. Portal vein thrombosis: prevalence, patient characteristics and lifetime risk: a population study based on 23,796 consecutive autopsies. World J Gastroenterol 2006;12(13):2115–9.
10. Amitrano L, Guardascione MA, Brancaccio V, et al. Risk factors and clinical presentation of portal vein thrombosis in patients with liver cirrhosis. J Hepatol 2004; 40(5):736–41.

11. Belli L, Romani F, Sansalone CV, et al. Portal thrombosis in cirrhotics. A retrospective analysis. Ann Surg 1986;203(3):286–91.
12. Nonami T, Yokoyama I, Iwatsuki S, et al. The incidence of portal vein thrombosis at liver transplantation. Hepatology 1992;16(5):1195–8.
13. Llovet JM, Bruix J. Prospective validation of the Cancer of the Liver Italian Program (CLIP) score: a new prognostic system for patients with cirrhosis and hepatocellular carcinoma. Hepatology 2000;32(3):679–80.
14. Pirisi M, Avellini C, Fabris C, et al. Portal vein thrombosis in hepatocellular carcinoma: age and sex distribution in an autopsy study. J Cancer Res Clin Oncol 1998;124(7):397–400.
15. Rabe C, Pilz T, Klostermann C, et al. Clinical characteristics and outcome of a cohort of 101 patients with hepatocellular carcinoma. World J Gastroenterol 2001;7(2):208–15.
16. Plessier A, Rautou PE, Valla DC. Management of hepatic vascular diseases. J Hepatol 2012;56(Suppl 1):S25–38.
17. Condat B, Vilgrain V, Asselah T, et al. Portal cavernoma-associated cholangiopathy: a clinical and MR cholangiography coupled with MR portography imaging study. Hepatology 2003;37(6):1302–8.
18. Rosu A, Searpe C, Popescu M. Portal vein thrombosis with cavernous transformation in myeloproliferative disorders: review update. In: Garbuzenko DV, editor. Portal hypertension - causes and complications. Rijeka (Croatia): InTech; 2012.
19. Valla DC, Condat B. Portal vein thrombosis in adults: pathophysiology, pathogenesis and management. J Hepatol 2000;32(5):865–71.
20. Crawford JM. Vascular disorders of the liver. Clin Liver Dis 2010;14(4):635–50.
21. Ponziani FR, Zocco MA, Campanale C, et al. Portal vein thrombosis: insight into physiopathology, diagnosis, and treatment. World J Gastroenterol 2010;16(2):143–55.
22. Dultz G, Kronenberger B, Azizi A, et al. Portal vein thrombosis as complication of romiplostim treatment in a cirrhotic patient with hepatitis C-associated immune thrombocytopenic purpura. J Hepatol 2011;55(1):229–32.
23. Afdhal NH, Giannini EG, Tayyab G, et al. Eltrombopag before procedures in patients with cirrhosis and thrombocytopenia. N Engl J Med 2012;367(8):716–24.
24. Garcia-Pagan JC, Valla DC. Portal vein thrombosis: a predictable milestone in cirrhosis? J Hepatol 2009;51(4):632–4.
25. Bayraktar Y, Harmanci O. Etiology and consequences of thrombosis in abdominal vessels. World J Gastroenterol 2006;12(8):1165–74.
26. Dahlback B. Progress in the understanding of the protein C anticoagulant pathway. Int J Hematol 2004;79(2):109–16.
27. Tripodi A, Mannucci PM. The coagulopathy of chronic liver disease. N Engl J Med 2011;365(2):147–56.
28. Zocco MA, Di Stasio E, De Cristofaro R, et al. Thrombotic risk factors in patients with liver cirrhosis: correlation with MELD scoring system and portal vein thrombosis development. J Hepatol 2009;51(4):682–9.
29. Kajihara M, Kato S, Okazaki Y, et al. A role of autoantibody-mediated platelet destruction in thrombocytopenia in patients with cirrhosis. Hepatology 2003;37(6):1267–76.
30. Lisman T, Bongers TN, Adelmeijer J, et al. Elevated levels of von Willebrand Factor in cirrhosis support platelet adhesion despite reduced functional capacity. Hepatology 2006;44(1):53–61.
31. Feys HB, Canciani MT, Peyvandi F, et al. ADAMTS13 activity to antigen ratio in physiological and pathological conditions associated with an increased risk of thrombosis. Br J Haematol 2007;138(4):534–40.

32. Tripodi A. Hemostasis abnormalities in chronic liver failure. In: Gines P, Kamath PS, Arroyo V, editors. Chronic liver failure: mechanisms and management. New York: Springer; 2010. p. 289–303.

33. Tripodi A, Primignani M, Chantarangkul V, et al. An imbalance of pro- vs anti-coagulation factors in plasma from patients with cirrhosis. Gastroenterology 2009;137(6):2105–11.

34. Tripodi A, Primignani M, Lemma L, et al. Detection of the imbalance of procoagu-lant versus anticoagulant factors in cirrhosis by a simple laboratory method. Hepatology 2010;52(1):249–55.

35. Caldwell SH, Hoffman M, Lisman T, et al. Coagulation disorders and hemostasis in liver disease: pathophysiology and critical assessment of current manage-ment. Hepatology 2006;44(4):1039–46.

36. Giannini EG, Savarino V. Thrombocytopenia in liver disease. Curr Opin Hematol 2008;15(5):473–80.

37. Lisman T, Leebeek FW, Mosnier LO, et al. Thrombin-activatable fibrinolysis inhibitor deficiency in cirrhosis is not associated with increased plasma fibrino-lysis. Gastroenterology 2001;121(1):131–9.

38. Colucci M, Binetti BM, Branca MG, et al. Deficiency of thrombin activatable fibri-nolysis inhibitor in cirrhosis is associated with increased plasma fibrinolysis. Hepatology 2003;38(1):230–7.

39. Dahlback B. Blood coagulation. Lancet 2000;355(9215):1627–32.

40. Esmon CT. Basic mechanisms and pathogenesis of venous thrombosis. Blood Rev 2009;23(5):225–9.

41. Yerdel MA, Gunson B, Mirza D, et al. Portal vein thrombosis in adults undergoing liver transplantation: risk factors, screening, management, and outcome. Trans-plantation 2000;69(9):1873–81.

42. Cazals-Hatem D, Hillaire S, Rudler M, et al. Obliterative portal venopathy: portal hypertension is not always present at diagnosis. J Hepatol 2011;54(3):455–61.

43. Condat B, Pessione F, Hillaire S, et al. Current outcome of portal vein thrombosis in adults: risk and benefit of anticoagulant therapy. Gastroenterology 2001; 120(2):490–7.

44. Tsochatzis EA, Senzolo M, Germani G, et al. Systematic review: portal vein throm-bosis in cirrhosis. Aliment Pharmacol Ther 2010;31(3):366–74.

45. Hoekstra J, Janssen HL. Vascular liver disorders (II): portal vein thrombosis. Neth J Med 2009;67(2):46–53.

46. Sogaard KK, Astrup LB, Vilstrup H, et al. Portal vein thrombosis; risk factors, clinical presentation and treatment. BMC Gastroenterol 2007;7:34.

47. Janssen HL, Wijnhoud A, Haagsma EB, et al. Extrahepatic portal vein thrombosis: aetiology and determinants of survival. Gut 2001;49(5):720–4.

48. Chandra R, Kapoor D, Tharakan A, et al. Portal biliopathy. J Gastroenterol Hepatol 2001;16(10):1086–92.

49. Chattopadhyay S, Nundy S. Portal biliopathy. World J Gastroenterol 2012;18(43): 6177–82.

50. Chawla Y, Duseja A, Dhiman RK. Review article: the modern management of portal vein thrombosis. Aliment Pharmacol Ther 2009;30(9):881–94.

51. Tessler FN, Gehring BJ, Gomes AS, et al. Diagnosis of portal vein thrombosis: value of color Doppler imaging. AJR Am J Roentgenol 1991;157(2):293–6.

52. Parvey HR, Raval B, Sandler CM. Portal vein thrombosis: imaging findings. AJR Am J Roentgenol 1994;162(1):77–81.

53. Van Gansbeke D, Avni EF, Delcour C, et al. Sonographic features of portal vein thrombosis. AJR Am J Roentgenol 1985;144(4):749–52.

54. Rossi S, Rosa L, Ravetta V, et al. Contrast-enhanced versus conventional and color Doppler sonography for the detection of thrombosis of the portal and hepatic venous systems. AJR Am J Roentgenol 2006;186(3):763–73.

55. Kapoor S, Pal S, Sahni P, et al. Thromboelastographic evaluation of coagulation in patients with extrahepatic portal vein thrombosis and non-cirrhotic portal fibrosis: a pilot study. J Gastroenterol Hepatol 2009;24(6):992–7.

56. Rossetto V, Spiezia L, Senzolo M, et al. Whole blood rotation thromboelastometry (ROTEM(R)) profiles in subjects with non-neoplastic portal vein thrombosis. Thromb Res 2013;132(2):e131–4.

57. Muller MC, Meijers JC, Vroom MB, et al. Utility of thromboelastography and/or thromboelastometry in adults with sepsis: a systematic review. Crit Care 2014;18(1):R30.

58. Condat B, Pessione F, Helene Denninger M, et al. Recent portal or mesenteric venous thrombosis: increased recognition and frequent recanalization on anticoagulant therapy. Hepatology 2000;32(3):466–70.

59. Handa P, Crowther M, Douketis JD. Portal vein thrombosis: a clinician-oriented and practical review. Clin Appl Thromb Hemost 2013;20(5):498–506.

60. Hall TC, Garcea G, Metcalfe M, et al. Management of acute non-cirrhotic and non-malignant portal vein thrombosis: a systematic review. World J Surg 2011;35(11):2510–20.

61. de Franchis R. Evolving consensus in portal hypertension. Report of the Baveno IV consensus workshop on methodology of diagnosis and therapy in portal hypertension. J Hepatol 2005;43(1):167–76.

62. Khanna R, Sarin SK. Non-cirrhotic portal hypertension - diagnosis and management. J Hepatol 2014;60(2):421–41.

63. Delgado MG, Seijo S, Yepes I, et al. Efficacy and safety of anticoagulation on patients with cirrhosis and portal vein thrombosis. Clin Gastroenterol Hepatol 2012;10(7):776–83.

64. Amitrano L, Guardascione MA, Menchise A, et al. Safety and efficacy of anticoagulation therapy with low molecular weight heparin for portal vein thrombosis in patients with liver cirrhosis. J Clin Gastroenterol 2010;44(6):448–51.

65. Francoz C, Belghiti J, Vilgrain V, et al. Splanchnic vein thrombosis in candidates for liver transplantation: usefulness of screening and anticoagulation. Gut 2005;54(5):691–7.

66. Maruyama H, Okugawa H, Takahashi M, et al. De novo portal vein thrombosis in virus-related cirrhosis: predictive factors and long-term outcomes. Am J Gastroenterol 2013;108(4):568–74.

67. Takatori H, Hayashi T, Sunagozaka H, et al. Danaparoid sodium monotherapy for portal vein thrombosis in cirrhotic patients is as effective as combination therapy with antithrombin III. Hepatology 2013;58:894A.

68. Copaci I, Ismail G, Micu L, et al. Anticoagulant therapy with sulodexidum for portal vein thrombosis in patients with liver cirrhosis. Hepatology 2013;58:867A–8A.

69. Werner KT, Sando S, Carey EJ, et al. Portal vein thrombosis in patients with end stage liver disease awaiting liver transplantation: outcome of anticoagulation. Dig Dis Sci 2013;58(6):1776–80.

70. Senzolo M, M Sartori T, Rossetto V, et al. Prospective evaluation of anticoagulation and transjugular intrahepatic portosystemic shunt for the management of portal vein thrombosis in cirrhosis. Liver Int 2012;32(6):919–27.

71. Bento L, Huerta AR, Pascual C, et al. Antithrombotic therapy in non-neoplastic chronic portal venous thrombosis in cirrhosis: recanalization and liver function evaluation. Blood 2011;118 [abstract: 3358].

72. Francoz C, Dondero F, Abdelrazek W, et al. Screening for portal vein thrombosis in candidates for liver transplantation and anticoagulation until transplantation: results of a prospective assessment. Liver Transpl 2008;14(Suppl S1):S245.
73. Qi X, Han G, Fan D. Management of portal vein thrombosis in liver cirrhosis. Nat Rev Gastroenterol Hepatol 2014;11(7):435–46.
74. Huard G, Bilodeau M. Management of anticoagulation for portal vein thrombosis in individuals with cirrhosis: a systematic review. Int J Hepatol 2012;2012:672986.
75. Garcia-Tsao G, Bosch J. Management of varices and variceal hemorrhage in cirrhosis. N Engl J Med 2010;362(9):823–32.
76. Sarin SK, Gupta N, Jha SK, et al. Equal efficacy of endoscopic variceal ligation and propranolol in preventing variceal bleeding in patients with noncirrhotic portal hypertension. Gastroenterology 2010;139(4):1238–45.
77. Primignani M. Portal vein thrombosis, revisited. Dig Liver Dis 2010;42(3):163–70.
78. Uflacker R. Applications of percutaneous mechanical thrombectomy in transjugular intrahepatic portosystemic shunt and portal vein thrombosis. Tech Vasc Interv Radiol 2003;6(1):59–69.
79. Francoz C, Valla D, Durand F. Portal vein thrombosis, cirrhosis, and liver transplantation. J Hepatol 2012;57(1):203–12.
80. Bauer J, Johnson S, Durham J, et al. The role of TIPS for portal vein patency in liver transplant patients with portal vein thrombosis. Liver Transpl 2006;12(10):1544–51.
81. Fanelli F. The evolution of transjugular intrahepatic portosystemic shunt: tips. ISRN Hepatol 2014;2014:1–12.
82. Boyer TD, Haskal ZJ, American Association for the Study of Liver Diseases. The role of transjugular intrahepatic portosystemic shunt (TIPS) in the management of portal hypertension: update 2009. Hepatology 2010;51(1):306.
83. Han G, Qi X, He C, et al. Transjugular intrahepatic portosystemic shunt for portal vein thrombosis with symptomatic portal hypertension in liver cirrhosis. J Hepatol 2011;54(1):78–88.
84. Juric I, Primorac D, Zagar Z, et al. Frequency of portal and systemic bacteremia in acute appendicitis. Pediatr Int 2001;43(2):152–6.
85. Kanellopoulou T, Alexopoulou A, Theodossiades G, et al. Pylephlebitis: an overview of non-cirrhotic cases and factors related to outcome. Scand J Infect Dis 2010;42(11–12):804–11.
86. Plemmons RM, Dooley DP, Longfield RN. Septic thrombophlebitis of the portal vein (pylephlebitis): diagnosis and management in the modern era. Clin Infect Dis 1995;21(5):1114–20.
87. Chang YS, Min SY, Joo SH, et al. Septic thrombophlebitis of the porto-mesenteric veins as a complication of acute appendicitis. World J Gastroenterol 2008;14(28):4580–2.
88. Baril N, Wren S, Radin R, et al. The role of anticoagulation in pylephlebitis. Am J Surg 1996;172(5):449–52 [discussion: 452–3].
89. Hoekstra J, Seijo S, Rautou PE, et al. Pregnancy in women with portal vein thrombosis: results of a multicentric European study on maternal and fetal management and outcome. J Hepatol 2012;57(6):1214–9.
90. Mehta N, Chen K, Powrie RO. Prescribing for the pregnant patient. Cleve Clin J Med 2014;81(6):367–72.
91. Martin P, DiMartini A, Feng S, et al. Evaluation for liver transplantation in adults: 2013 practice guideline by the American Association for the Study of Liver Diseases and the American Society of Transplantation. Hepatology 2014;59(3):1144–65.

Moving?

Make sure your subscription moves with you!

To notify us of your new address, find your **Clinics Account Number** (located on your mailing label above your name), and contact customer service at:

Email: journalscustomerservice-usa@elsevier.com

800-654-2452 (subscribers in the U.S. & Canada)
314-447-8871 (subscribers outside of the U.S. & Canada)

Fax number: 314-447-8029

Elsevier Health Sciences Division
Subscription Customer Service
3251 Riverport Lane
Maryland Heights, MO 63043

*To ensure uninterrupted delivery of your subscription, please notify us at least 4 weeks in advance of move.

Printed and bound by CPI Group (UK) Ltd, Croydon, CR0 4YY

07/10/2024

01040499-0004